TEXTBOOK OF

Nutrigenetics & Nutrigenomics

Dr.Shanthi Lakshmi Duraimani

notionpress.com

INDIA • SINGAPORE • MALAYSIA

ISBN

Hardcase 979-8-90431-905-2
Paperback 979-8-90176-738-2

DEDICATION

With the boundless grace of my beloved Lord Krishna, I walk this journey of life.
Every breath, every thought, every word I write is a gift from Him,
a gentle reminder of the eternal presence of the Divine.

I bow in deep reverence to
Sri Kanchi Mahaperiyava, Sri Swami Samarth, and Maharishi Mahesh Yogi
whose wisdom and compassion have been my guiding light,
illuminating my path through moments of doubt and darkness,
and nurturing in me the strength to pursue truth and knowledge.

This book is not mine alone;
it is a humble offering to the Almighty,
to the eternal source of wisdom and love,
whose unseen hands shape every step of my existence.

Contents

I owe my deepest gratitude to my parents, **C. Duraimani** and **D. Jansi Rani**, for their immeasurable support throughout my life. Their unwavering encouragement and, above all, their commitment to giving me a strong education laid the foundation for everything I have achieved in my career.

I also wish to acknowledge my brother, **C. D. Arun Kumar**, who supported me during the early days of my education and played an important role in shaping my path.

Since my teenage years, I have looked up to my friend, who eventually became my life partner, my husband, **R. K. Yesudasan**. He has been a source of strength and inspiration throughout every stage of my life: teenage, adulthood, and the present. I remain grounded because of him, and any peak I have reached in my career is a result of his constant and selfless support.

My heartfelt thanks extend to my father-in-law, **R. Kannadasan**, and mother-in-law, **K. Banumathi**, who have always treated me as their own daughter. Their constant support, especially after the birth of my daughter, has been invaluable. I am also grateful to my sister-in-law, **R. K. Rajalakshmi**, and my brother, **Jagajeev,** for their encouragement and kindness.

Finally, to my little princess, **Yaalini Yera**, you are the love of my life and the driving force that inspires me to move forward with courage and determination. Your presence fills my days with joy and purpose, and I dedicate this journey to you as well.

During my master's degree in human genetics, I first encountered the story of **Rosalind Franklin** and her pioneering work on the discovery of the DNA double helix. As I read about her struggles, I often wondered how challenging it must have been, in those times, to balance the expectations of society, the weight of professional ambition, and the responsibilities of being a woman in science. Her remarkable X-ray diffraction images laid out the foundation for understanding the very structure of life, yet her contributions were overshadowed, and she did not receive the Nobel Prize she so rightfully deserved. This realization left me heartbroken, but it also ignited a deep fire within me. Rosalind Franklin became my greatest inspiration—not only for her scientific brilliance, but also for her resilience, quiet strength, and the grace with which she pursued truth in the face of adversity. She taught me that recognition may not always come immediately, but the impact of sincere work and dedication is eternal.

My second great inspiration has been **Kiran Mazumdar-Shaw,** the visionary founder of **Biocon**. I was in awe when I first learned that she established a biotechnology company at a time when genetics and biotechnology were only beginning to take shape in India. With courage, foresight, and determination, she transformed challenges into opportunities, paving the way for India to emerge as a global player in biotechnology. Her journey symbolizes the power of perseverance, innovation, and leadership. As a woman entrepreneur and scientist, she broke barriers, proving that women can not only participate in but also lead and redefine the scientific and business landscapes.

Both Rosalind Franklin and Kiran Mazumdar-Shaw remain guiding lights for me, reminding me to pursue science with integrity, to remain steadfast in the face of challenges, and to contribute meaningfully to the fields of genetics and biotechnology with both courage and compassion.

This textbook has also benefited from the invaluable support of colleagues who added their skills and creativity. **Malvika Dalvi**, a nutrigenomics expert serving as the **editor**, played an essential role in refining the manuscript and ensuring clarity, flow, and precision throughout the chapters.

I would also like to acknowledge **Clinical Nutritionist Abinaya Selvanathan** and **Raganiyanthri**, **Biotechonologist and Graphic designer** whose talent and dedication brought scientific concepts to life through the creation of drawings and images. Their work has made the content more engaging, visually clear, and accessible to readers.

Together, their contributions have added depth and polish to this work, and I am deeply grateful for their efforts.

Dr. **Shanthi Lakshmi** is a molecular geneticist, educator, and life sciences consultant with over a decade of experience at the intersection of genetics, health, and wellness. With a master's degree in human genetics and a strong foundation in molecular biology, she has dedicated her career to advancing nutrigenetics, nutrigenomics, and personalized nutrition.

As an **independent Life Sciences Consultant**, Dr. Shanthi Lakshmi has collaborated with leading biotech companies such as **Janssen Biotech** and a range of innovative startups. Her career spans diverse domains, including **Laboratory Information Management Systems (LIMS)**, molecular biology, artificial intelligence in healthcare, and the development of nutrigenomic products and services.

In her role as a **LIMS Specialist** at GVW, Dr. Shanthi Lakshmi led the implementation and optimization of LIMS for Janssen Biotech, ensuring seamless integration and enhanced operational efficiency. She also spearheaded global efforts in **molecular biology standardization,** establishing unified techniques across laboratories to improve research reproducibility and scientific rigor.

Her entrepreneurial spirit is reflected in the creation of **health and wellness applications**, ranging from habit-forming and mindfulness meditation apps to digital nutrition and mental health solutions. By combining **digital marketing strategies** with scientific innovation, Dr. Shanthi Lakshmi successfully drove product adoption and revenue growth.

At **NuGenomics,** where she served as Chief Scientific Officer, Dr. Shanthi Lakshmi led teams in R&D, product development, health coaching, and operations. She has trained more than **100 nutritionists in nutrigenetics** and guided over **3,000 clients** toward better health outcomes using personalized genetic insights. Her dedication to education also extends to training clinicians, dietitians, and healthcare providers to integrate nutrigenomics into clinical practice.

Currently, Dr. Shanthi Lakshmi works as an **independent consultant**, providing services in:

LIMS implementation and optimization, molecular biology technique standardization, health and wellness app development with digital marketing integration, nutrigenetic product development and health coaching, nutrigenetics and microbiome panel development, nutrigenetics training and workforce development, and AI-based healthcare product innovation and integration.

Dr. Shanthi Lakshmi's career reflects a commitment to bridging science and practice—transforming complex genomic data into actionable insights that empower individuals to achieve optimal health. Her work continues to advance the integration of genetics, nutrition, and technology in shaping the future of personalized medicine.

About the Editor

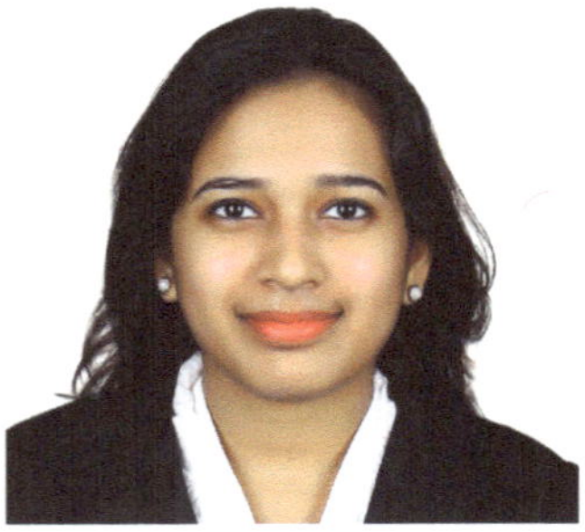

Malvika Dalvi is a dedicated researcher in nutrition, nutrigenomics, and microbiome science, with a strong academic foundation and a passion for advancing personalized healthcare. She holds a Master of Science in Nutrition and Dietetics (Specialization in Nutrigenomics) from the Symbiosis Institute of Health Sciences. Prior to that, she completed her Bachelor's degree in Biotechnology at Vivekanand Education Society's College of Arts, Science & Commerce, University of Mumbai.

Malvika has extensive experience in nutrigenomics, microbiome research, and the development of personalized health solutions. Her academic training and professional work reflect a deep interest in understanding how genetic and microbial factors interact with nutrition to influence human health. She has published peer-reviewed review articles and contributed educational content covering key health areas such as obesity, sports nutrition, and diabetes.

Beyond research, Malvika has a strong background in science communication and educational content creation, bringing clarity and accessibility to complex topics. Her editorial work ensures precision, coherence, and impact, while her creative contributions help make scientific knowledge more engaging for students and professionals alike.

Her goal is to advance the field of nutrigenomics and microbiome science through innovative research and meaningful contributions that bridge laboratory discoveries with practical applications in health and wellness.

This textbook is an essential guide for students pursuing a career in nutrigenetics. This comprehensive resource provides an in-depth exploration of the fascinating fields of nutrigenetics and nutrigenomics, offering a solid foundation for understanding the intricate relationship between genetics, nutrition, and human health.

The textbook begins with an introductory section that highlights the importance of nutrigenetics and nutrigenomics in the field of nutrition. Students will gain insights into how these disciplines contribute to our understanding of how genetic variations influence nutrient metabolism and the response to dietary interventions. By emphasizing the concept of personalized nutrition, students will discover how tailoring dietary recommendations based on an individual's genetic makeup can optimize health outcomes.

Throughout the textbook, students will embark on a captivating journey through the fundamentals of genetics, unraveling the complexities of DNA, genes, and chromosomes. They will delve into Mendelian inheritance patterns, genetic variations, and how gene expression and regulation influence nutrient metabolism. With a solid grasp of the basics, students will be well-equipped to explore the realm of nutrigenetics and nutrigenomics.

The textbook features dedicated chapters that extensively cover both nutrigenetics and nutrigenomics. In the nutrigenetics section, students will learn about the influence of genetic variations on nutrient metabolism, including single gene-nutrient interactions and gene-diet interactions. Through real-life examples and case studies, students will comprehend how genetic variations can affect an individual's response to specific dietary components.

Moving into nutrigenomics, students will explore the realm of gene expression and transcriptomics, gaining insights into the high-throughput technologies employed in studying gene expression profiles. They will explore the impact of nutrients and diet on gene expression and understand how omics data integration contributes to our understanding of nutrition and health.

The textbook also delves into practical applications of nutrigenetics and nutrigenomics. Students will gain familiarity with nutrigenetic testing methods, interpretation of genetic data, and the utilization of online databases and resources. Through practical exercises and case studies, students will develop skills to apply this knowledge in real-world scenarios.

Furthermore, the textbook presents an outlook on future perspectives and emerging trends in the fields of nutrigenetics and nutrigenomics. Students will gain an understanding of the advancements in genetic research and technology and how these advancements may shape the future of personalized nutrition and clinical practice.

Ultimately, the textbook aims to equip nutrition students with a comprehensive understanding of nutrigenetics and nutrigenomics, empowering them to incorporate this knowledge into their future careers. With its engaging content, practical exercises, and relevant case studies, this textbook serves as an invaluable resource for students seeking to navigate the dynamic and exciting fields of nutrigenetics and nutrigenomics.

When it comes to writing style, I have opted for an unconventional approach compared to traditional textbooks. To engage students, each chapter is structured in a storytelling format, with carefully selected analogies to enhance comprehension. My primary goal was to create an engaging learning experience, avoiding monotony often found in traditional textbooks.

A New Frontier in Nutrition: Nutrigenetics and Nutrigenomics

Imagine standing at the edge of a field, ready to run. The wind is cool against your skin, and you feel the earth beneath your feet, solid and reassuring. Now imagine you have a map of that field, detailing every bump, every divot, every advantage, and every challenge you'll face. With this map, wouldn't your run be more efficient and focused? This is what nutrigenetics and nutrigenomics offer us: a personalized map of our genetic makeup that guides us on how to fuel our bodies effectively.

Nutrigenetics and nutrigenomics are emerging fields that explore the intricate relationship between our genes and the nutrients we consume. While these terms are often used interchangeably, they have distinct aspects. Nutrigenetics focuses on how individual genetic variations influence a person's response to nutrients, whereas nutrigenomics looks at how nutrients and dietary components affect gene expression.

Before exploring nutrigenetics and nutrigenomics, it's important to understand basic genetics—how DNA is structured, how genes function and are expressed, how genetic differences arise, and how these differences interact with diet and lifestyle. Additionally, understanding the role of epigenetics, genetic mutations, and polymorphisms can provide deeper insights into how individual genetic profiles influence nutrient metabolism and overall health.

In this chapter, we embark on a journey through the foundational aspects of genetics, which form the basis for the study of **nutrigenomics** and **nutrigenetics**. Our exploration begins with the **historical overview of genetics,** tracing the evolution of genetic thought from early observations of heredity to modern breakthroughs that have transformed our understanding of how genes influence biological traits. This historical perspective lays the groundwork for understanding the genetic factors that affect human health and nutrition.

We then delve into Mendelian genetics, where Gregor Mendel's pioneering research on inheritance patterns first unveiled the principles by which traits are passed from one generation to the next. The classical framework provides the foundation for understanding how genetic variation influences both health and disease, as well as the intricate patterns of inheritance observed in populations.

Building upon these principles, we explore the patterns of inheritance, focusing on how genetic variations manifest in individuals and populations, influencing physical traits and disease susceptibility. This leads us to the central dogma of molecular biology: the conceptual framework that explains the flow of genetic information from DNA to RNA to proteins. These molecular processes are fundamental to cellular function and metabolism.

To understand these processes in greater depth, we break down the mechanisms of replication, transcription, and translation, which illustrate how genetic instructions are copied, transcribed into RNA, and then translated into functional proteins. These processes are essential to understanding how genetic instructions are carried out at the molecular level and how they direct the cellular machinery.

The chapter concludes with a discussion of the Human Genome Project, a monumental achievement that mapped the entire human genome. This groundbreaking project has unlocked vast new possibilities for personalized medicine, including the fields of nutrigenetics and nutrigenomics, by providing scientists with the tools to identify and understand genetic variations that affect nutrient metabolism, disease risk, and health outcomes.

Together, these foundational concepts in classical and molecular genetics provide an essential background for exploring the dynamic and evolving fields of nutrigenetics and nutrigenomics. This chapter sets the stage for personalized health interventions, where the interaction between genes and nutrition offers the potential for highly individualized approaches to health and disease prevention.

The Evolution of Genetics: A Historical Journey

The study of genetics—focused on genes, heredity, and variation in living organisms—provides fundamental insights into the mechanisms of life. For centuries, humanity has sought to understand how traits are transmitted from one generation to the next. This journey through the history of genetics reveals how humanity transitioned from rudimentary ideas about heredity to the groundbreaking discoveries of the 20th century.

Early Theories and Observations

The story of genetics began long before the term "**genetics**" was even coined. Ancient civilizations, including the Greeks and the Romans, pondered how traits were inherited. Hippocrates, a Greek physician, suggested that "seeds" from all parts of the body were transmitted to offspring. Although inaccurate, this theory highlighted early attempts to explain inheritance.

One of the earliest recorded theories of inheritance came from the **Greek philosopher Aristotle**. He proposed that traits were inherited through a mixture of male and female fluids. While this idea lacked scientific rigor, it laid out a conceptual foundation for future inquiries into heredity. However, it wasn't until much later that more scientific approaches to studying inheritance emerged.

Early Hereditary Theories

Before **Charles Darwin**, several notable figures made significant contributions to the understanding of heredity. One of the earliest was **Carolus Linnaeus**, a Swedish botanist, physician, and zoologist, who developed the binomial nomenclature system for classifying organisms. While Linnaeus' focus was not on genetics, his classification framework helped shape the study of biological relationships.

Another key figure was **Jean-Baptiste Lamarck, a French naturalist**, who proposed the **theory of inheritance** of acquired characteristics. According to **Lamarck**, organisms could pass on traits acquired during their lifetime to their offspring. Although later disproven, Lamarck's ideas marked a significant step toward understanding heredity.

Charles Darwin and the Theory of Natural Selection

Charles Darwin, the renowned naturalist, though not directly involved in genetics, profoundly influenced the field through his theory of evolution by natural selection. In his seminal work, **"On the Origin of Species" (1859)**, Darwin proposed that species evolve through a process of natural selection, where individuals with advantageous traits are more likely to survive and reproduce, driving species evolution

While Darwin's theory explained how species evolved, it did not explain the mechanisms of heredity. Darwin himself acknowledged this gap in his theory and proposed the concept of "**pangenesis**," which suggested that particles called "**gemmules**" carried hereditary information from all parts of the body to the reproductive organs. Although pangenesis was later disproven, it exemplified Darwin's efforts to integrate heredity into evolutionary theory.

Gregor Mendel: The Father of Modern Genetics

The true **father of modern genetics is Gregor Mendel**, an **Austrian monk** who conducted groundbreaking experiments in the mid-19th century. Mendel's work with pea plants in the monastery garden led to the discovery of the **fundamental principles of inheritance**. By crossbreeding pea plants with different traits, Mendel observed patterns in the way traits were passed down through generations.

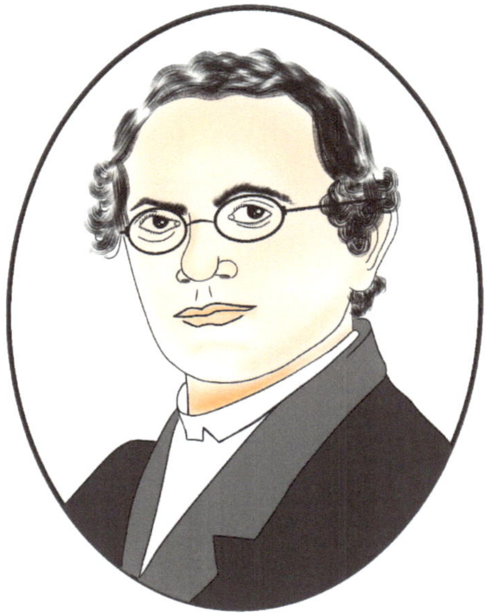

Through meticulous experiments, Mendel discovered that traits are passed down in discrete units—what we now call genes. He formulated the **laws of inheritance, including the Law of Segregation and the Law of Independent Assortment,** which explained how traits are inherited independently of each other.

Despite the groundbreaking nature of his findings, Mendel's work was largely ignored during his lifetime and only gained recognition at the dawn of the 20th century.

The Rediscovery of Mendel's Work and the Rise of Genetics

Around 1900, scientists like **Hugo de Vries, Carl Correns, and Erich von Tschermak** independently rediscovered Mendel's findings, sparking renewed interest in heredity. This marked the birth of genetics as a formal scientific discipline. The term **"genetics"** was coined by the British biologist William Bateson in 1905, solidifying the field's distinct identity.

The early 20th century saw rapid advancements in genetics research. **Thomas Hunt Morgan**, an American geneticist, conducted experiments with fruit flies (***Drosophila melanogaster***) that demonstrated the existence of chromosomes as carriers of genes. Morgan's work provided crucial evidence for the **chromosomal theory of inheritance**, which proposed that genes are located on chromosomes and that these chromosomes are the vehicles of genetic inheritance.

Coining Key Terms in Genetics

The terminology used in genetics today has its roots in the early 20th century:

- **Gene:** The term **"gene"** was coined by the **Danish botanist Wilhelm Johannsen in 1909**. He used it to describe the **fundamental units of heredity.**
- **Genetics:** Introduced by **William Bateson in 1905** to define **the study of heredity and variation**.

- **Genome:** The term **"genome,"** which refers to the complete set of genes or genetic material in an organism, was first used by **Hans Winkler, a German botanist, in 1920.**
- **Genotype and Phenotype:** Wilhelm Johannsen also introduced these terms. **"Genotype"** refers to the **genetic makeup of an organism**, while **"phenotype"** refers to the **observable characteristics.**

Genetics Before the 20th Century: Ancient Practices and Early Insights

While the 20th century brought significant advancements in genetics, there were early practices and insights that hinted at an understanding of heredity. Selective breeding of plants and animals has been practiced for thousands of years. Ancient farmers and breeders observed that certain traits could be enhanced through careful selection and mating of individuals with desirable characteristics.

For example, ancient Egyptians selectively bred animals like dogs and cattle, while early civilizations in the Americas domesticated crops such as maize and potatoes through selective breeding. These practices, though not based on a scientific understanding of genetics, demonstrated an intuitive grasp of heredity and trait inheritance.

Historical texts also provide evidence of early insights into genetic inheritance. The ancient Indian text ***"Charaka Samhita,"*** written around **300 BCE**, contains references to hereditary conditions and the transmission of traits from parents to offspring. Similarly, ancient Chinese texts also contain discussions about hereditary traits and breeding practices.

Timeline of Key Discoveries in Genetics

- **Ancient Civilizations:** Early theories and practices of heredity, including selective breeding and philosophical theories by Hippocrates and Aristotle.
- **1707-1778:** Carolus Linnaeus develops the binomial nomenclature system for classifying organisms.
- **1809:** Jean-Baptiste Lamarck proposes the theory of inheritance of acquired characteristics.
- **1859:** Charles Darwin publishes ***"On the Origin of Species,"*** introducing the theory of natural selection.
- **1866:** Gregor Mendel publishes his experiments on pea plants, formulating the laws of inheritance.
- **1900:** Mendel's work is rediscovered by Hugo de Vries, Carl Correns, and Erich von Tschermak.
- **1905:** William Bateson coined the term "genetics."
- **1909:** Wilhelm Johannsen introduces the term "gene."
- **1920:** Hans Winkler coins the term "genome."
- **1910-1920s:** Thomas Hunt Morgan's experiments with fruit flies confirm the chromosomal theory of inheritance.

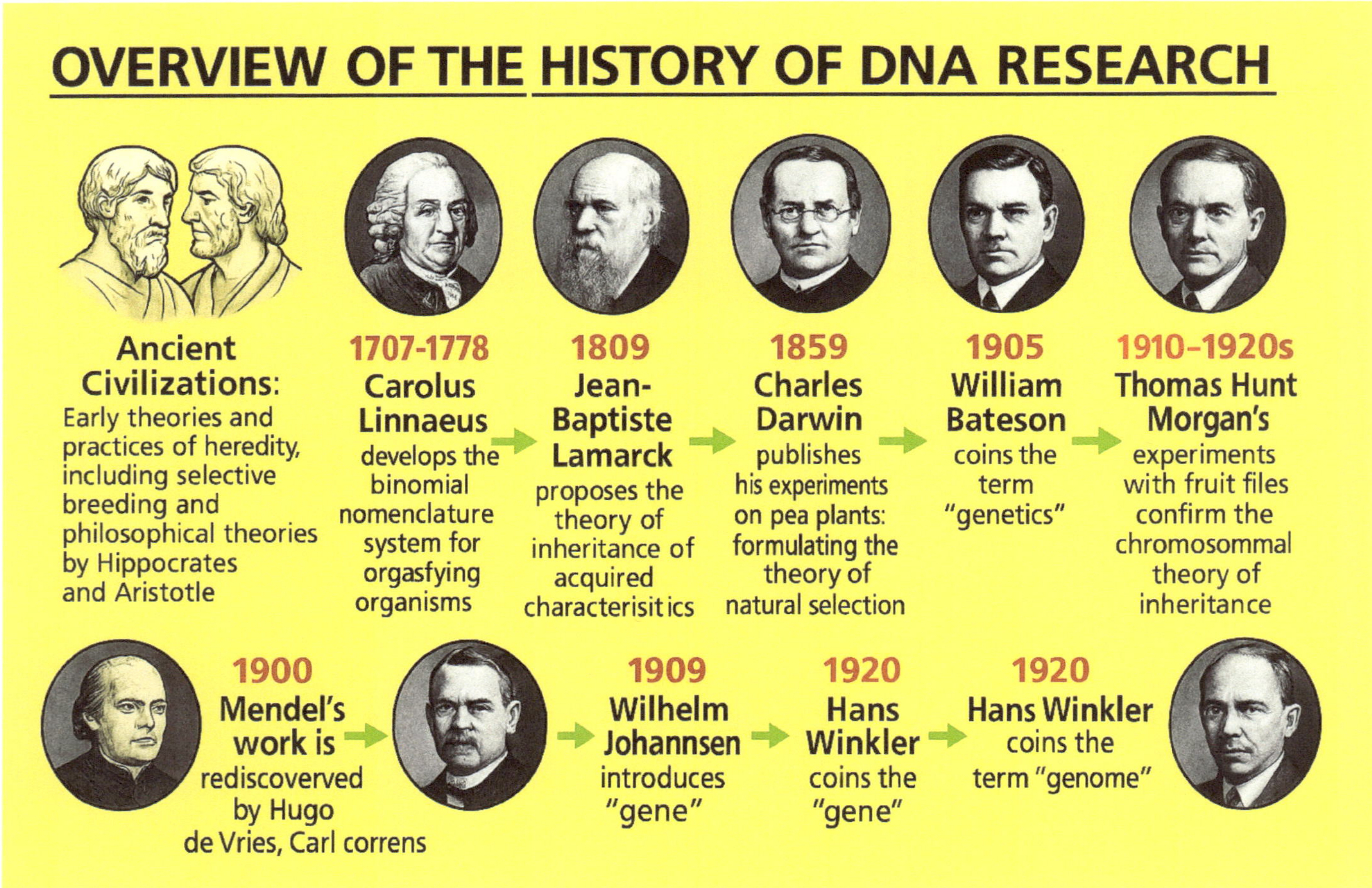

Conclusion

The history of genetics is a testament to humanity's relentless curiosity about the natural world. From ancient observations and theories to the groundbreaking discoveries of the 20th century, the field of genetics has transformed our understanding of life. The foundational work of pioneers like Mendel and subsequent discoveries of the 20th century have provided a comprehensive framework for modern genetics. With this historical context in mind, the next chapter delves into the pivotal discoveries of Mendelian genetics.

Mendelian Genetics

Introduction

Gregor Mendel, often referred to as the **"Father of Genetics,"** made groundbreaking contributions to the field of genetics through his meticulous experiments with pea plants. His work laid the foundation for our understanding of heredity and genetic inheritance, principles now known as Mendelian Genetics. This section provides a brief overview of Mendel's personal life, his journey into genetics, and a detailed explanation of his genetic theories, including simple examples for clarity.

Personal Life and Background

Gregor Johann Mendel was born on July 20, 1822, in Heinzendorf, Austria (now Hynčice, Czech Republic). He was raised in a modest farming family, which instilled in him a strong appreciation for nature and plant life. His early education took place in local schools, where he exhibited a keen interest in science and mathematics.

Mendel entered the Augustinian Abbey of St. Thomas in Brno (then Brünn), where he was ordained as a priest in 1847. The abbey provided him with an environment conducive to scientific study, and he later became a teacher. Mendel's scientific journey was significantly influenced by his studies at the University of Vienna, where he attended courses in physics and botany.

Journey into Genetics

Mendel's interest in genetics was sparked by his desire to understand how traits were inherited from one generation to the next. At the abbey, he began his experiments with **garden peas (*Pisum sativum*)** around 1856. Peas were an ideal choice due to their various **distinct traits (such as flower color and seed shape)** and their ability to self-pollinate or be cross-pollinated manually.

Mendelian Experiments

Mendel conducted his experiments over eight years, meticulously cross-breeding pea plants and recording the traits of their offspring. He observed over **28,000 pea plants**, which provided a statistically significant basis for his conclusions. His attention to detail and systematic approach allowed him to identify patterns of inheritance that had previously gone unnoticed. He focused on seven distinct traits, including **seed shape (round or wrinkled), seed color (yellow or green), flower color (purple or white), and pod shape (inflated or constricted).**

His methodical approach allowed him to observe how these traits were passed from one generation to the next. Through careful analysis, Mendel formulated three foundational principles of inheritance: **the Law of Segregation, the Law of Independent Assortment, and the Law of Dominance.**

The Law of Segregation

Mendel's Law of Segregation states that each individual has two alleles for each trait, one inherited from each parent. These alleles separate (or segregate) during the formation of gametes (sperm and egg cells), ensuring that each gamete carries only one allele for each trait.

Example: Imagine you have a pair of socks, one red and one blue. When you pack them into two separate bags, each bag will end up with only one sock. Similarly, during reproduction, the pair of alleles separates so that each gamete gets only one allele.

In Mendel's experiments, when he cross-bred pea plants with round seeds (dominant) and wrinkled seeds (recessive), he found that the first generation (F1) plants all had round seeds. When these F1 plants were self-pollinated, the second generation (F2) showed a 3:1 ratio of round to wrinkled seeds.

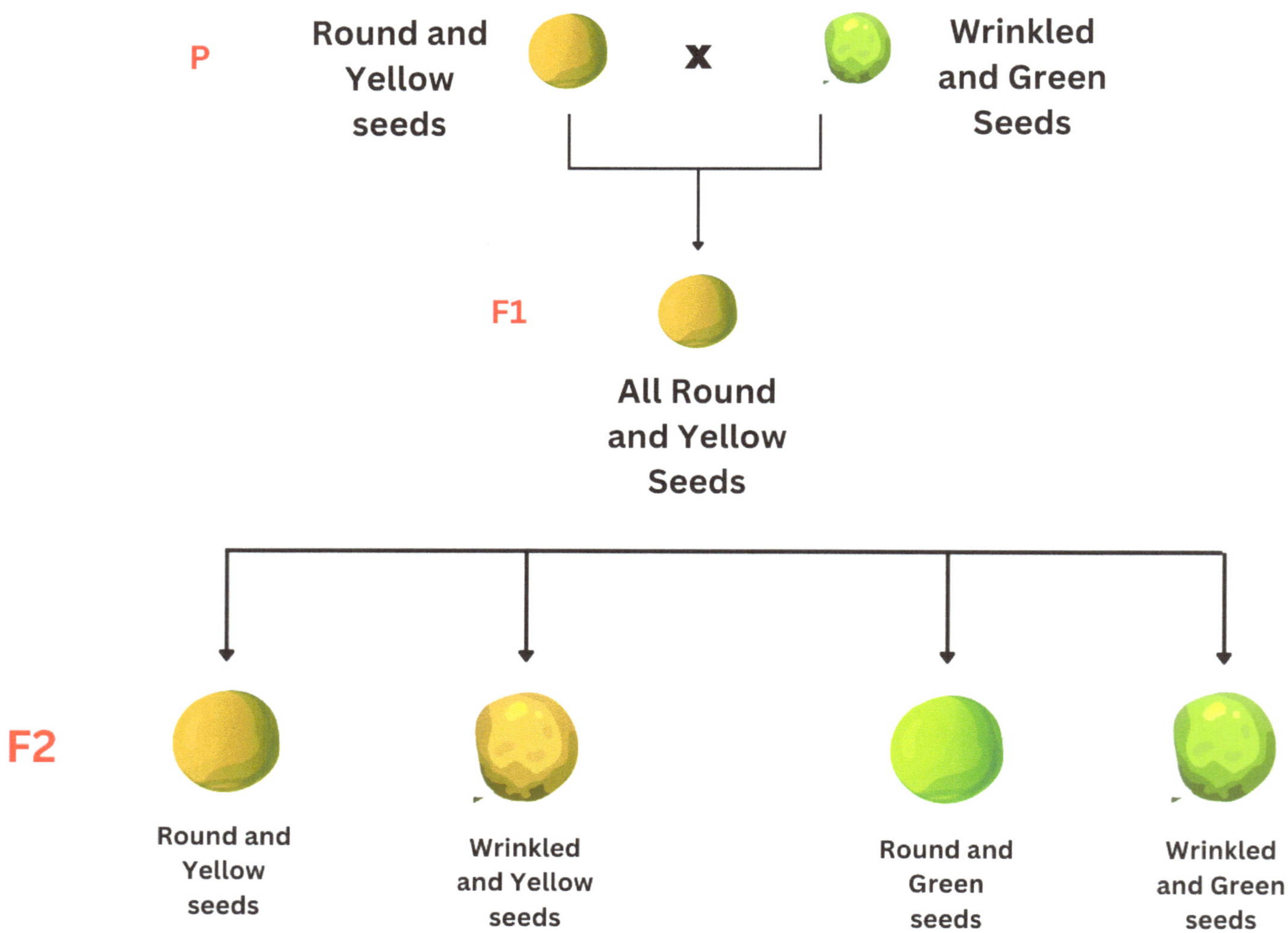

Law of Segregation

Monohybrid Cross

A monohybrid cross involves the mating of individuals that are heterozygous (having two different alleles) for a single trait. This type of cross helps to predict the inheritance pattern of a single trait.

Example: Let's cross two pea plants, each heterozygous for seed shape (Rr). The possible gametes they can produce are 'R' and 'r.' When these gametes combine, the resulting offspring will have the following genotypic and phenotypic ratios:

- **Genotype Ratio:** 1:2:1 (*RR*: *Rr*: *rr*)
- **Phenotype Ratio:** 3:1 (round seeds to wrinkled seeds)

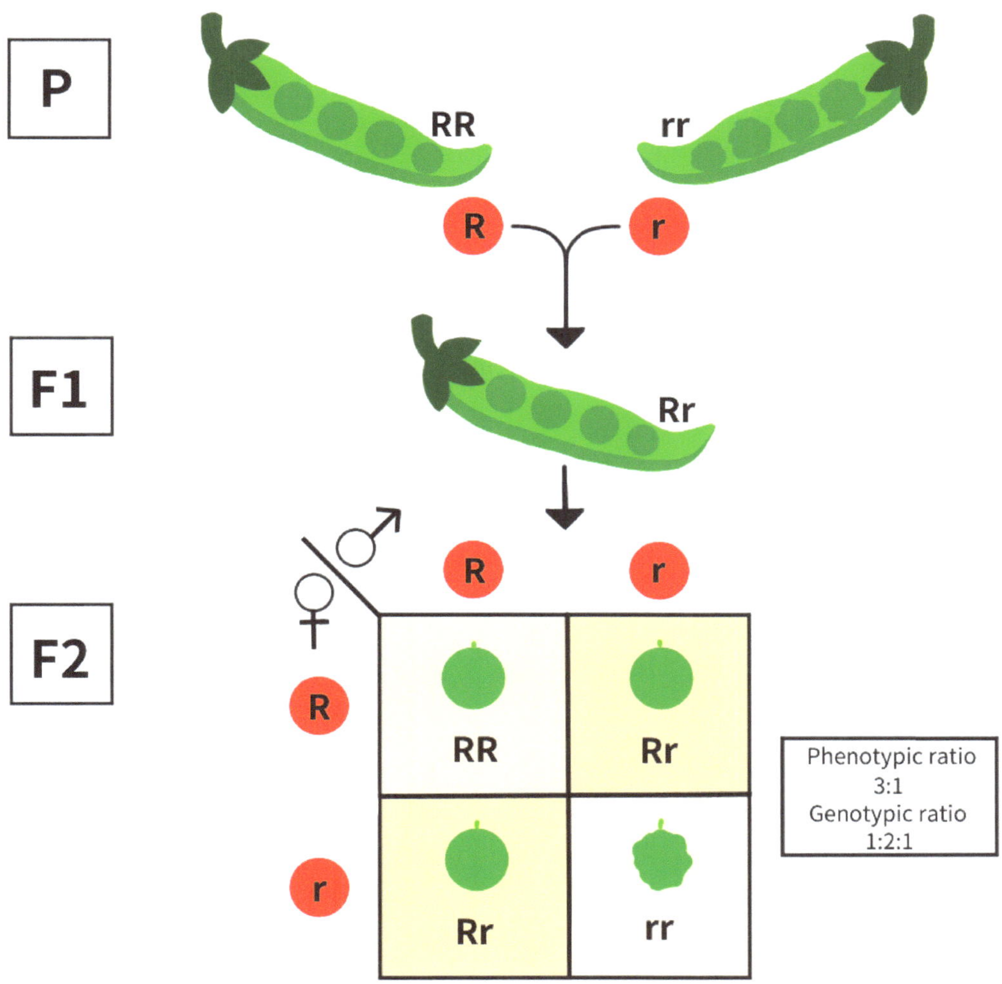

Law of Dominance

In Mendelian genetics, **dominance** refers to the relationship between two alleles of a gene, where one allele masks or suppresses the expression of the other in a heterozygous individual. The expressed allele is known as the **dominant allele**, while the hidden or unexpressed allele is called the **recessive allele**.

Mendel formalized this concept through what is now known as the **Law of Dominance**, which states that when two different alleles are present in an individual, the dominant allele determines the observable trait (phenotype), and the recessive allele is expressed only when both alleles are recessive.

Imagine a flashlight powered by two batteries—one strong and one weak. As long as the strong battery is present, the flashlight shines brightly. The weak battery is still there, but its effect is masked. Similarly, in genetics, the presence of a dominant allele masks the expression of the recessive allele.

Example:

In Mendel's pea plant experiments, the allele for **round seeds (R)** is dominant over the allele for **wrinkled seeds (r)**. Plants with genotypes **RR** or **Rr** produce round seeds because the dominant allele **R** determines the phenotype. Only plants with two recessive alleles (**rr**) express the wrinkled seed trait. This classic pattern clearly illustrates the principle of dominance in inheritance

Recessive Traits

Recessive traits are expressed phenotypically only when an individual inherits two copies of the recessive allele (rr). **Example:** Continuing with Mendel's pea plant experiments, the allele for wrinkled seeds (r) is recessive to the allele for round seeds (R). A pea plant with the genotype RR or Rr will have round seeds because the dominant allele 'R' suppresses the expression of the recessive allele 'r'. Only pea plants with the genotype rr (homozygous recessive) will exhibit wrinkled seeds.

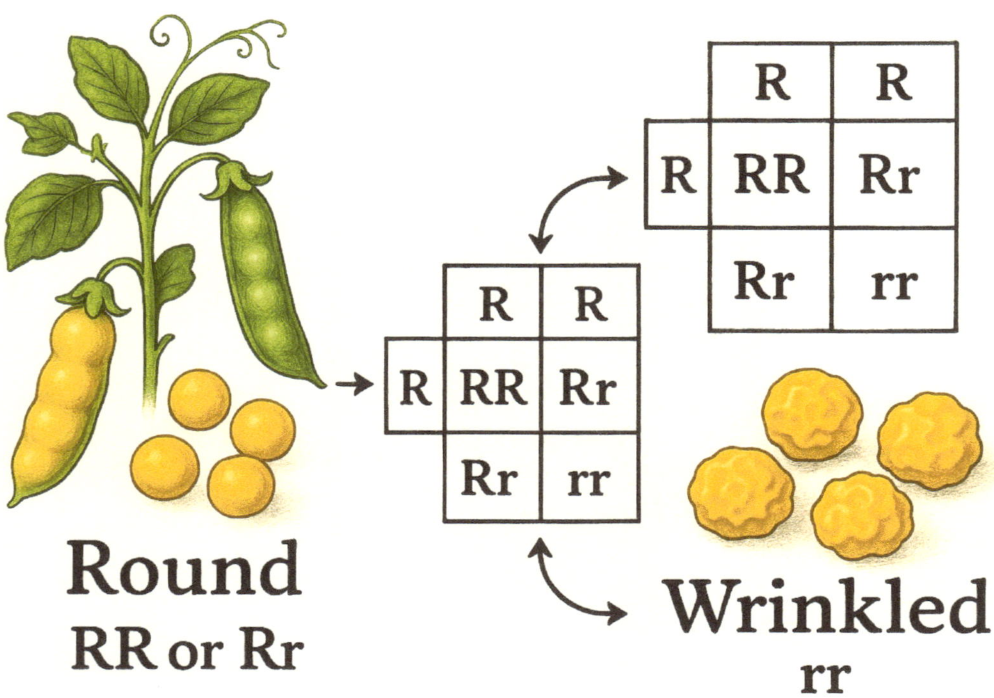

Codominance

Codominance is a genetic phenomenon where two different alleles of a gene are both expressed in the heterozygous condition, resulting in a combined phenotype that shows both traits distinctly.

Example: An excellent example of codominance is found in the ABO blood group system. In this system, there are three alleles involved: I^A, I^B, and i. The I^A and I^B alleles are codominant. If an individual inherits both I^A and I^B alleles (genotype I^AI^B), they will express both A and B antigens on their red blood cells, resulting in blood type AB. This demonstrates how both alleles are expressed equally and distinctly in the phenotype of the heterozygous individual.

Genotype	Ag present	Phenotype
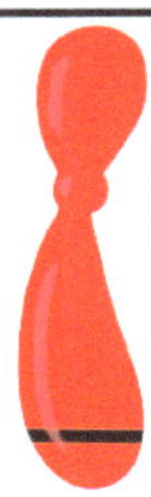 I^AI^A/I^Ai	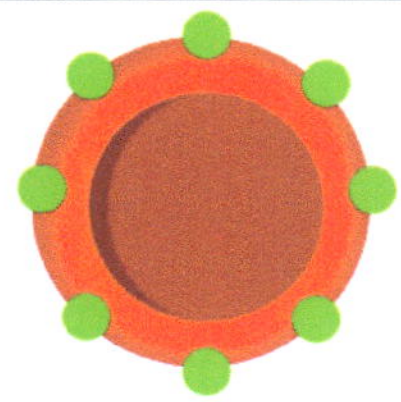 Antigen A	Blood group A
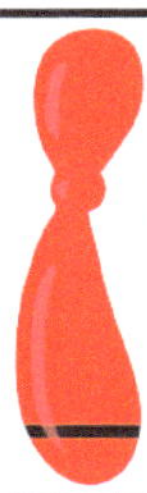 I^BI^B/I^Bi	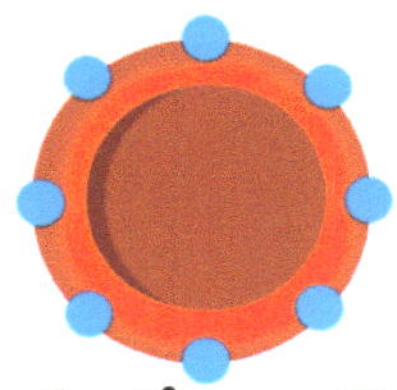 Antigen B	Blood group B
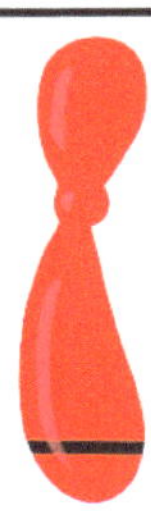 I^AI^B	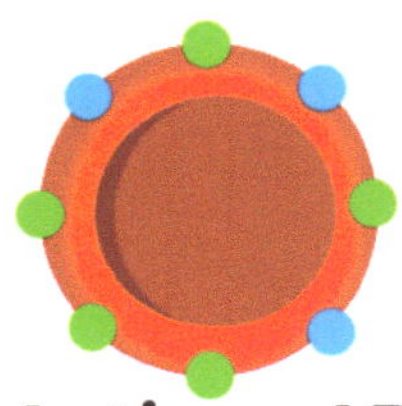 Antigen AB	Blood group AB

Codominance

Incomplete Dominance (Semidominance)

Incomplete dominance, also known as **Semidominance,** occurs when the phenotype of the heterozygous individual is intermediate between the phenotypes of the two homozygous individuals. Neither allele is dominant over the other, resulting in a blending of traits.

Example: In snapdragons, flower color is determined by two alleles: R (red) and r (white). If a plant is heterozygous (Rr), it will produce pink flowers. This intermediate color shows how neither allele is fully dominant, and the phenotype is a mixture of the two homozygous phenotypes.

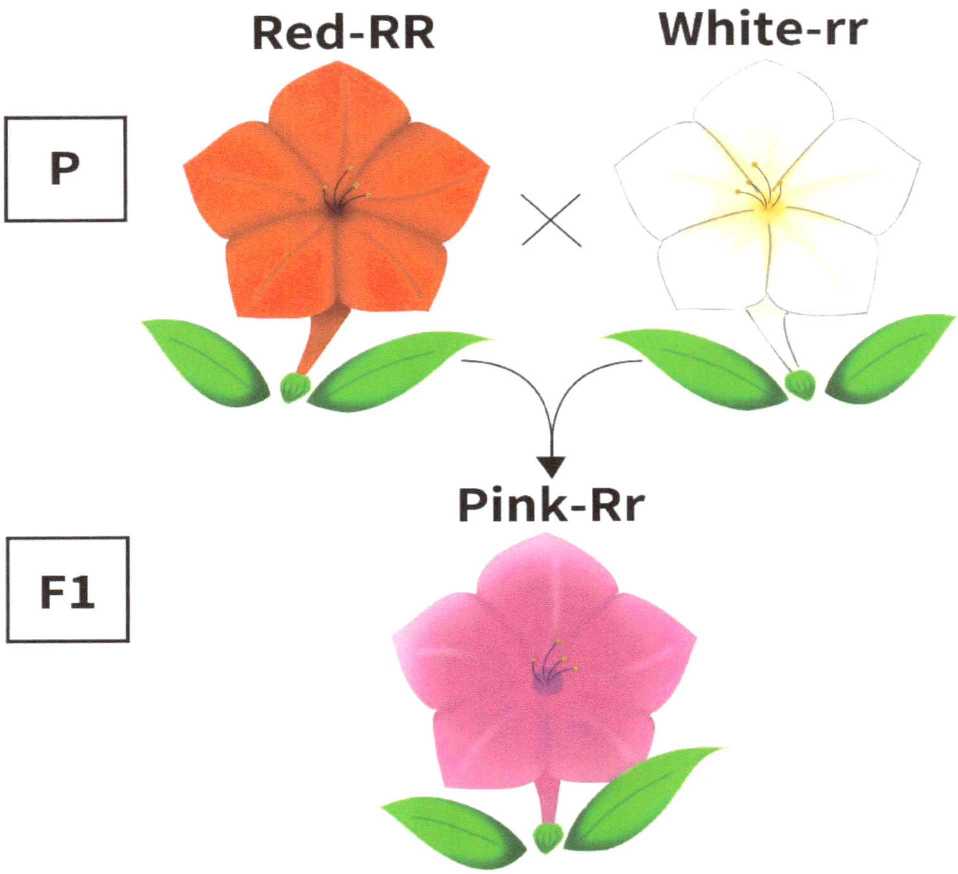

Incomplete Dominance (Semi-Dominance)

Lethal Alleles

Lethal alleles are mutations of genes that can cause the death of an organism, often before birth, when expressed homozygously.

Example: One example of a lethal allele in humans is Tay-Sachs disease. It is caused by a mutation in the *HEXA gene*, leading to the accumulation of harmful substances in the brain and nervous system. Individuals homozygous for the recessive allele (hh) typically do not survive past early childhood due to severe neurological impairment. In this case, the lethal allele is only expressed when present in a homozygous condition, highlighting the recessive nature of lethal alleles.

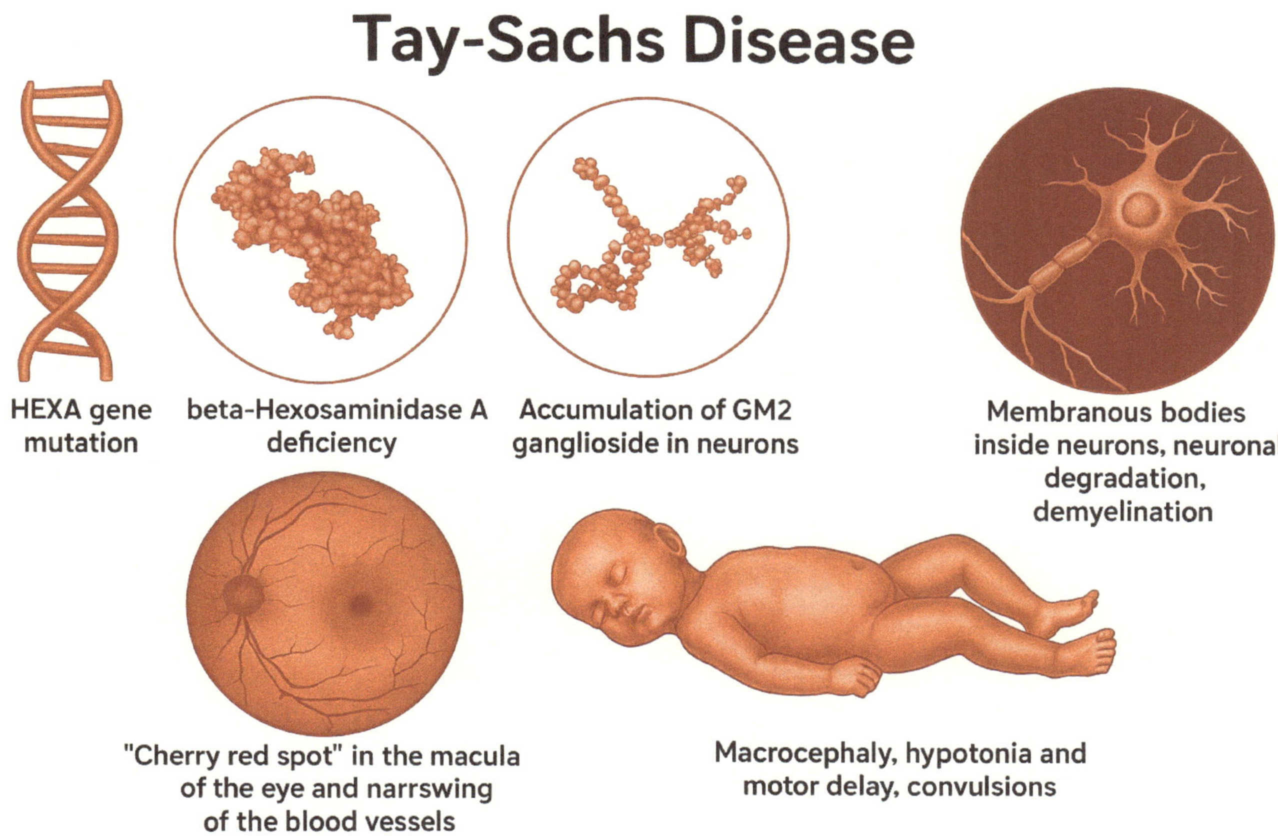

The Law of Independent Assortment

The Law of Independent Assortment states that alleles for different traits are distributed to gametes independently of one another. This means the inheritance of one trait does not influence the inheritance of another trait.

Example: Think of it like flipping two coins at the same time. The outcome of one coin (heads or tails) does not affect the outcome of the other coin. Each coin flip is an independent event.

Mendel demonstrated this principle by conducting dihybrid crosses, where he analyzed the inheritance of two traits simultaneously. For instance, when crossing plants with yellow round seeds and green wrinkled seeds, he observed that the traits assorted independently, resulting in a **9:3:3:1** ratio in the F2 generation.

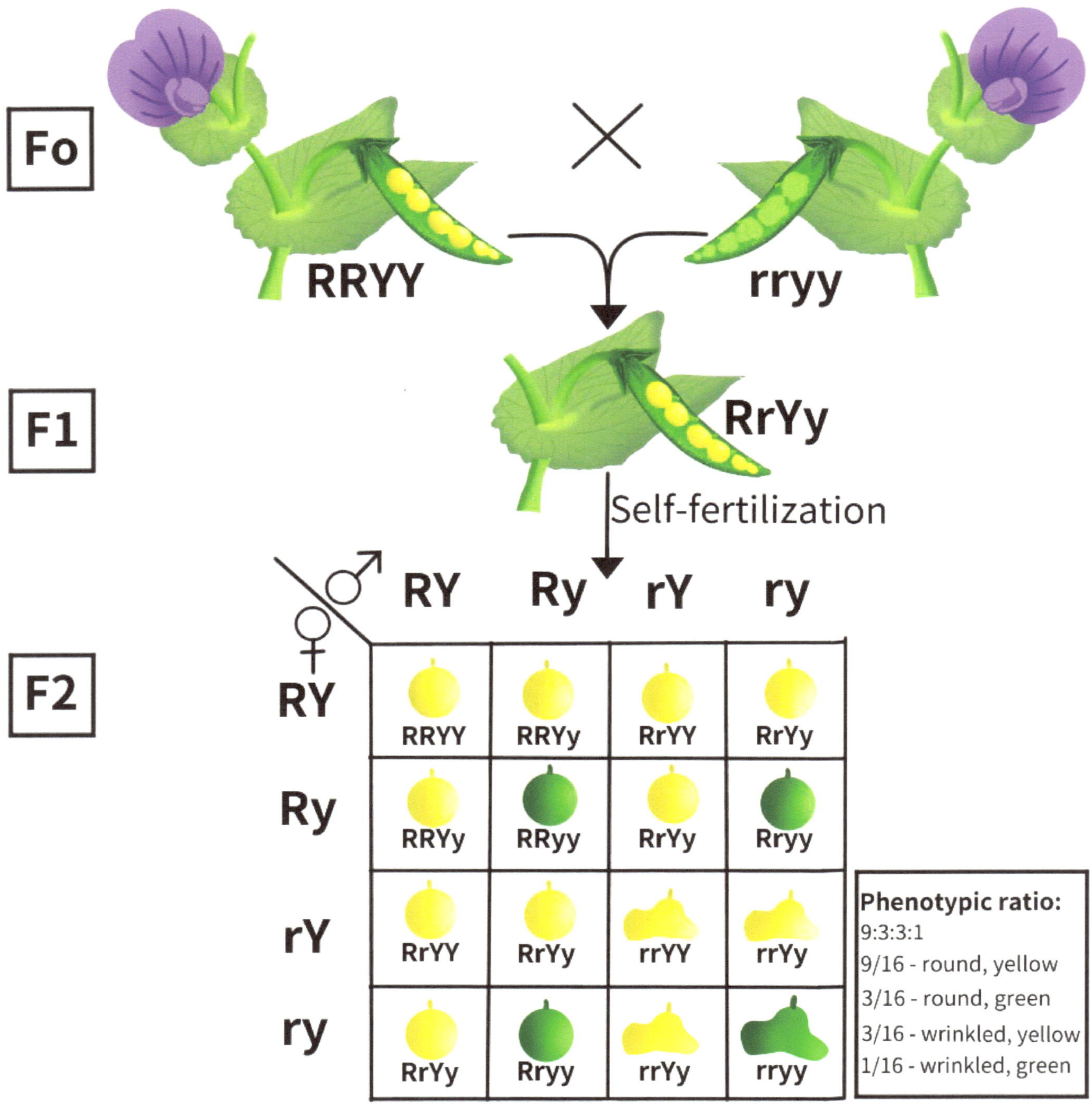

Impact and Rediscovery

Mendel's work was published in 1866 in the proceedings of the Natural History Society of Brünn, but it remained largely unnoticed by the scientific community during his lifetime. It wasn't until 1900 that Hugo de Vries, Carl Correns, and Erich von Tschermak independently rediscovered Mendel's work. This rediscovery marked the beginning of modern genetics, and Mendel's principles became widely recognized and foundational to the field.

Conclusion

Gregor Mendel's meticulous experiments and keen observations revolutionized our understanding of heredity. His laws of segregation, independent assortment, and dominance remain central to genetics, shaping our comprehension of genetic inheritance and variation. Mendel's legacy continues to influence modern research, underscoring the importance of his contributions to the field of genetics.

Unraveling the Mysteries of Genetics: Gene Interactions, Epistasis, and Blood Type Inheritance

Gene Interactions

Gene interactions occur when two or more genes influence a single trait. These interactions can significantly complicate the inheritance patterns observed by Gregor Mendel. Unlike Mendelian inheritance, where one gene controls one trait, gene interactions demonstrate the complexity of genetic regulation.

Example: Consider the coat color in Labrador Retrievers, a classic example of gene interaction. Two genes are involved: one gene (B) determines whether the coat is **black (B)** or **brown (b),** while another gene (E) determines whether the pigment is deposited in the fur. If a dog has the ee genotype, it will be yellow regardless of its B gene alleles because the E gene is epistatic to the B gene. This interaction results in three possible coat colors: **black**, **brown**, and **yellow.**

In this case, the B gene influences pigment color, but the expression of this pigment is controlled by the E gene. When a Labrador Retriever has at least one dominant E allele (EE or Ee), the B gene's effect on coat color (black or brown) is visible. However, if the Labrador has two recessive e alleles (ee), it will have a yellow coat, masking the effect of the B gene alleles entirely.

- **BB or Bb, EE/Ee: Black coat**
- **bb, EE/Ee: Brown coat**
- **Any B gene with ee: Yellow coat**

This illustrates how gene interactions can lead to unexpected and diverse outcomes in genetic inheritance.

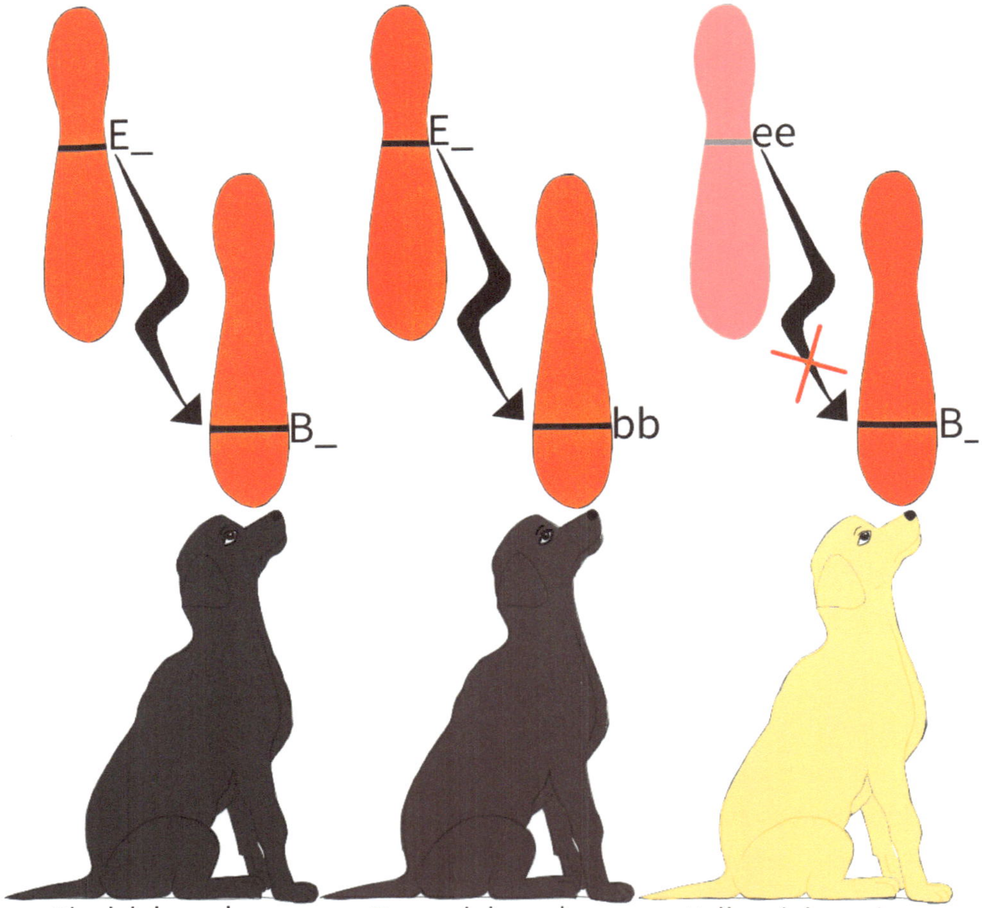

Epistasis

Epistasis is a specific type of gene interaction where one gene masks or suppresses the expression of another gene. This can significantly alter phenotypic ratios from what Mendelian genetics would predict.

Example: Returning to the Labrador Retriever example, the **E locus is epistatic to the B locus**, and the B locus is **hypostatic**. A dog with the genotype ee will have a yellow coat, regardless of whether it carries alleles for black (BB or Bb) or brown (bb) pigment. This means that the presence of the ee genotype at the E gene masks the expression of the B gene, resulting in a yellow coat. This kind of interaction can lead to modified phenotypic ratios, such as the **9:3:4 (instead of 9:3:3:1) ratio** observed in certain dihybrid crosses involving epistatic genes.

Epistasis can also be observed in other species and traits. For instance, in mice, the gene for coat color can be influenced by a separate gene that determines whether pigment is produced at all. If the mice carry the recessive allele for no pigment, they will be albino regardless of their coat color genes. Such examples underscore the importance of understanding gene interactions in predicting and explaining genetic outcomes.

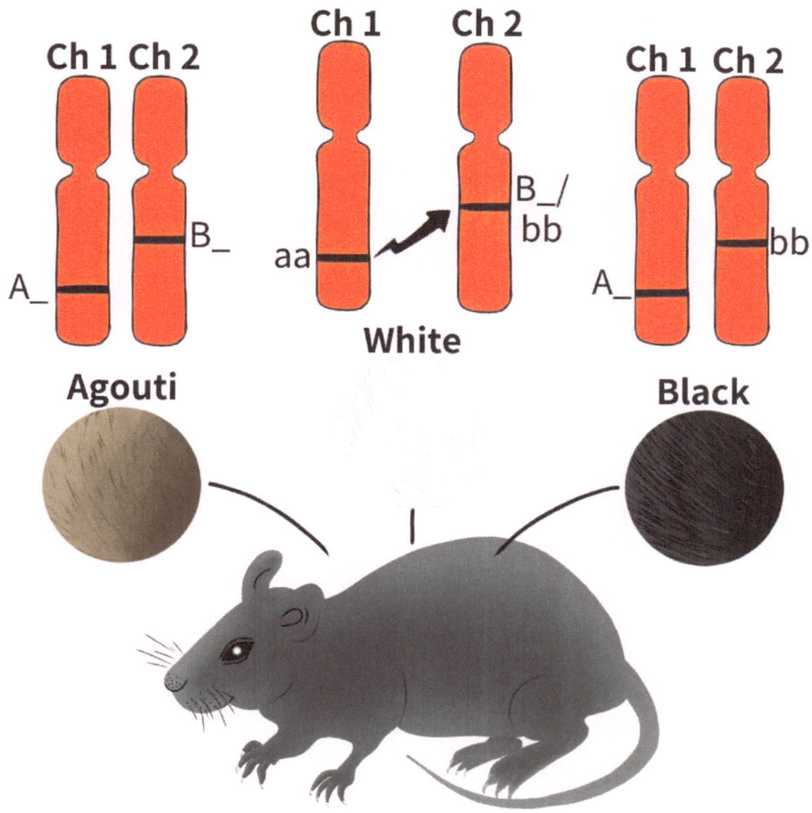

Gene vs. Environmental Effects

While genes play a crucial role in determining traits, the environment can also significantly influence an organism's phenotype. The interplay between genetic and environmental factors is essential in shaping the characteristics of living organisms.

Examples: Consider height in humans. While genes largely determine height, environmental factors such as nutrition and health during childhood can impact a person's final height. A person with genes for tall stature may not reach their potential height if they experience poor nutrition during their growth years. Conversely, a person with genes for shorter stature might achieve a taller height if they receive optimal nutrition and healthcare.

Another example is the **color of hydrangea flowers**. The color of these flowers is influenced by the **pH level of the soil** in which they are grown. In **acidic soil, hydrangea flowers tend to be blue, while in alkaline soil, they are more likely to be pink.** This demonstrates how environmental factors can directly influence the expression of genetic traits.

In humans, the development of certain diseases can also be influenced by both genetic predisposition and environmental factors. For instance, someone may carry genes that increase their risk for type 2 diabetes, but lifestyle factors such as diet and exercise can play a crucial role in whether they actually develop the condition. This complex interplay between genes and the environment highlights the need to consider both factors in understanding and predicting phenotypic outcomes.

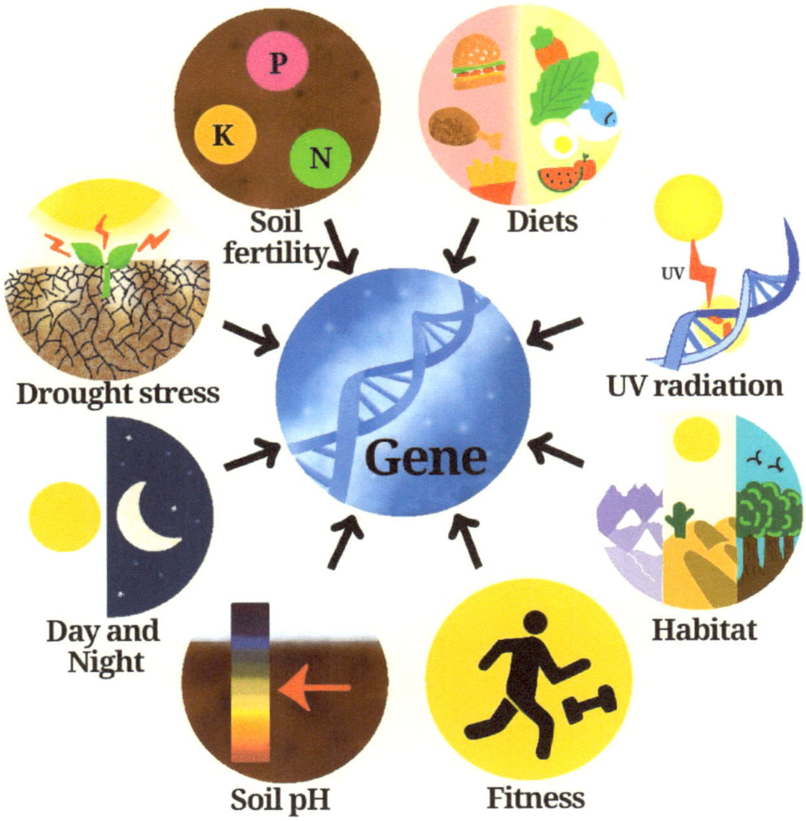

Multiple Alleles

Multiple alleles refer to the presence of more than two alleles for a particular gene within a population, even though an individual can only have two alleles (one from each parent). This concept expands the diversity of possible genetic combinations and phenotypes within a population.

Example: The ABO blood type system in humans is controlled by three alleles: I^A, I^B, and i. The I^A and I^B alleles are co-dominant, meaning that both alleles are expressed equally if present. The i allele is recessive to both I^A and I^B.

- I^AI^A or I^Ai: Blood type A
- I^BI^B or I^Bi: Blood type B
- I^AI^B: Blood type AB (both antigens are present)
- ii: Blood type O (neither antigen is present)

Genotype	Blood Type
I^AI^A or I^Ai	A
I^BI^B or I^Bi	B
I^AI^B	AB
ii	O

Blood type is determined by the presence or absence of specific antigens on the surface of red blood cells. Individuals with blood type A have A antigens, those with blood type B have B antigens, those with blood type AB have both A and B antigens, and those with blood type O have neither antigen. The ABO system shows how multiple alleles create a variety of phenotypes, each significant for blood transfusion compatibility and other medical considerations.

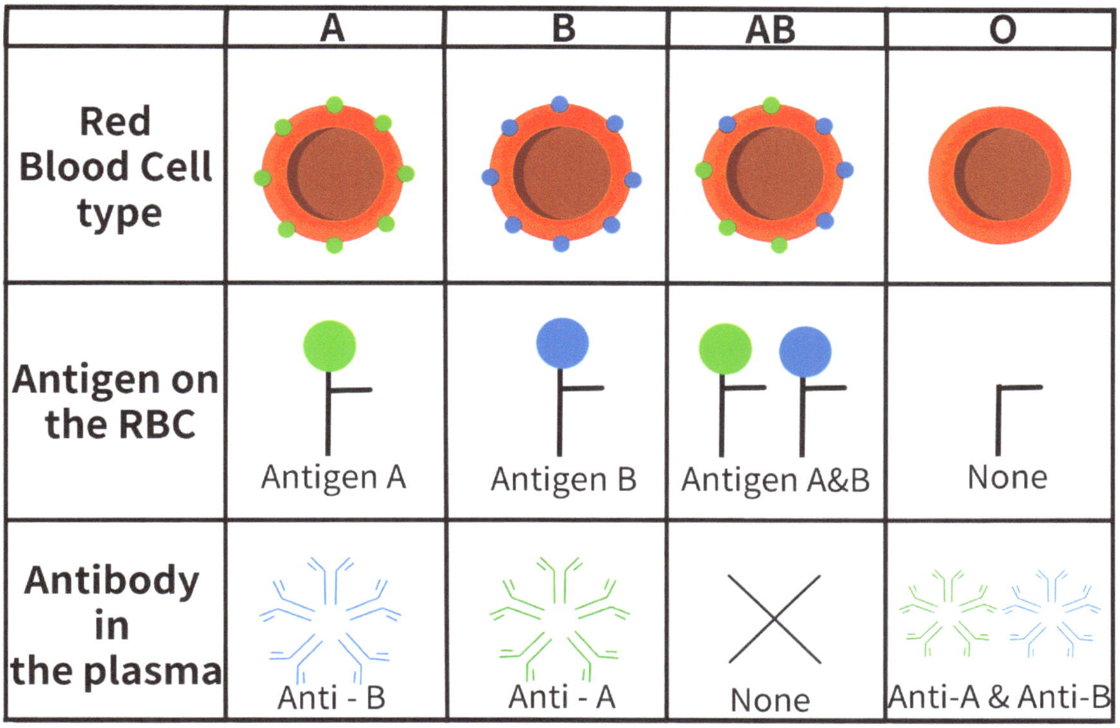

ABO blood group antigens are present on red blood cells, and IgM antibodies are present in the serum

Bombay Phenotype: When the Switch Controls the Lights

The Bombay phenotype is a fascinating example of how one gene can override another. In most people, the ABO blood group is determined by the alleles I^A, I^B, or i, which dictate whether A, B, AB, or O antigens appear on red blood cells. However, before these antigens can be displayed, the body first needs a basic structure called the H antigen, which acts like a foundation. Individuals with the hh genotype are unable to produce this H antigen. Without this foundation, even if a person carries the I^A or I^B alleles, the A or B antigens cannot be expressed. As a result, the person appears to have blood type O, even if genetically they should be A, B, or AB.

Analogy:

Imagine building a signboard with glowing letters. The A and B letters represent the ABO alleles, bright, colorful, and ready to shine. But there's a catch: the letters can only light up if the power switch is turned on. The H antigen is that switch. In the Bombay phenotype, the switch is missing. So even if the letters are in place, they remain dark. To anyone looking, it appears like there are no letters at all, just a blank sign. In the same way, a person with the Bombay phenotype looks like blood type O, but genetically, they may carry A or B alleles that simply cannot be expressed.

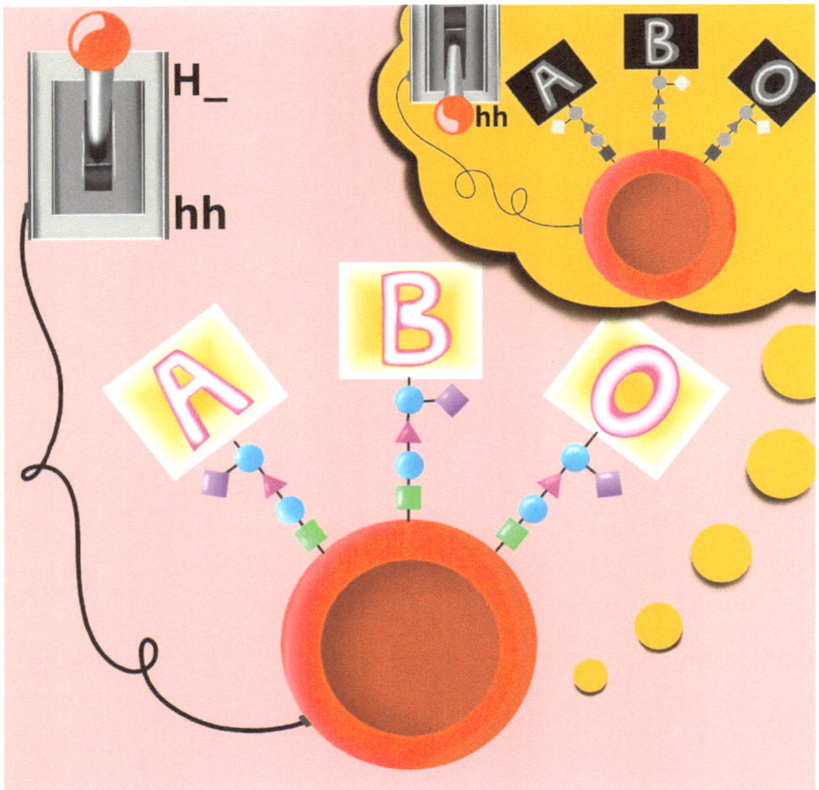

Rh Factor Alleles

The Rh factor is another important blood group system in humans, determined by the presence (Rh+) or absence (Rh-) of the Rh antigen on red blood cells. It is controlled by a single gene with two alleles:

- **D (dominant) – presence of the Rh antigen (Rh^+)**
- **d (recessive) – absence of the Rh antigen (Rh^-)**

Genotype	Rh Factor
DD or Dd	Rh-positive (Rh^+)
dd	Rh-negative (Rh^-)

Example: A person with the genotype Dd will be Rh-positive, as the D allele is dominant over the d allele, ensuring the expression of the Rh antigen.

The **Rh factor is particularly important in pregnancy**. If **an Rh-negative mother carries an Rh-positive fetus, her immune system may recognize the baby's Rh antigen as foreign and produce antibodies** against it. This immune response can lead to hemolytic disease of the newborn (HDN) in future pregnancies.

To prevent complications, Rh-negative mothers are given **Rh immunoglobulin (RhoGAM) injections,** which prevent their immune system from developing antibodies against Rh-positive blood cells.

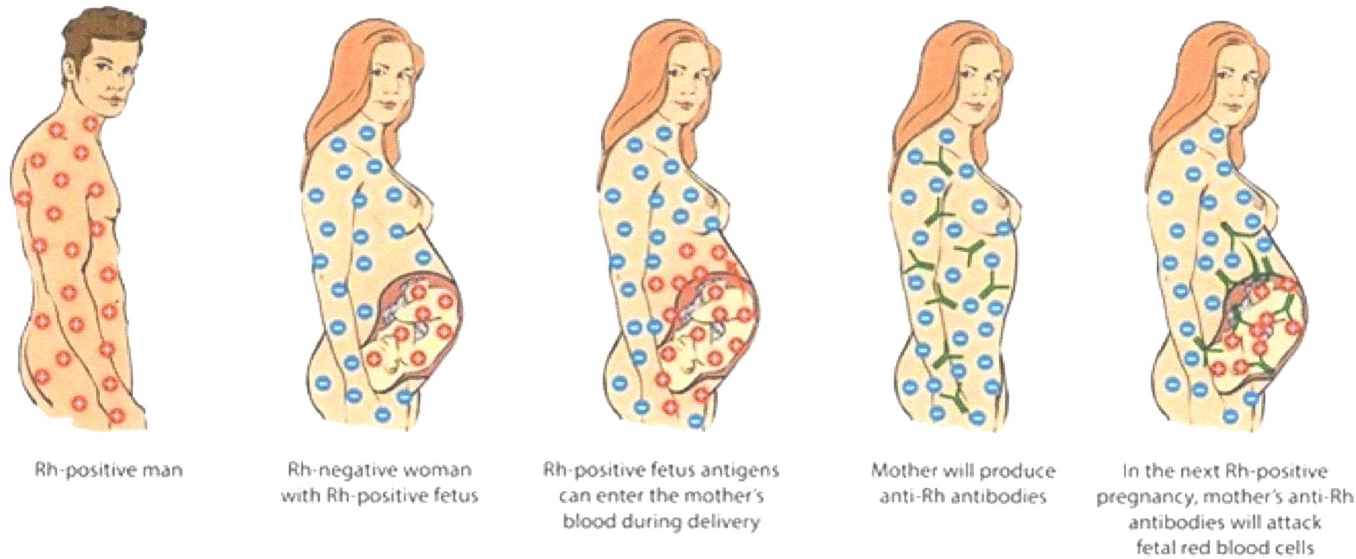

Pedigree Analysis and Type of Inheritance

Understanding Pedigree Analysis in Genetics

Pedigree analysis is a fundamental tool in genetics used to study the inheritance of traits across generations. It involves the creation and interpretation of **pedigree charts**, which are graphical representations of a family tree that display the relationships among family members and indicate which individuals exhibit or carry a particular trait. By analyzing these charts, geneticists can:

- Identify patterns of inheritance (dominant, recessive, X-linked, mitochondrial, etc.).
- Detects carriers of genetic conditions.
- Predict the likelihood of traits appearing in future generations.

Importance and Applications

Pedigree analysis has critical applications in both medical and research settings:

- **Clinical Genetics:** Helps genetic counselors assess the risk of inherited disorders (e.g., hemophilia, cystic fibrosis) and guide family planning.
- **Medical Research:** Aids in identifying genes responsible for hereditary conditions, advancing treatments, and developing targeted therapies.
- **Complex Traits & Multifactorial Inheritance:** Beyond single-gene disorders, pedigree analysis helps researchers study traits influenced by multiple genes and environmental factors.

By examining pedigrees, researchers can gain insights into the genetic basis of these traits and their inheritance patterns, facilitating the study of polygenic and multifactorial traits.

Basic Symbols in Pedigree Charts

1. **Individual Symbols:**
    - **Male:** ♂ or ■ (square)
    - **Female:** ♀ or ○ (circle)
    - **Unknown Sex:** ◊ (diamond)
2. **Trait Symbols:**
    - **Affected Individual:** ■ (shaded square) or ● (shaded circle)
    - **Unaffected Individual:** □ (unshaded square) or ○ (unshaded circle)
    - **Carrier (for recessive traits):** ◐ (half-shaded square or circle) or a dot inside the symbol (● in a circle or square)
3. **Relationship Symbols:**
    - **Mating Line:** Horizontal line connecting a male and female symbol (♂–♀ or □–○)
    - **Sibling Line:** Horizontal line connecting sibling symbols, descending from parents
    - **Offspring Line:** Vertical line from the mating line, connecting to offspring
4. **Generations:**
    - **Generations are labeled with Roman numerals:** I, II, III, etc.
5. **Other Symbols:**
    - **Proband:** Individual from whom the pedigree is initiated, marked with an arrow (→) pointing to the symbol
    - **Deceased Individual:** A diagonal line through the symbol
    - **Consanguinity (mating between relatives):** Double horizontal line connecting the mating pair
    - **Adoption:**
        - **Adopted In:** Dotted line around the individual symbol
        - **Adopted Out:** Brackets around the individual symbol
    - **Twins:**
        - **Monozygotic (identical) Twins:** A horizontal line connecting two symbols with an additional horizontal line between them (□–○–□)
        - **Dizygotic (fraternal) Twins:** A horizontal line connecting two symbols without an additional line between them (□–○)

Example Pedigree Chart Symbols

- **Male:** □
- **Female:** ○

- **Affected Male:** ■
- **Affected Female:** ●
- **Carrier Male (Recessive Trait):** ◐ (half-shaded square)
- **Carrier Female (Recessive Trait):** ◐ (half-shaded circle)
- **Deceased Individual:** ⊗ (symbol with a diagonal line through it)
- **Consanguineous Mating:** Double horizontal line between two symbols (□═○)
- **Proband:** Symbol with an arrow pointing to it (→□ or →○)
- **Adopted In:** □ (square with dashed border) or ○ (circle with dashed border)
- **Adopted Out:** □ (square with brackets) or ○ (circle with brackets)
- **Monozygotic (Identical) Twins:** □–○–□ (additional horizontal line between the twins)
- **Dizygotic (Fraternal) Twins:** □–○ (no additional line between the twins)

Constructing a Pedigree

Constructing a pedigree involves several systematic steps to ensure that family relationships and the inheritance of traits are accurately represented. Below are detailed steps for creating a pedigree, gathering family history information, and representing different family members and their relationships.

Steps in Creating a Pedigree

- **Identify the Proband**
  - The proband, also known as the index case, is the individual from whom the pedigree analysis begins. It is the starting point of the pedigree analysis. This person usually seeks genetic counseling or testing due to a health concern or trait of interest.
  - Example: In a family concerned about a hereditary form of cancer, the proband might be the first family member diagnosed with the condition.
- **Collect Comprehensive Family History**
  - Gather detailed information about the proband's family, including health histories and genetic traits. This involves talking to family members and reviewing medical records when possible.
  - **Example:** When studying a hereditary cardiovascular condition, ask about occurrences of heart disease, high cholesterol, and strokes in both immediate and extended family members.
- **Document Each Family Member**
  - Record the names, birthdates, and other relevant details of each family member.
  - Example: For each individual, note their health status, known genetic conditions, and ages at diagnosis or death.

- **Determine Relationships and Generation Levels**
  - Organize the family members into generations, typically labeled with **Roman numerals** (I, II, III, etc.), with the oldest generation at the top.
  - Example: Grandparents are labelled as **Generation I**, their children as **Generation II**, and their grandchildren as **Generation III**.
- **Draw the Pedigree Using Standard Symbols**
  - Use standardized symbols to represent males (squares), females (circles), and unknown sex (diamonds). Connect family members with appropriate lines to show relationships.
  - Example: Use horizontal lines for marriages and vertical lines to connect parents to their offspring.
- **Indicate Individuals with the Trait of Interest**
  - Shade symbols of individuals who exhibit the trait of interest and leave unshaded those who do not.
  - Example: In a pedigree for an autosomal dominant trait like Huntington's disease, affected individuals would have shaded symbols.
- **Label Each Individual**
  - Label each person with a unique identifier, such as a combination of generation number and individual number (e.g., II-1, II-2).
  - Example: The first child in Generation II could be labeled as **II-1**, the second child as **II-2**, and so on.

Gathering Family History Information

Gathering accurate family history information is crucial for constructing a reliable pedigree. Here are the steps to gather this information effectively:

- **Interview the Proband and Family Members**
  - Conduct interviews with the proband and as many family members as possible. Use structured questionnaires to ensure consistency.
  - Example: Ask about known **medical conditions, ages of onset, and causes of death** for each family member.
- **Obtain Medical Records and Genetic Test Results**
  - Review **medical records and genetic test results** when available to confirm self-reported information.
  - Example: Verify a reported case of breast cancer with medical records detailing diagnosis and treatment.

- **Identify Patterns of Inheritance**
  - Look for patterns of inheritance that suggest whether a trait is **autosomal dominant, autosomal recessive, X-linked, or mitochondrial.**
  - Example: Multiple affected individuals in successive generations may suggest an autosomal dominant inheritance pattern.
- **Include Environmental and Lifestyle Factors**
  - Note environmental and lifestyle factors that may influence the expression of genetic traits.
  - Example: Record information about **smoking habits, diet, and physical activity**, which can impact conditions like heart disease.
- **Document Incomplete Information**
  - Clearly document any **gaps or uncertainties** in the family history to avoid misinterpretation.
  - Example: If the health history of a distant relative is unknown, indicate this with a note on the pedigree.

Pedigree analysis is a powerful tool for understanding inheritance patterns and genetic risk. By following a structured approach, geneticists and healthcare professionals can accurately assess familial traits, predict genetic risks, and support informed medical decisions.

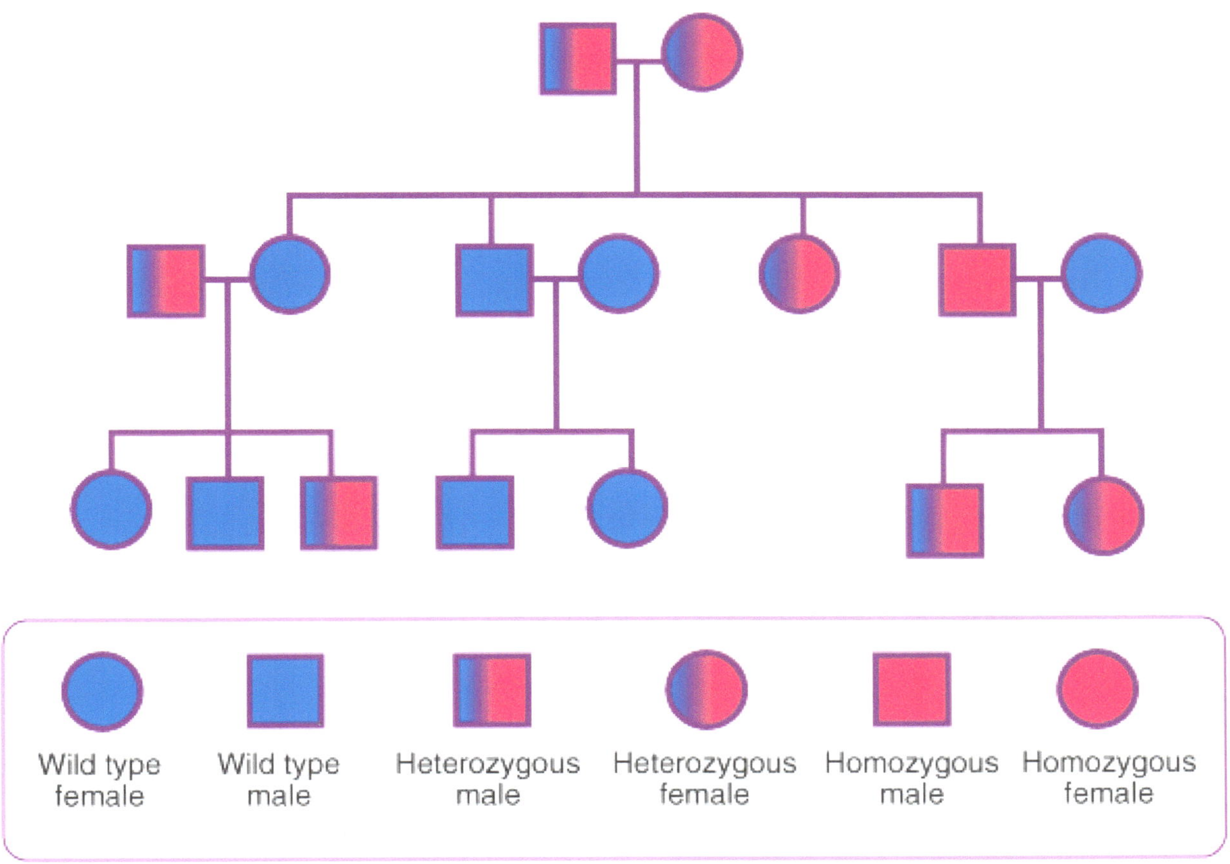

Overview of Inheritance Patterns

Inheritance patterns describe how genetic traits and disorders are passed from parents to offspring. These patterns provide insights into the likelihood of a trait appearing in a family, the mechanism behind its transmission, and the genetic basis of various conditions. Understanding these patterns is fundamental in genetics, helping to predict and diagnose genetic disorders, counsel patients, and develop personalized treatment plans.

Autosomal Dominant Inheritance

Definition and Characteristics

Autosomal dominant inheritance refers to a pattern where only one copy of a mutant allele (from either parent) is sufficient to cause the expression of a trait or disorder. This type of inheritance typically manifests in **every generation**, and affected individuals have a **50%** chance of passing the mutant allele to their offspring.

Characteristics of Autosomal Dominant Inheritance:

1. Vertical Transmission: Traits appear in consecutive generations.
2. Equal Sex Distribution: Both males and females are equally affected.
3. Variable Expressivity: The severity of symptoms can vary among affected individuals.
4. Reduced Penetrance: Some individuals with the mutant allele may not show symptoms.

Example: Familial Hypercholesterolemia

Familial Hypercholesterolemia (FH) is a genetic disorder characterized by high levels of **low-density lipoprotein (LDL) cholesterol**, leading to an increased risk of cardiovascular disease. It is inherited in an autosomal dominant manner.

Genetic Basis:

- Mutations in the ***LDLR, APOB,* or *PCSK9*** genes disrupt the regulation of cholesterol levels.

Clinical Features:

- Elevated LDL cholesterol levels from a young age.
- Increased risk of early-onset cardiovascular disease.
- Physical signs such as **xanthomas** (cholesterol deposits in the skin) and **corneal arcus** (cholesterol deposits in the eyes).

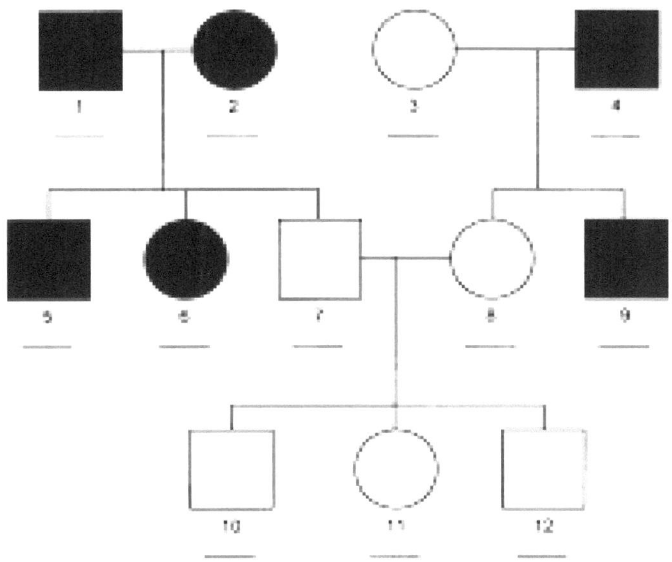

Autosomal Recessive Inheritance

Definition and Characteristics

Autosomal recessive inheritance requires **two copies** of a mutant allele (one from each parent) for a trait or disorder to be expressed. Individuals with only one copy of the mutant allele are carriers and do not exhibit symptoms. This pattern is often seen in cases where both parents are **carriers**, and the trait may **skip generations**.

Characteristics of Autosomal Recessive Inheritance:

1. Horizontal Transmission: Traits may appear in siblings but not necessarily in every generation.
2. Equal Sex Distribution: Both males and females are equally affected.
3. Carrier Parents: Parents of affected individuals are typically carriers.
4. 25% Risk: Offspring of two carrier parents have a **25% chance** of being affected.

Example: Phenylketonuria (PKU)

Phenylketonuria (PKU) is a metabolic disorder caused by a deficiency in the enzyme **phenylalanine hydroxylase**, leading to an accumulation of phenylalanine and its toxic metabolites.

Genetic Basis:

- Mutations in the **PAH** gene result in enzyme deficiency.

Clinical Features:

- Intellectual disability if untreated.
- Seizures, behavioral problems, and skin disorders.
- Manageable with a strict low-phenylalanine diet to prevent complications.

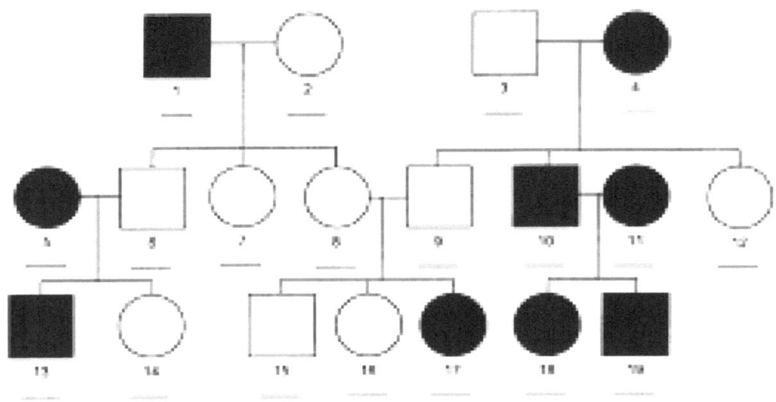

X-Linked Dominant Inheritance

Definition and Characteristics

X-linked dominant inheritance occurs when a mutation in a gene on the X chromosome is sufficient to cause the trait or disorder. Both males and females can be affected, but males often experience more severe symptoms due to having only one X chromosome.

Characteristics of X-Linked Dominant Inheritance:

1. No Male-to-Male Transmission: Affected males cannot pass the trait to their sons.
2. Affected Females: Females can pass the trait to both sons and daughters.
3. Variable Severity: Males are usually more severely affected than females.
4. Vertical Transmission: Traits appear in consecutive generations.

Example: Vitamin D-resistant Rickets

Vitamin D-resistant Rickets (Hypophosphatemic Rickets) is a disorder characterized by impaired **phosphate reabsorption** in the kidneys, leading to bone deformities.

Genetic Basis:

- **Mutations in the *PHEX* gene on the X chromosome.**

Clinical Features:

- Bone deformities similar to **rickets**.
- Growth retardation.
- **Hypophosphatemia** (low phosphate levels in the blood).

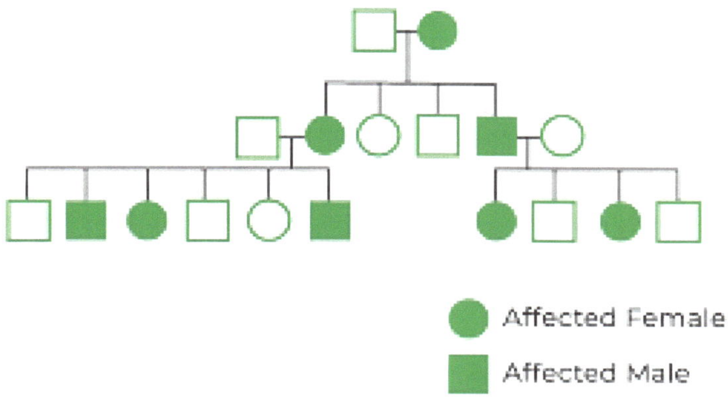

X-Linked Recessive Inheritance

Definition and Characteristics

X-linked recessive inheritance occurs when a mutation in a gene on the X chromosome causes the trait or disorder. Males are more frequently affected due to having only one X chromosome, while **females are usually carriers** and may not show symptoms.

Characteristics of X-Linked Recessive Inheritance:

1. No Male-to-Male Transmission: Affected males cannot pass the trait to their sons.
2. Carrier Females: Females with one mutant allele are carriers and can pass the trait to their offspring.
3. Affected Males: Males with the mutant allele are affected.
4. Higher Male Prevalence: Males are more commonly affected than females.

Example: Hemophilia

Hemophilia is a **bleeding disorder** caused by deficiencies in clotting factors, leading to prolonged bleeding.

Genetic Basis:

- Mutations in the F8 (Hemophilia A) or F9 (Hemophilia B) genes on the X chromosome.

Clinical Features:

- Excessive or prolonged bleeding from minor injuries as well as easy bruising.
- Spontaneous bleeding into joints and muscles.
- Manageable with clotting factor replacement therapy.

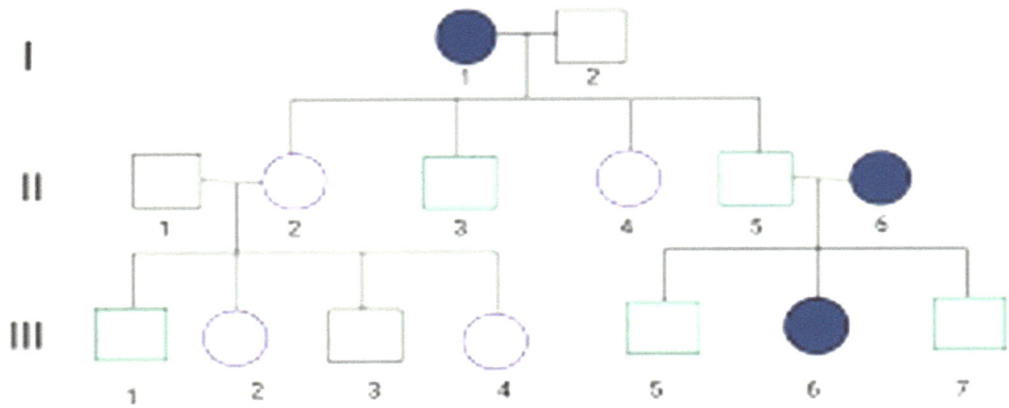

Mitochondrial Inheritance

Definition and Characteristics

Mitochondrial inheritance involves genes located in the mitochondria, which are inherited exclusively from the mother. This pattern affects **both males and females**, but only females can pass the traits to their offspring.

Characteristics of Mitochondrial Inheritance:

1. **Maternal Inheritance:** Traits are passed from **mother to all offspring**.
2. **Equal Sex Distribution:** Both males and females are affected.
3. **Variable Expressivity:** The severity of symptoms can vary widely among affected individuals.

Example: Leber's Hereditary Optic Neuropathy (LHON)

Leber's Hereditary Optic Neuropathy (LHON) is a mitochondrial disorder causing vision loss due to degeneration of the optic nerve.

Genetic Basis:

- Mutations in **mitochondrial DNA (mtDNA)**, often in the ***ND4*, *ND1*, or *ND6*** genes.

Clinical Features:

- Sudden, painless vision loss in young adulthood.
- Central vision is primarily affected, leading to legal blindness.
- Males are more commonly affected than females.

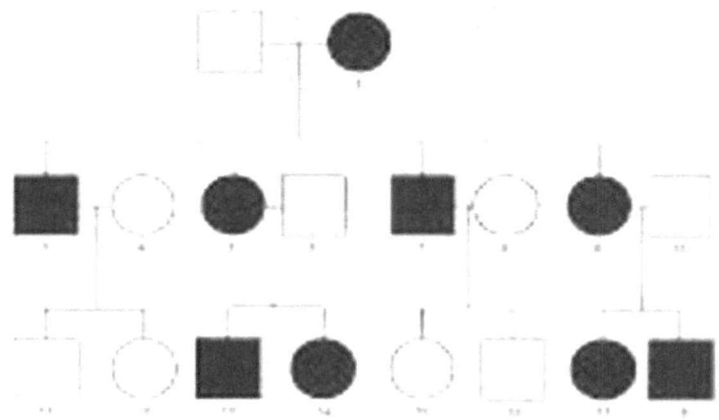

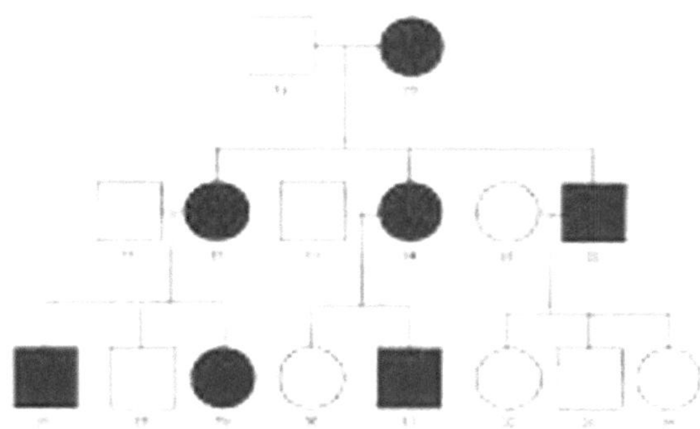

Conclusion

Understanding autosomal, X-linked, and mitochondrial inheritance is crucial in genetics, as these patterns determine how traits and disorders are passed down through generations. Autosomal inheritance (dominant and recessive) affects both sexes equally and follows predictable inheritance patterns, while X-linked traits often impact males more severely. Mitochondrial inheritance, passed exclusively from the mother, can lead to varying symptom severity among individuals. Recognizing these patterns helps in diagnosing genetic conditions, counseling families on inheritance risks, and developing targeted treatments for genetic disorders.

Simple Questions

1. Who is known as the "Father of Genetics"?
2. When and where was Gregor Mendel born?
3. What influenced Mendel's interest in plants and genetics?
4. Where did Mendel conduct his famous experiments?
5. What organism did Mendel use in his genetic experiments?
6. What are the key traits Mendel studied in pea plants?
7. How many generations did Mendel observe in his experiments?
8. What is the Law of Segregation?
9. Explain Mendel's observation in the F1 and F2 generations regarding seed shape.
10. What is a monohybrid cross, and how does it work?
11. What does the genotype ratio 1:2:1 mean in a monohybrid cross?
12. What is meant by a dominant allele?
13. Give an example of a dominant trait in Mendel's experiments.
14. What is a recessive trait?
15. How is codominance different from simple dominance?
16. What is an example of codominance in humans?
17. What is semidominance (or incomplete dominance)?
18. Give an example of semidominance in plants.
19. What is a lethal allele? Provide an example.
20. What is the Law of Independent Assortment?
21. How did Mendel demonstrate the Law of Independent Assortment?
22. What is the Law of Dominance?
23. Why was Mendel's work largely ignored during his lifetime?
24. What is epistasis?
25. Can you give an example of epistasis in animals?
26. What is the difference between gene interaction and epistasis?
27. How can environmental factors influence the expression of genetic traits?
28. What is the significance of multiple alleles in the ABO blood group system?
29. What is the Rh factor, and why is it important in pregnancy?
30. How are X-linked traits inherited differently from autosomal traits?

Answers

1. Gregor Mendel is known as the "Father of Genetics."
2. He was born on July 20, 1822, in Heinzendorf, Austria (now Hynčice, Czech Republic).
3. Mendel's interest in plants and genetics was influenced by his rural upbringing and early exposure to farming.
4. Mendel conducted his experiments in the Augustinian Abbey of St. Thomas in Brno, Austria.
5. Mendel used garden pea plants (*Pisum sativum*) in his genetic experiments.
6. Mendel studied traits such as seed shape, seed color, flower color, and pod shape.
7. Mendel observed over 28,000 pea plants, across several generations.
8. The Law of Segregation states that each individual has two alleles for each trait, which segregate during gamete formation.
9. In the F1 generation, all seeds were round, but in the F2 generation, there was a 3:1 ratio of round to wrinkled seeds.
10. A monohybrid cross is a genetic cross between individuals that differ in a single trait, such as seed shape.
11. The 1:2:1 ratio means one homozygous dominant, two heterozygous, and one homozygous recessive individual.
12. A dominant allele is one that masks the effect of the other allele in a heterozygous individual.
13. The round seed allele (R) was dominant over the wrinkled seed allele (r).
14. A recessive trait is only expressed when an individual has two recessive alleles.
15. In codominance, both alleles are expressed equally in the heterozygous condition, unlike simple dominance.
16. An example of codominance is the ABO blood group system, where both A and B antigens are expressed in AB individuals.
17. Semidominance, or incomplete dominance, occurs when the heterozygous phenotype is a blend of the two homozygous phenotypes.
18. In snapdragons, the heterozygous genotype (Rr) results in pink flowers, an intermediate color.
19. A lethal allele is one that can cause death when present in a homozygous condition, such as in Tay-Sachs disease.
20. The Law of Independent Assortment states that genes for different traits are inherited independently of each other.
21. Mendel demonstrated the Law of Independent Assortment by conducting dihybrid crosses, showing independent inheritance of traits.
22. The Law of Dominance states that one allele may mask the effect of another allele, with the dominant allele being expressed.
23. Mendel's work was ignored during his lifetime due to its lack of immediate practical application and because it conflicted with the prevailing scientific views.
24. Epistasis is a gene interaction where one gene masks or suppresses the expression of another gene.

25. In Labrador Retrievers, the E gene (epistasis) can mask the coat color determined by the B gene, leading to a yellow coat.
26. Gene interaction involves multiple genes influencing a single trait, whereas epistasis is a form of gene interaction where one gene masks the effects of another.
27. Environmental factors, like nutrition, can influence the expression of genetic traits, such as height or disease susceptibility.
28. The ABO blood group system has multiple alleles (I^A, I^B, and i), resulting in various possible blood types based on their combinations.
29. The Rh factor is a protein found on red blood cells. It is important in pregnancy because an Rh-negative mother carrying an Rh-positive baby may develop antibodies that attack the baby's red blood cells.
30. X-linked traits are inherited through the X chromosome and affect males more often, as they have only one X chromosome, whereas autosomal traits are inherited through non-sex chromosomes and affect both sexes equally.

Problem-Solving Questions

1. In pea plants, the allele for tall (T) is dominant over the allele for short (t). If a heterozygous tall plant (Tt) is crossed with a homozygous short plant (tt), what are the possible genotypes and phenotypes of their offspring?
2. In a monohybrid cross, a homozygous dominant plant (RR) is crossed with a homozygous recessive plant (rr). What will be the genotype and phenotype ratios of the F1 generation?
3. If two heterozygous pea plants (Rr) for seed color are crossed, where R is the dominant allele for round seeds and r is the recessive allele for wrinkled seeds, what is the expected phenotypic ratio in the F2 generation?
4. In a flowering plant species, the allele C produces red flowers and is dominant over the allele c, which results in white flowers. If a plant with the genotype Cc (heterozygous red) is crossed with a plant that is cc (homozygous white), what are the expected genotypic and phenotypic ratios of their offspring?
5. In pea plants, the allele for round seeds (R) is dominant over the allele for wrinkled seeds (r). If a homozygous round-seeded plant (RR) is crossed with a homozygous wrinkled-seeded plant (rr), what will be the expected genotype and phenotype of the F_1 generation?
6. In pea plants, round seeds (R) are dominant over wrinkled seeds (r), and yellow seed color (S) is dominant over green seed color (s). If two plants that are heterozygous for both traits (RrSs × RrSs) are crossed, what is the expected phenotypic ratio of the F_2 offspring?
7. A woman who is a carrier for hemophilia (X^HX^h) marries a man who has hemophilia (X^hY). What are the chances of their children having hemophilia? Provide the genotype and phenotype of the children.
8. A red-flowered snapdragon (RR) is crossed with a white-flowered snapdragon (rr). If the F1 generation produces pink-flowered snapdragons, what type of inheritance pattern is this an example of, and what are the possible genotypes and phenotypes of the F2 generation?
9. In humans, the allele for blood type A (I^A) is dominant over blood type O (i). If a man with blood type A (I^A i) marries a woman with blood type O (ii), what are the chances of their children having blood type A, B, or O?
10. If a pea plant with genotype AaBb is crossed with another pea plant with genotype aabb, what are the expected genotypes and phenotypes of their offspring?

Answers

1.
   a. Genotypes of offspring: 50% Tt, 50% tt
   b. Phenotypes of offspring: 50% tall, 50% short
2.
   a. Genotypes of F1 generation: 100% Rr
   b. Phenotypes of F1 generation: 100% tall (since R is dominant over r)
3.
   a. Genotypic ratio: 1 RR: 2 Rr: 1 rr
   b. Phenotypic ratio: 3 round seeds: 1 wrinkled seed
4.
   a. Genotypic Ratio: 1 Cc: 1 cc;
   b. Phenotypic Ratio: 1 red-flowered plant: 1 white-flowered plant
5.
   a. Genotype of the F_1 generation: 100% Rr (heterozygous)
   b. Phenotype of the F_1 generation: 100% round seeds, because the dominant allele R masks the recessive **r** allele.
6. Expected Phenotypic Ratio: 9 round yellow: 3 round green: 3 wrinkled yellow: 1 wrinkled green
7.
   a. Genotypes of children: 50% X^HX^h (carrier females), 50% X^hY (hemophiliac males)
   b. Phenotypes of children: 50% carrier females (no hemophilia), 50% hemophiliac males
8.
   a. Inheritance pattern: Incomplete dominance (semidominance)
   b. Genotypes of F1 generation: 100% heterozygous (Rr)
   c. Phenotypes of F1 generation: 100% pink flowers
   d. F2 generation genotypes: 1 RR: 2 Rr: 1 rr
   e. F2 generation phenotypes: 1 red: 2 pink: 1 white
9.
   a. Genotypic ratio of children: 50% I^A i (blood type A): 50% ii (blood type O)
   b. Phenotypic ratio of children: 50% blood type A, 50% blood type O
10.
   a. Genotypic ratio of offspring: 1 AaBb:1 Aabb:1 aaBb:1 aabb
   b. Phenotypic ratio of offspring: 1:1:1:1

References

1. Bateson, W. (1909). *Mendel's principles of heredity*. Cambridge University Press.
2. Darwin, C. (1859). *On the origin of species by means of natural selection*. John Murray.
3. Dean, L. (2005). The ABO blood group. In *Blood groups and red cell antigens*. National Center for Biotechnology Information (US). Retrieved May 1, 2025, from https://www.ncbi.nlm.nih.gov/books/NBK2267/
4. Dean, L. (2005). The Rh blood group. In *Blood groups and red cell antigens* (Chapter 7). National Center for Biotechnology Information (US). https://www.ncbi.nlm.nih.gov/books/NBK2269/
5. Griffiths, A. J. F., Wessler, S. R., Carroll, S. B., & Doebley, J. (2000). *Introduction to genetic analysis* (7th ed.). W. H. Freeman.
6. Henig, R. M. (2000). *The monk in the garden: The lost and found genius of Gregor Mendel, the father of genetics*. Houghton Mifflin Harcourt.
7. Johannsen, W. (1909). The genotype conception of heredity. *The American Naturalist, 43*(505), 129–159. https://doi.org/10.1086/279040
8. Linnaeus, C. (1758). *Systema naturae* (10th ed.). Laurentius Salvius.
9. Meunier, H., & Stern, C. (1913). A case of semi-dominance. *Genetics, 6*(6), 627–658.
10. Morgan, T. H. (1910). Sex limited inheritance in *Drosophila*. *Science, 32*(812), 120–122. https://doi.org/10.1126/science.32.812.120
11. National Center for Biotechnology Information. (2021). *Blood groups and red cell antigens*. NCBI Bookshelf. https://www.ncbi.nlm.nih.gov/books/NBK2261/
12. Scriver, C. R., Beaudet, A. L., Sly, W. S., & Valle, D. (Eds.). (2001). *The metabolic and molecular bases of inherited disease* (8th ed.). McGraw-Hill.
13. Sturtevant, A. H. (1965). *A history of genetics*. Harper & Row.
14. Tippett, P. (1983). Codominance. *Nature, 304*(5924), 115. https://doi.org/10.1038/304115a0
15. Winkler, H. (1920). *The genome: An introduction*. Gustav Fischer.

CHAPTER 2

MOLECULAR ARCHITECTURE OF DNA AND RNA: FOUNDATIONS OF GENETIC INFORMATION

Introduction: The Blueprint of Life

At the heart of every living cell lies a **blueprint**—a master plan that dictates an organism's structure and function. This blueprint is encoded in two fundamental molecules: **DNA (Deoxyribonucleic Acid) and RNA (Ribonucleic Acid)**. The discovery and understanding of these molecules have been one of the most thrilling sagas in the history of science. Our journey begins with the pioneers who unveiled the secrets of DNA and RNA, leading to a detailed exploration of their structures and functions.

The History: Unraveling the Double Helix

In the early 20th century, scientists were on a quest to understand the molecular basis of inheritance. Among these trailblazers were Rosalind Franklin, James Watson, and Francis Crick, whose contributions led to the revelation of DNA's iconic **double-helix** structure.

The Legacy of Rosalind Franklin: Pioneer of DNA

Early Life and Education

Rosalind Elsie Franklin was born on July 25, 1920, in London, England, into an influential Jewish family. From an early age, Franklin exhibited a keen interest in science and mathematics. Her educational journey was filled with notable achievements that paved the way for her scientific career.

She attended St. Paul's Girls' School, a prestigious institution known for its rigorous academic environment. Here, she excelled in science and math, encouraged by teachers who recognized her potential. Her early academic success laid the foundation for her future studies and career.

In 1938, Franklin entered Newnham College, Cambridge, where she studied chemistry. At Cambridge, she was influenced by renowned chemists and developed a strong interest in physical chemistry. Despite the male-dominated environment of the time, Franklin's determination and intellectual prowess enabled her to thrive.

She earned her PhD in physical chemistry in 1945 under the supervision of **Ronald Norrish, a future Nobel laureate.** Her doctoral research on the properties of coal and carbon later influenced her work on DNA structure.

After completing her PhD, Franklin moved to Paris to work at the Laboratoire Central des Services Chimiques de l'État. Here, she conducted pioneering research on the microstructures of carbon and coal, using **X-ray diffraction techniques**. Her research on carbon structures earned her scientific recognition and sharpened her expertise in X-ray crystallography.

King's College London: The DNA Project

In 1951, Franklin returned to England to join the Biophysics Unit at **King's College London**. It was here that she began her groundbreaking research on the structure of DNA. Working **alongside Maurice Wilkins, Raymond Gosling**, and other researchers, Franklin applied her expertise **in X-ray diffraction to study DNA fibers.**

The DNA Research: A Closer Look

Franklin's precise experimentation at King's College led to critical discoveries that reshaped our understanding of DNA's structure.

X-ray Diffraction Techniques

X-ray diffraction is a technique used to study the atomic and molecular structure of crystals. When X-rays strike a crystalline sample, they scatter in specific patterns. By analyzing these patterns, scientists can infer the arrangement of atoms within the crystal. Franklin's expertise in this technique was instrumental in her study of DNA.

Photograph 51: The Key Discovery

One of Franklin's most groundbreaking contributions was capturing the now-**famous X-ray diffraction image, Photograph 51.** This image offered undeniable proof of DNA's helical structure. Photograph 51 showed a distinct pattern of spots that suggested a double helix with a regular repeating structure.

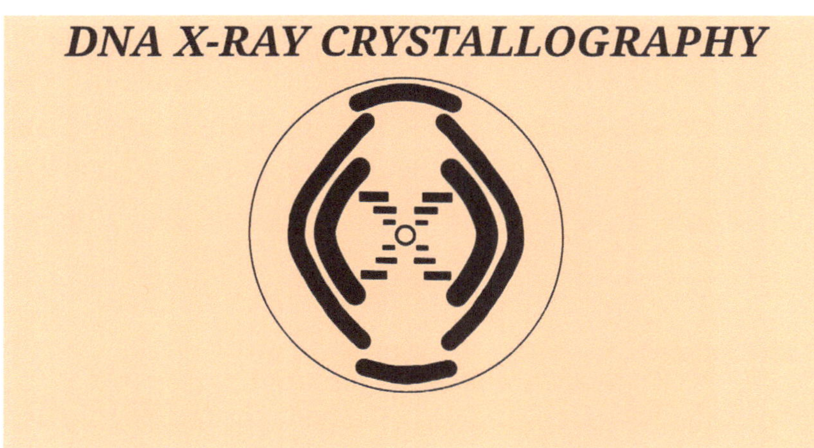

Interpretation of Data

Franklin's meticulous analysis of X-ray diffraction data provided critical insights into the structure of DNA. Her findings revealed several key characteristics:

1. **Helical Structure**: The diffraction pattern indicated that DNA had a helical structure.
2. **Phosphate Backbone**: Franklin deduced that the phosphate groups were located on the outside of the helix, with the bases oriented inward.
3. **Repetitive Nature**: The consistent spacing of diffraction spots suggested a uniform, repeating unit within the helical structure.

Determining DNA's structure from diffraction patterns was like piecing together the shape of a sculpture using only the shadows it casts. Just as shadows reveal hidden contours, Franklin's meticulous analysis of diffraction patterns uncovered the intricate architecture of DNA.

The Double Helix: Watson, Crick, and Franklin's Legacy

Franklin's groundbreaking research was pivotal in the race to uncover DNA's structure, a competition that involved multiple scientists working independently and sometimes contentiously. James Watson and Francis Crick, working at the Cavendish Laboratory in Cambridge, were also striving to solve the DNA puzzle.

The Race to Discover DNA's Structure

Watson and Crick were aware of Franklin's work through various channels, including discussions with Maurice Wilkins and seeing Photograph 51 without Franklin's direct knowledge. Drawing from Franklin's data, particularly her X-ray diffraction images—alongside findings from other researchers, **Watson and Crick constructed a DNA model featuring the now-famous double helix and complementary base pairing.**

Publication and Recognition

In 1953, Watson and Crick published their model of the DNA double helix in the journal ***Nature*.** Franklin's own work on the structure of DNA was published in the same issue, providing supporting evidence for the helical model. Despite Franklin's critical contributions, Watson and Crick received the majority of the recognition, leaving her role largely overshadowed for decades.

Franklin's Later Work and Legacy

Following her groundbreaking research on DNA, Franklin turned her focus to virology, applying her expertise in **X-ray crystallography to study virus structures.**

Research on Viruses

In 1953, Franklin moved to Birkbeck College, where she studied the structure of viruses, including the **tobacco mosaic virus (TMV) and the poliovirus.** Her research on viral structures helped uncover fundamental principles of virus assembly, deepening scientific understanding of their molecular organization.

Tragic End

Rosalind Franklin passed away from **ovarian cancer in 1958 at the age of 37**, before she could witness the full recognition of her contributions. Despite her untimely death, her scientific achievements have left an indelible mark on the field of molecular biology.

Recognition and Tribute

Although initially overlooked, Franklin's contributions have since been widely acknowledged, solidifying her place in scientific history.

Posthumous Recognition

Rosalind Franklin did not receive the Nobel Prize, as it is not awarded posthumously. However, Franklin's legacy endures through numerous awards and honors, such as the **Rosalind Franklin University of Medicine and Science in Chicago and the Rosalind Franklin Medal from the Royal Society.**

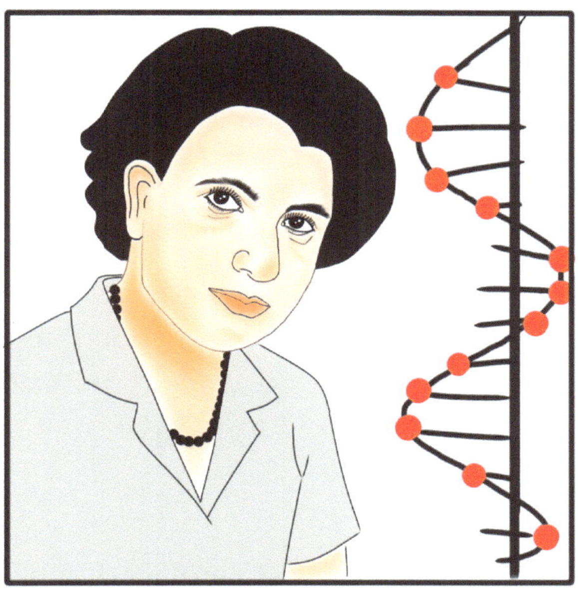

James Watson and Francis Crick: The Dynamic Duo

While Rosalind Franklin's work provided critical insights into the structure of DNA, the narrative would be incomplete without acknowledging the efforts of James Watson and Francis Crick. At the Cavendish Laboratory in Cambridge, they played a **pivotal role in deciphering the DNA double helix.** This chapter examines their backgrounds, scientific journey, and the role of Franklin's research in their discovery.

Early Lives and Academic Journeys

James Watson: The Young Prodigy

James Dewey Watson was born on April 6, 1928, in Chicago, Illinois. From a young age, Watson showed a keen interest in ornithology and genetics. He attended the University of Chicago, where he pursued his undergraduate studies, followed by a PhD in zoology from Indiana University. His early academic journey showcased a deep curiosity about life's fundamental mechanisms.

Francis Crick: The Interdisciplinary Scholar

Francis Harry Compton Crick was born on June 8, 1916, in Northampton, England. Crick's academic path was diverse; he started with physics at University College London and later transitioned to biology. His background in physics and mathematics provided him with a unique perspective on biological problems, laying out the foundation for his collaboration with Watson.

The Road to Cambridge: Forming a Partnership

Crick's Shift to Biology

Crick's transition from physics to biology was influenced by the interdisciplinary nature of the emerging field of molecular biology. During World War II, he worked on magnetic mines for the British Admiralty, but his passion for understanding life's fundamental processes led him to the Strangeways Laboratory in Cambridge, where he studied the physical properties of cytoplasm.

Watson's Early Research in Europe

After completing his PhD, Watson embarked on a research fellowship in Copenhagen, Denmark, where he studied bacterial genetics. It was during this period that Watson became intrigued by the problem of DNA's structure, a fascination that would eventually lead him to the Cavendish Laboratory in Cambridge.

Meeting at Cavendish

In 1951, Watson arrived at the Cavendish Laboratory, where he met Crick. Despite their different backgrounds, the two scientists were united by a single goal: unraveling the structure of DNA. Their collaboration thrived on the fusion of Watson's genetics expertise and Crick's knowledge of X-ray diffraction and theoretical biology.

The Influence of Rosalind Franklin's Research

Franklin's Data: A Crucial Contribution

Rosalind Franklin's X-ray diffraction work at King's College London was crucial to Watson and Crick's breakthrough. Although they did not work directly with Franklin, they gained access to her data through various channels, including discussions with Maurice Wilkins, a colleague of Franklin's who was also working on DNA. These data, particularly her diffraction images, played a decisive role in Watson and Crick's formulation of the double helix model.

Photograph 51: The Definitive Evidence

One of the most significant pieces of evidence was Photograph 51, an X-ray diffraction image of DNA captured by Franklin and her student, Raymond Gosling. This photograph provided clear evidence of a helical structure, with distinct patterns indicating the periodicity and symmetry of the helix.

Interpretation and Analysis

Watson and Crick recognized the importance of Franklin's photograph and her analysis, which suggested that the phosphate groups were on the outside of the helix and that the bases were stacked inside. This insight was pivotal in guiding their construction of the DNA model.

Building the Model: The Double Helix Emerges

The Hypothetical Model

Armed with the clues from Franklin's data, Watson and Crick began constructing a physical model of DNA. Their approach was to use trial and error, guided by the chemical and structural constraints revealed by the X-ray diffraction patterns. They hypothesized that DNA was composed of two strands forming a helical structure.

Unraveling the Code: Base Pairing as the Key

One of the key challenges was figuring out how the bases paired within the helix. **Watson and Crick proposed the idea of complementary base pairing, where Adenine (A) pairs with Thymine (T) and Guanine (G) pairs with Cytosine (C).** This base-pairing mechanism explained the uniform width of the helix and the specific patterns observed in the diffraction data.

Finalizing the Model

By integrating Franklin's data with their hypotheses, **Watson and Crick constructed a model that depicted DNA as a right-handed double helix.** The two strands were arranged in an **antiparallel orientation,** with base pairs positioned at the core and the **phosphate-sugar backbone** forming the outer framework. This model explained DNA's structural stability.

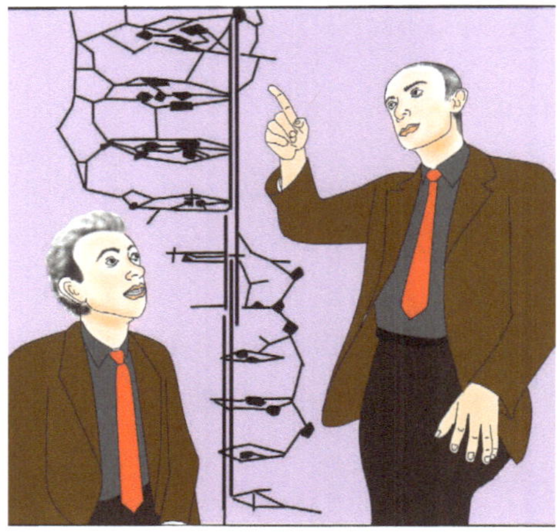

The Publication and Aftermath

The 1953 Breakthrough Paper

In April 1953, Watson and Crick published their model of DNA in the journal ***Nature*.** Their paper, titled **"A Structure for Deoxyribose Nucleic Acid,"** was succinct yet revolutionary, proposing the now-iconic double-helix model and its implications for genetic replication. This revelation marked a paradigm shift in molecular biology, laying the foundation for modern genetics.

Franklin's Supporting Paper

In the same issue of ***Nature*, Franklin and her colleague, Raymond Gosling**, published their own paper detailing the X-ray diffraction data that supported the helical structure.

Nobel Prize and Recognition

In 1962, **James Watson, Francis Crick, and Maurice Wilkins were awarded the Nobel Prize in Physiology or Medicine** for their discoveries concerning the molecular structure of nucleic acids.

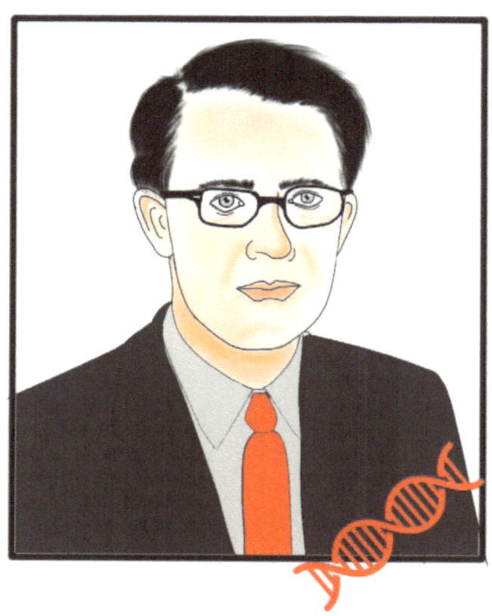

Maurice Wilkins

Conclusion: The Collaborative Triumph

The discovery of the DNA double helix was a collaborative effort that combined the talents and insights of multiple scientists. While Watson and Crick are often credited with the breakthrough, the contributions of Rosalind Franklin and Maurice Wilkins were equally indispensable. This discovery not only revolutionized our understanding of genetics but also underscored the importance of collaboration and the open exchange of scientific knowledge.

The Story of DNA Structure: A Double Helix Tale

Imagine a vast library where the books are not just stored but intricately woven into a spiral staircase. Each step of this staircase represents a pair of bases, held together by hydrogen bonds, while the railings are formed by two intertwining strands of nucleotides. This is the elegant double helix of DNA—nature's blueprint for life.

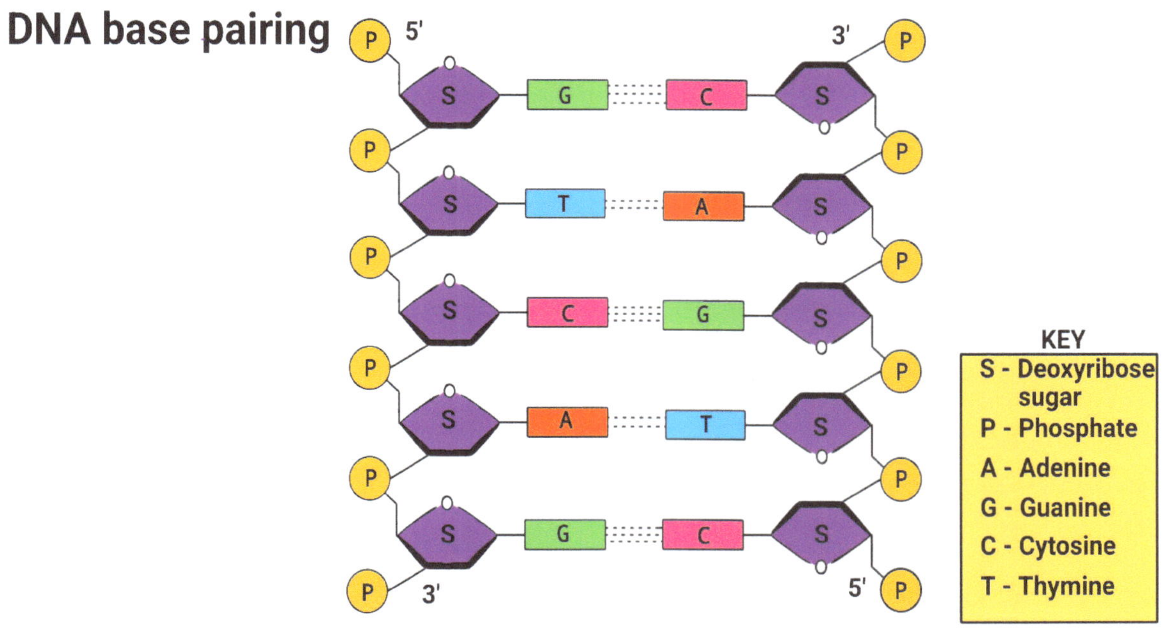

The Building Blocks: Nucleotides

At the core of DNA is the **nucleotide,** a molecule made up of three components: a phosphate group, a deoxyribose sugar, and a nitrogenous base. DNA contains **four nitrogenous bases—Adenine (A), Thymine (T), Guanine (G), and Cytosine (C). These bases pair in a highly specific manner (A with T, G with C), forming the rungs of the DNA ladder.**

The Strands: Sugar-Phosphate Backbone

The sides of the DNA ladder are formed by alternating sugar and phosphate groups, known as the sugar-phosphate backbone. Each nucleotide is connected to the next by covalent bonds between the phosphate of one nucleotide and the sugar of the next. This creates a stable yet flexible structure that can twist into the double helix.

The Helix: A Spiraling Masterpiece

DNA's double helix follows a right-handed spiral, meaning it twists in a clockwise direction. The two strands run in opposite orientations, a feature known as **antiparallelism,** which is crucial for DNA replication and transcription. This orientation ensures that genetic information is precisely copied and utilized by cellular machinery.

Example: *Picture a twisted ladder where each rung is a pair of nitrogenous bases and the sides are formed by sugar-phosphate backbones. The specific pairing of bases ensures that the genetic information is accurately copied and transmitted.*

The Details of DNA Structure

To delve deeper into the structure of DNA, we must explore the specifics of its components and their interactions.

Nitrogenous Bases and Base Pairing

In the early 1950s, biochemist **Erwin Chargaff** made a crucial discovery that greatly advanced our understanding of DNA. Through his experiments, Chargaff found that in any given DNA sample, the amount of adenine (A) always equaled the amount of thymine (T), and the amount of guanine (G) always equaled the amount of cytosine (C). This observation, known as ***Chargaff's Rule,*** formed the foundation for understanding how the nitrogenous bases pair in the DNA double helix. His work, published in 1950, led to the realization that the base pairing in DNA is highly specific and follows a precise pattern.

DNA contains four nitrogenous bases: Adenine (A), Thymine (T), Guanine (G), and Cytosine (C). These bases are categorized into two groups:

- **Purines** (Adenine and Guanine) – larger, double-ring structures.
- **Pyrimidines** (Thymine and Cytosine) – smaller, single-ring structures.

The base pairing between these nitrogenous bases is highly specific and governed by hydrogen bonds:

- **Adenine (A) pairs with Thymine (T)** through **two hydrogen bonds.**
- **Guanine (G) pairs with Cytosine (C)** through **three hydrogen bonds, making the G-C pair more stable than the A-T pair.**

This complementary base pairing is essential for maintaining the uniform width of the DNA helix and plays a critical role in genetic fidelity during DNA replication, ensuring the accurate transmission of genetic information.

Phosphodiester Bonds and Strand Directionality

The nucleotides are linked together by **phosphodiester** bonds, which form between the 3' hydroxyl group of one sugar and the 5' phosphate group of the next. This establishes **directionality** in the DNA strand:

- The **5' end** has a free **phosphate group**.
- The **3' end** has a free **hydroxyl group**.

This polarity is crucial for processes like DNA replication and transcription, as enzymes recognize and operate along the strand in a **5' to 3' direction**.

Major and Minor Grooves: Binding Sites for Proteins

The helical twist of DNA creates two alternating grooves along its surface:

- The **major groove** is **wider** and provides easier access for proteins that regulate gene expression, such as transcription factors.
- The **minor groove** is **narrower** but still plays a role in interactions with small molecules and some regulatory proteins.

These grooves act as docking sites for **enzymes and regulatory proteins**, influencing processes such as DNA replication, repair, and transcription.

DNA Supercoiling: Compacting Genetic Material

Given the immense length of DNA, it must be efficiently packaged within cells. This is achieved through **supercoiling**, where the double helix twists upon itself to form a more compact structure. Supercoiling ensures that DNA fits within the **nucleus** while remaining accessible for cellular processes.

RNA Structure: The Versatile Molecule

RNA (Ribonucleic Acid) is a crucial biomolecule that serves as both a carrier of genetic information and a functional molecule in cellular processes. While RNA shares similarities with DNA, its distinct structural differences make it more flexible and functionally diverse.

The Building Blocks: Ribonucleotides

RNA is composed of **ribonucleotides**, each consisting of:

- A **ribose sugar**, which differs from DNA's deoxyribose by having a hydroxyl (-OH) group at the **2' position**, making RNA **more chemically reactive and less stable**.
- A **phosphate group**, forming the backbone of the molecule.

- A **nitrogenous base**, with RNA using **uracil (U) instead of thymine (T)**. Like thymine, uracil pairs specifically with **adenine (A)**.

These differences allow RNA to perform a wider range of cellular functions beyond genetic storage.

Single-Stranded Structure

Unlike the double-stranded DNA, RNA is typically **single-stranded.** This single-stranded nature allows RNA to fold into complex three-dimensional shapes, enabling it to perform a variety of functions within the cell.

RNA Types and Functions

RNA exists in multiple forms, each specialized for distinct cellular functions. While DNA stores genetic information, RNA serves as both a messenger and an active participant in gene expression and protein synthesis.

1. **mRNA (Messenger RNA):** mRNA carries genetic information from DNA to the ribosomes, where proteins are synthesized. It serves as a **template for translation**, ensuring the correct sequence of amino acids in a protein.
2. **tRNA (Transfer RNA):** tRNA functions as the **molecular adapter** in translation, delivering specific amino acids to the ribosome. Each tRNA contains an **anticodon** that pairs with a complementary mRNA codon, ensuring accurate protein assembly.
3. **rRNA (Ribosomal RNA):** rRNA is a structural component of ribosomes, the cellular machinery that synthesizes proteins. rRNA helps to catalyze the formation of peptide bonds between amino acids.
4. **snRNA (Small Nuclear RNA):** snRNA plays a key role in **pre-mRNA splicing**, removing non-coding regions (**introns**) and joining coding sequences (**exons**) to create functional mRNA.
5. **miRNA (MicroRNA) and siRNA (Small Interfering RNA):** These are **regulatory RNAs** modulate gene expression by binding to mRNA, either **blocking translation or triggering mRNA degradation**, ensuring precise control of protein production.

Types of RNA

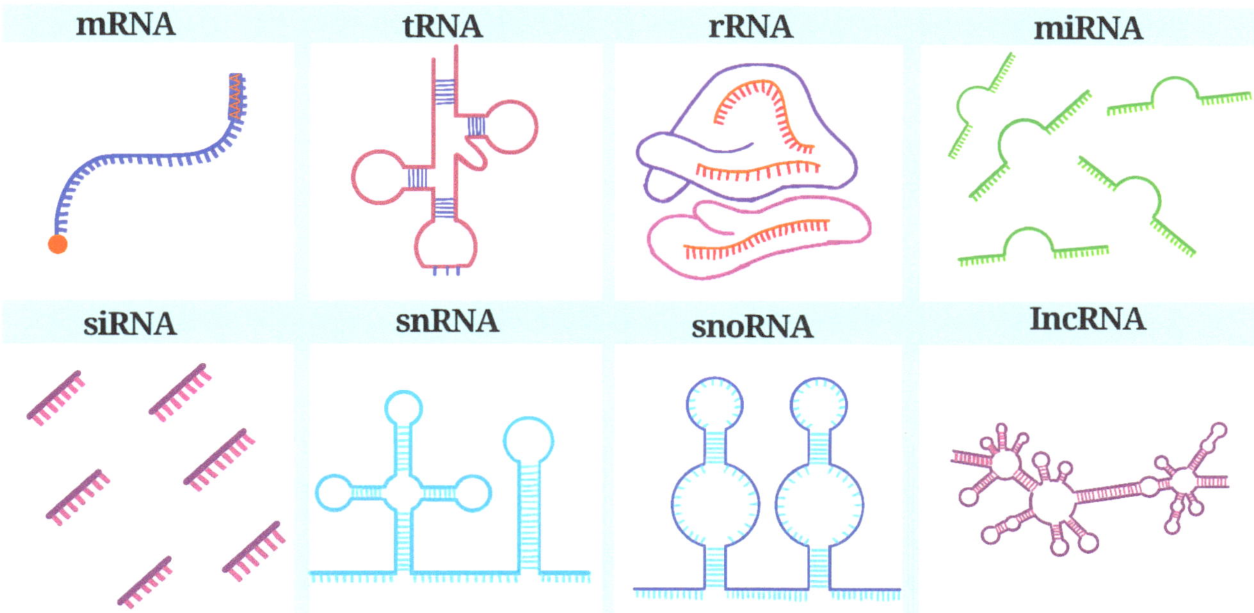

The Story of RNA Structure

Imagine RNA as a versatile artist, capable of taking on different shapes and forms to perform a variety of tasks. Unlike DNA, which remains a stable double helix, RNA's **single-stranded nature and ribose sugar** grants it remarkable flexibility. This allows it to fold into **functional structures essential for catalysis, binding, and regulation**.

Primary Structure: The Linear Code

The primary structure of RNA is its linear sequence of ribonucleotides. Each ribonucleotide consists of a ribose sugar, a phosphate group, and one of four nitrogenous bases—**Adenine (A), Uracil (U), Guanine (G), and Cytosine (C).** The sequence of these bases encodes genetic information and serves as the foundation for RNA folding.

Secondary Structures: Molecular Framework

RNA can form secondary structures such as **hairpins, loops, and bulges.** These structures are created by intramolecular base pairing, where complementary regions of the RNA strand fold and pair with each other. These secondary structures serve as **the foundation for more complex folding**.

Tertiary Structures: The Functional Forms

The secondary structures can further fold into intricate three-dimensional structures, stabilized by interactions such as **hydrogen bonds, van der Waals forces, and ionic bonds**. These tertiary shapes are essential for the function of RNA molecules, especially those involved in catalysis and binding.

Analogy: *Picture a long ribbon that can fold into intricate shapes and loops. Each fold and twist enables the ribbon to perform a different function, just as RNA folds allow it to act in various cellular processes. The way it folds determines whether it acts as a scaffold, an enzyme, or a messenger—just as RNA's structure defines its function in the cell.*

DNA vs. RNA: A Comparative Tale

While DNA and RNA share some similarities, their differences are crucial for their respective roles in the cell.

Stability: Longevity vs. Adaptability

DNA is built for **stability and permanence**, thanks to the absence of a 2′ hydroxyl group in its sugar. This structural advantage allows DNA to **preserve genetic information** across generations.

In contrast, RNA contains a reactive 2′ hydroxyl group, making it **more prone to degradation.** This inherent instability is not a flaw—it is a **feature** that enables RNA to function **temporarily**, adapting quickly to the cell's needs.

Structure: Rigidity vs. Flexibility

DNA exists as a **rigid double-stranded helix**, providing **error-resistant storage** for genetic instructions. This structure ensures that information is accurately passed on during cell division.

RNA, however, is **single-stranded**, allowing it to **bend, fold, and twist into complex shapes**. This flexibility is essential for RNA's diverse functions, from catalysis to gene regulation.

Functions: The Blueprint vs. The Workforce

DNA serves as the **genetic blueprint**, storing and transmitting hereditary information.

RNA is the **active executor**, translating these instructions into action. Whether as **messenger RNA (mRNA)** carrying genetic code, **transfer RNA (tRNA)** assembling proteins, or **ribosomal RNA (rRNA)** forming cellular machinery, RNA **drives the processes that sustain life**.

Analogy: The Architect and the Builders

Imagine DNA as the master architect's blueprint, carefully drafted to ensure the perfect design. RNA, in turn, is the construction crew, interpreting the plan, assembling the structure, and making real-time adjustments.

Simple Questions

1. What is the blueprint of life?
2. Who were the pioneers in DNA research?
3. What did Rosalind Franklin contribute to the discovery of DNA?
4. What is X-ray diffraction used for?
5. What is Photograph 51?
6. What did the X-ray diffraction pattern of DNA reveal?
7. What did Franklin deduce about DNA's structure from X-ray data?
8. Who are James Watson and Francis Crick?
9. How did Watson and Crick contribute to DNA's structure?
10. What was Watson and Crick's model of DNA?
11. Why is the discovery of DNA's structure important?
12. What is the sugar-phosphate backbone in DNA?
13. What are the nitrogenous bases in DNA?
14. How do the nitrogenous bases pair in DNA?
15. What is the function of the double helix structure of DNA?
16. What is Chargaff's Rule?
17. What is the difference between purines and pyrimidines in DNA?
18. What is the structure of DNA's double helix?
19. What is DNA replication?
20. What is the role of DNA in genetic inheritance?
21. What are the primary building blocks of RNA?
22. How does RNA differ from DNA?
23. What is mRNA, and what is its function?
24. What is tRNA, and what is its function?
25. What is rRNA, and what role does it play in protein synthesis?
26. What is snRNA, and why is it important?
27. What are miRNA and siRNA?
28. What is the primary structure of RNA?
29. How does RNA fold into secondary and tertiary structures?
30. Why is RNA more flexible than DNA?

Answers

1. The blueprint of life is the genetic information encoded in DNA.
2. The pioneers in DNA research were Rosalind Franklin, James Watson, and Francis Crick.
3. Rosalind Franklin captured the crucial X-ray diffraction image that provided evidence of DNA's helical structure.
4. X-ray diffraction is a technique used to study the atomic structure of molecules by analyzing patterns formed when X-rays are directed at crystals.
5. Photograph 51 is a famous X-ray diffraction image that revealed DNA's helical structure.
6. The X-ray diffraction pattern of DNA revealed that DNA had a helical structure with repeating units.
7. Franklin deduced that DNA had a helical structure with phosphate groups on the outside and bases inside.
8. James Watson and Francis Crick were the scientists who proposed the double helix model of DNA.
9. Watson and Crick used Franklin's X-ray data and other findings to construct the double helix model of DNA.
10. Watson and Crick's model showed DNA as a double helix with complementary base pairing.
11. The discovery of DNA's structure is important because it explains how genetic information is stored and transmitted in cells.
12. The sugar-phosphate backbone is formed by alternating sugar and phosphate groups, providing structural support for DNA.
13. The nitrogenous bases in DNA are Adenine (A), Thymine (T), Guanine (G), and Cytosine (C).
14. Adenine pairs with Thymine, and Guanine pairs with Cytosine through hydrogen bonds.
15. The double helix structure of DNA provides stability and facilitates the accurate transmission of genetic information.
16. Chargaff's Rule states that in any DNA sample, the amount of Adenine equals Thymine, and the amount of Guanine equals Cytosine.
17. Purines (Adenine and Guanine) are larger, double-ring structures, while Pyrimidines (Thymine and Cytosine) are smaller, single-ring structures.
18. DNA's double helix consists of two intertwined strands of nucleotides that spiral around each other.
19. DNA replication is the process by which DNA is copied before cell division.
20. DNA stores genetic instructions, which are inherited by offspring, ensuring the continuity of life.
21. RNA is composed of ribonucleotides, which consist of a ribose sugar, a phosphate group, and a nitrogenous base.

22. RNA is single-stranded, uses uracil (U) instead of thymine, and is chemically more reactive than DNA.
23. mRNA carries genetic information from DNA to the ribosome for protein synthesis.
24. tRNA acts as an adapter during translation, bringing amino acids to the ribosome to build proteins.
25. rRNA is a key component of the ribosome, where it helps catalyze the formation of peptide bonds between amino acids.
26. snRNA plays a role in splicing pre-mRNA by removing introns and joining exons.
27. miRNA and siRNA are small RNA molecules that regulate gene expression by degrading mRNA or inhibiting translation.
28. The primary structure of RNA is its linear sequence of ribonucleotides.
29. RNA folds into secondary structures, such as hairpins, by base pairing within the molecule, and further folds into tertiary structures for functional roles.
30. RNA is more flexible than DNA because it is single-stranded and can adopt various three-dimensional shapes to perform diverse functions.

Problem-Based Questions

1. A researcher is studying a DNA sequence and finds that the amount of Adenine (A) is 25%. What percentage of Thymine (T) would be present in the same DNA sample according to Chargaff's Rule?
2. In a DNA sample, the ratio of Guanine (G) to Cytosine (C) is 1:1. If the concentration of Guanine is 40%, what is the concentration of Cytosine?
3. A researcher analyzes an X-ray diffraction image of DNA and observes that the spots are spaced at regular intervals. What structural feature of DNA does this pattern suggest?
4. In an experiment, DNA is heated to 95°C and then slowly cooled. The researcher observes that the two strands of DNA separate. What does this observation indicate about the structure of DNA?
5. A mutation occurs in the DNA sequence that changes a guanine (G) to adenine (A). How might this change affect the DNA structure and function?
6. If a DNA molecule has a sequence of bases: AAGCTG, what would the complementary strand of this DNA be?
7. In a study of RNA, it is observed that a molecule of mRNA carries the codon sequence AUG-UCU-AGG. What would the corresponding anticodons on tRNA be?
8. A strand of RNA is given as 5'-AUGGCUUA-3'. What is the sequence of the corresponding DNA strand?
9. In a hypothetical organism, the RNA polymerase is mutated such that it cannot correctly bind to the promoter region. What would be the result of this mutation on transcription?
10. A researcher observes that the structure of rRNA closely resembles the shape of a ribosome. Why is this feature important for its function?
11. If the RNA molecule contains the sequence AUGCGU, what will be the sequence of the polypeptide chain formed during translation?
12. If a molecule of RNA is found to contain uracil (U), what does this indicate about the type of molecule it is?
13. A researcher measures the ratio of purines to pyrimidines in a sample of DNA and finds the ratio is 1:1. What can be concluded about the base composition of the DNA?
14. What is the complementary DNA strand for a segment of RNA with the sequence 5'-AUGGCU-3'?
15. A mutation occurs that changes a thymine (T) to guanine (G) in a DNA sequence. What effect would this have on protein synthesis?
16. In RNA processing, a segment of the mRNA is spliced out and discarded. What is this segment called?
17. A researcher finds that DNA from a certain organism is 40% guanine. What is the percentage of thymine in the DNA?
18. In RNA transcription, what would be the RNA sequence transcribed from the DNA template strand 3'-TACGGT-5'?
19. A researcher observes that the DNA strand is 5'-ATGCAT-3'. What is the corresponding RNA sequence that would be transcribed from this strand?
20. If DNA polymerase makes an error during DNA replication, how would this impact the resulting strand?

Answers

1. According to Chargaff's Rule, the amount of Adenine (A) equals the amount of Thymine (T). Therefore, if A is 25%, T will also be 25%.
2. According to Chargaff's Rule, G equals C. Therefore, if G is 40%, C will also be 40%. The regular spacing of the diffraction spots suggests that DNA has a helical structure, as identified in the double helix model.
3. This observation indicates that the two strands of DNA are held together by hydrogen bonds, and the DNA strands can separate when heated, as seen in DNA denaturation.
4. A mutation that changes G to A can alter base pairing. Normally, G pairs with C, but if G changes to A, it could result in incorrect base pairing, leading to mutations that affect DNA replication and transcription.
5. The complementary strand of AAGCTG would be TTCGAC, following the base pairing rules (A pairs with T, C pairs with G).
6. The corresponding anticodons would be UAC-AGA-UCC, as tRNA anticodons are complementary to the mRNA codons.
7. The corresponding DNA strand would be 3'-TACCGAAT-5', as RNA uses uracil (U) instead of thymine (T) and pairs with adenine (A) in the DNA.
8. If RNA polymerase cannot bind to the promoter region, transcription would be inhibited, preventing the synthesis of mRNA from the DNA template.
9. The structural similarity of rRNA to the ribosome allows rRNA to be a key structural component of ribosomes, facilitating protein synthesis by catalyzing peptide bond formation.
10. The polypeptide chain will be formed from the amino acids corresponding to the codons: Methionine (AUG), Arginine (CGU). The sequence would be "Methionine Arginine."
11. The presence of uracil (U) indicates that the molecule is RNA, as uracil replaces thymine (T) in RNA and pairs with adenine (A).
12. A 1:1 ratio of purines (A and G) to pyrimidines (T and C) indicates that the DNA follows Chargaff's Rule, with equal amounts of A to T and G to C.
13. The complementary DNA strand would be 3'-TACCGA-5', as uracil in RNA replaces thymine in DNA.
14. The mutation may cause a change in the protein synthesized, as the incorrect base pairing could lead to the wrong amino acid being incorporated during translation.
15. The discarded segment of mRNA is called an intron. The remaining segments that are spliced together are called exons.
16. If the DNA contains 40% guanine (G), it must also contain 40% cytosine (C) due to base pairing. This leaves 20% for adenine (A) and thymine (T), meaning thymine is 20%.
17. The RNA sequence transcribed from this DNA template would be 5'-AUGCCA-3', as RNA is synthesized in the 5' to 3' direction, complementary to the DNA template.
18. The corresponding RNA sequence would be 5'-AUGCAU-3', where uracil (U) replaces thymine (T) in RNA.
19. If DNA polymerase makes an error, it could introduce a mutation in the newly synthesized strand, potentially altering the genetic code and leading to changes in protein function or disease.

References

1. Watson, J. D., & Crick, F. H. C. (1953). Molecular structure of nucleic acids: A structure for deoxyribose nucleic acid. *Nature, 171*(4356), 737–738.
2. Franklin, R. E., & Gosling, R. G. (1953). Molecular configuration in sodium thymonucleate. *Nature, 171*(4369), 740–741.
3. Cobb, M., & Comfort, N. (2023, April 25). What Rosalind Franklin truly contributed to the discovery of DNA's structure. *Nature.*
4. Science History Institute. (n.d.). *Francis Crick, Rosalind Franklin, James Watson, and Maurice Wilkins*. Retrieved July 13, 2025, from https://www.sciencehistory.org/education/scientific-biographies/james-watson-francis-crick-maurice-wilkins-and-rosalind-franklin
5. Alberts, B., Johnson, A., Lewis, J., Raff, M., Roberts, K., & Walter, P. (2015). *Molecular biology of the cell* (6th ed.). Garland Science.
6. Travers, A., & Muskhelishvili, G. (2015). DNA structure and function. *FEBS Journal*, *282*(12), 2279–2295. https://doi.org/10.1111/febs.13307
7. Portin, P. (2014). The birth and development of the DNA theory of inheritance: Sixty years since the discovery of the structure of DNA. *Journal of Genetics, 93*(1), 293–302.
8. King's College London. (n.d.). *The story behind Photograph 51*. Retrieved July 13, 2025, from https://www.kcl.ac.uk/the-story-behind-photograph-51

The Story of the Cell Cycle

Imagine a bustling city. This city is like no other; it's alive. Each building represents a living cell, and the activities inside these buildings are the processes that keep the cell, and ultimately the city, functioning smoothly. Just as a city follows predictable routines, morning rush hours, midday work, and nighttime repairs, cells progress through distinct phases to grow, prepare, and divide. This entire process is known as the cell cycle.

The cell cycle is a series of stages that a cell goes through to divide and produce new cells. This process is crucial for growth, development, and repair in all living organisms. Let's embark on a journey to explore this fascinating cycle.

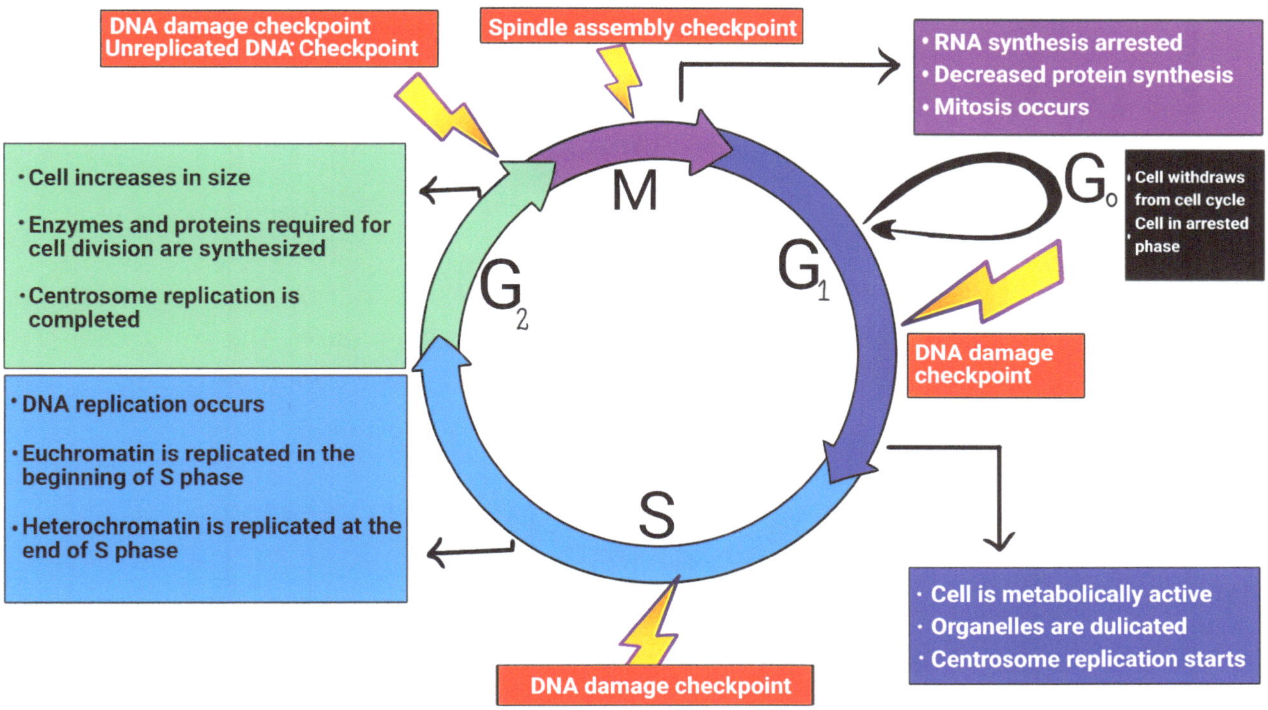

G1 Phase: The Growth Phase

Our journey begins in the **G1 phase**—the first gap phase. Picture a **newly constructed building**, awaiting furnishing and essential utilities before it can function properly. Similarly, during G1, the **cell grows in size, synthesizes proteins, and produces organelles** needed for its future tasks.

But before proceeding, the cell performs **critical checks**, assessing whether its environment is suitable for division. If conditions are unfavorable, the process **pauses for repairs**—just as a city might halt construction if materials are lacking or safety regulations aren't met.

Analogy: *A young plant seedling first absorbs water and nutrients, strengthening its structure before expanding its leaves and growing taller. Likewise, in G1, a cell gathers resources to ensure a successful future division.*

S Phase: The Synthesis Phase

Now, the cell enters the **S phase**, where it embarks on its most **critical task: DNA replication**. Imagine a **grand library** tasked with making an exact copy of every book in its collection. Similarly, during this phase, the cell **duplicates its entire genome**, ensuring that each future cell receives a complete set of genetic instructions.

This process is **highly precise**:

- **Helicase enzymes** unwind the DNA double helix, like a librarian carefully unfolding old manuscripts.
- **DNA polymerase** then meticulously **adds complementary nucleotides**, ensuring that two identical DNA molecules are formed.

The final result? Each **daughter cell** will inherit an **exact genetic blueprint** of the parent cell.

Analogy: *Picture a chef preparing for a grand banquet. To maintain consistency, they meticulously copy each recipe, ensuring that every dish tastes the same, no matter how many times it's made.*

G2 Phase: The Second Growth Phase

With DNA replication complete, the cell enters the G2 **phase**—a final **preparatory stage** before division. This phase is akin to a **final inspection before a spaceship launch**. The cell **grows further, synthesizes essential proteins, and assembles key organelles** necessary for division.

A crucial aspect of G2 is **quality control**:

- The cell **checks for DNA replication errors** and **activates repair mechanisms** if needed.
- It also begins organizing the **structures required for mitosis**, ensuring a smooth transition into cell division.

Analogy: *Think of a student submitting their thesis. Before handing it in, they carefully proofread the content, verify all references, and check that figures and diagrams are correctly placed—just as the cell ensures everything is in order before progressing.*

M Phase: The Mitotic Phase

The M phase (mitotic phase) is the **final act** of the cell cycle, where the cell **splits into two identical daughter cells**. Like a carefully choreographed **stage performance**, this phase unfolds in distinct steps, each playing a crucial role in ensuring accurate division.

Prophase: The Curtains Rise

- The **chromatin condenses** into distinct **chromosomes**, making them visible under a microscope.
- The **nuclear envelope begins to break down**, signaling that the cell is ready for division.
- **Spindle fibers**—rope-like structures—start forming, emerging from the centrioles at opposite ends of the cell.

Metaphase: The Center Stage

- The **chromosomes align** at the cell's equator, forming the **metaphase plate**.
- Each chromosome is attached to the spindle fibers, ensuring **equal distribution** to the daughter cells.

Anaphase: The Grand Split

- The sister chromatids separate, pulled toward opposite poles by the spindle fibers.
- Each chromatid is now an independent chromosome, ensuring equal genetic distribution.
- It's like a tug-of-war, where each side pulls with precision, ensuring the teams (chromosomes) are evenly split.

Telophase: The Final Bow

- **The chromosomes decondense back into chromatin.**
- **A new nuclear envelope forms around each set of chromosomes, creating two new nuclei.**
- **The spindle fibers disassemble, marking the end of mitosis.**

Cytokinesis: The Grand Finale

- **The cell membrane pinches inward, splitting the cytoplasm in two.**
- **This results in two identical daughter cells, each with a complete set of DNA.**

Analogy: *Imagine a baker preparing a batch of bread. After carefully mixing the dough (S phase) and letting it rise to perfection (G2 phase), the baker skillfully divides it into equal portions (M phase). Each portion is then baked into identical loaves, ensuring consistency—just as the cell divides to create two genetically identical daughter cells.*

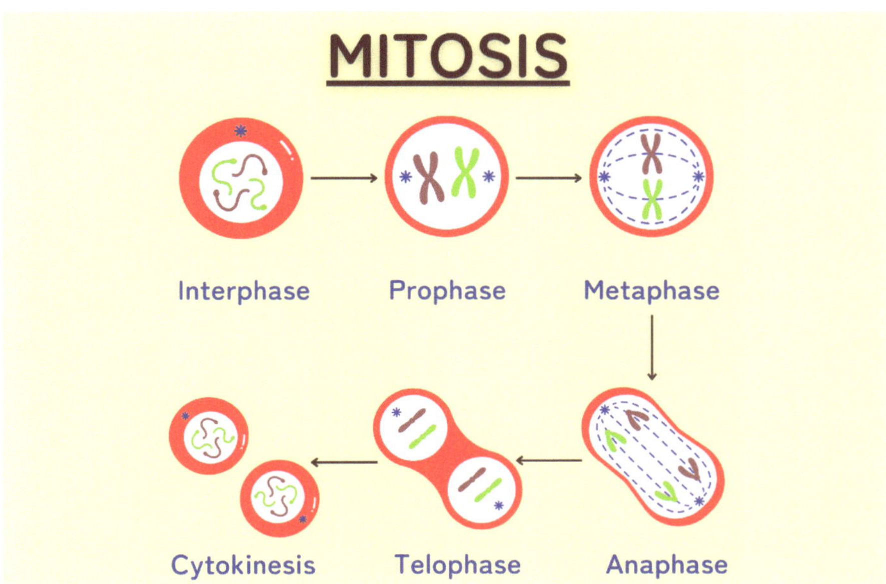

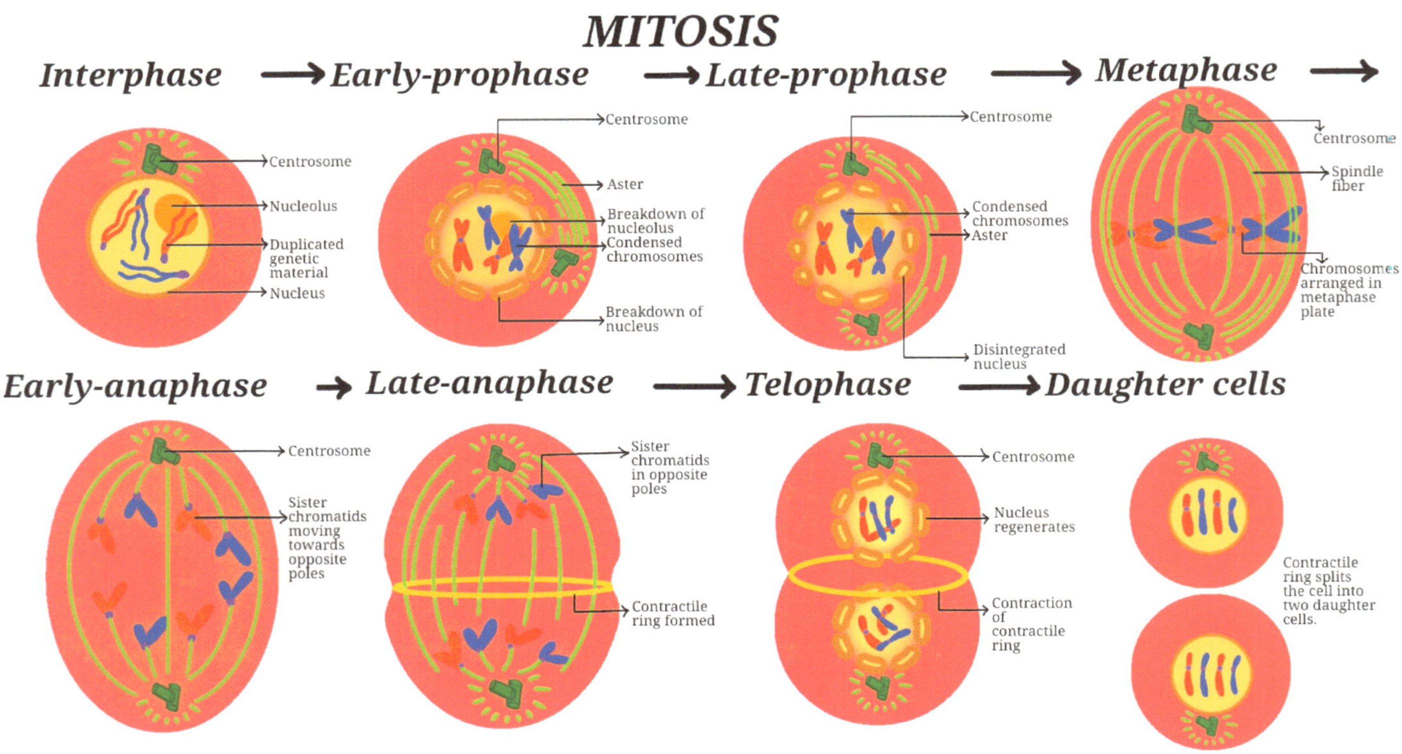

Regulation of the Cell Cycle

Like a well-organized system, the cell cycle has built-in checkpoints to ensure everything proceeds correctly. These checkpoints are regulated by proteins called **cyclins** and enzymes known as **cyclin-dependent kinases (CDKs)**, which act like security officers at an airport. They inspect passengers (cells) at key points, ensuring they are cleared for departure (division) or held back for further checks if something isn't right.

If these checkpoints fail, the result can be **uncontrolled cell division**, a defining characteristic of **cancer**. When cells bypass these regulatory mechanisms, they divide without restriction, leading to the formation of tumors. This makes proper cell cycle regulation essential for maintaining healthy growth and preventing disease.

Analogy: *Imagine a factory producing high-quality electronics. At different stages, inspectors examine each device to ensure there are no malfunctions. If a defect is found, production is paused until the issue is corrected. Without this quality control, faulty products could flood the market—just as unchecked cell division can lead to harmful consequences in the body.*

Conclusion: The Never-Ending Cycle

The cell cycle is a **continuous and self-sustaining process**, with each new cell embarking on its own journey of growth and division. It is the foundation of life, enabling organisms to grow, heal, and reproduce.

Much like a bustling city or a finely tuned assembly line, the cell cycle operates through precise coordination and regulation. By understanding its mechanisms, we gain deeper insight into the fundamental **processes that sustain life and maintain cellular health.**

The Tale of Meiosis

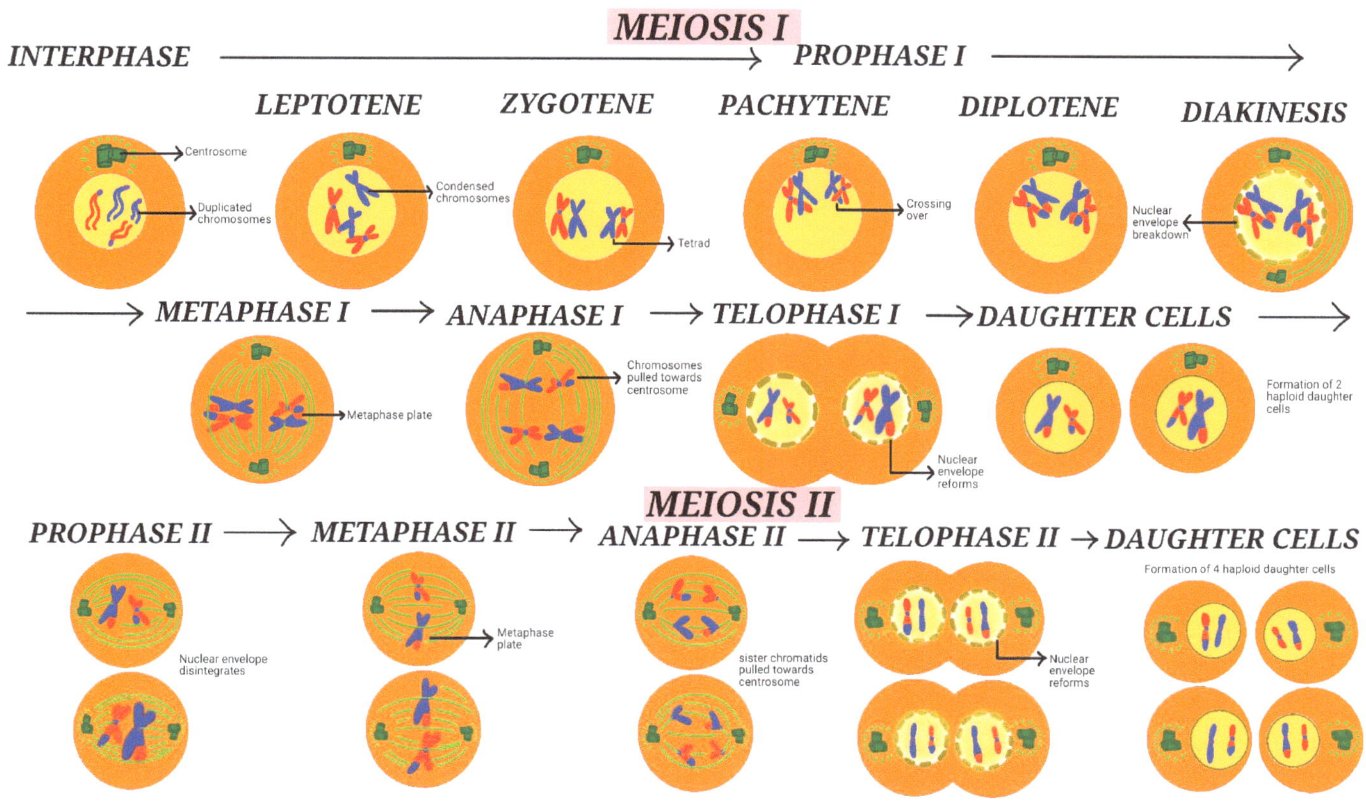

Introduction: The Secret of Life's Diversity

In a grand biological kingdom, the future of every generation depends on a remarkable event—a division unlike any other. This **sacred process** does not merely copy life; it **reshapes it, weaving new patterns of genetic uniqueness**. This enchanting process is **meiosis**, the key to diversity in sexually reproducing organisms.

Meiosis ensures that each new generation inherits **just the right number of chromosomes**, preventing an exponential increase across generations. It accomplishes this by **halving the chromosome count**, producing four genetically unique daughter cells. These specialized cells—**gametes (sperm in males, eggs in females)**—carry the blueprint of life and ensure variation among individuals.

Let's embark on this epic journey through meiosis, where chromosomes engage in a **carefully orchestrated dance**, setting the stage for life's endless diversity.

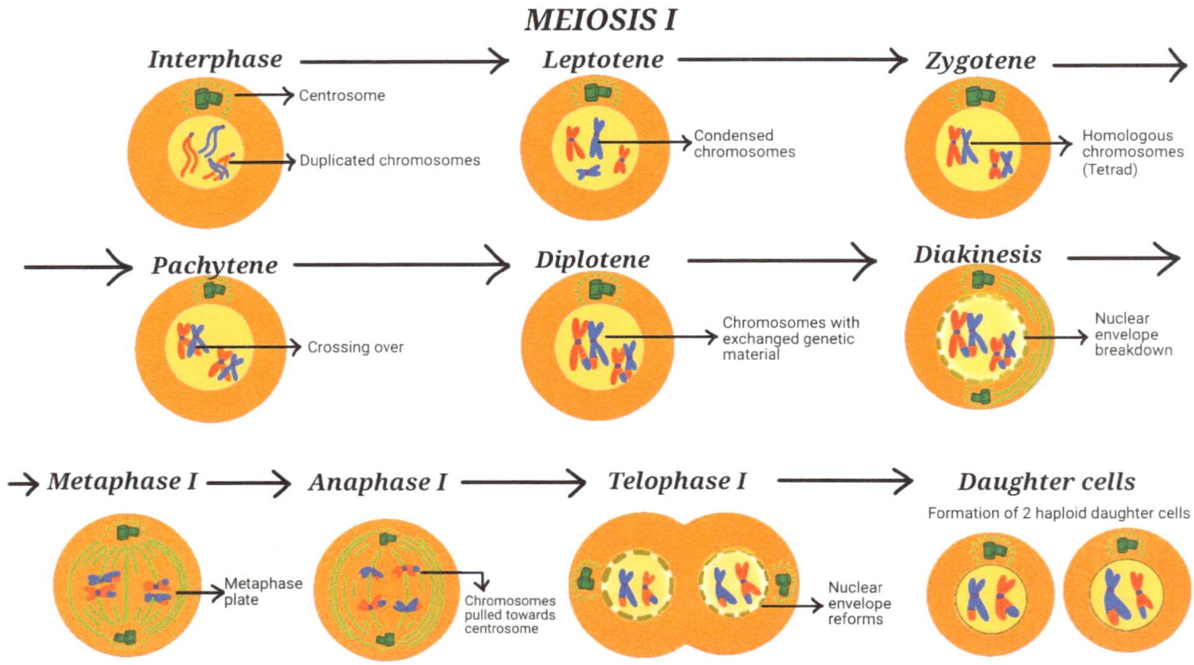

Meiosis I: The First Division

Our story begins in a cell brimming with potential, where chromosomes **gather in pairs**, preparing for a special event. Unlike ordinary cell division, **meiosis I is all about mixing and matching, ensuring genetic diversity**.

Prophase I: The Grand Ball

In the kingdom of the cell, a **grand ball** is held, where all the nobles—**homologous chromosomes**—elegantly pair up to dance. This pairing, known as **synapsis**, is a **momentous occasion**, as it allows the chromosomes to align closely with their partners.

But the real **magic** happens on the dance floor. As they twirl and sway, the **chromosomes exchange pieces of themselves**, a phenomenon called **crossing over**. This exchange ensures that when the ball ends, no dancer (chromosome) leaves the same as they arrived. The newly **recombinant chromosomes** now carry a **unique combination of genetic traits**, setting the stage for endless variation in future generations.

Analogy: *Imagine two dancers trading not just hats and scarves, but parts of their outfits—one swaps a shimmering blue sleeve for a golden one, while another trades a patterned sash for a velvet belt. By the end of the night, each dancer wears a unique ensemble, reflecting a blend of both original styles.*

Metaphase I: The Grand Lineup

The moment has arrived for the **chromosome pairs** to take their places. Like nobles **preparing for a grand procession**, they align along the **center of the ballroom (cell)**. However, this lineup is **not**

predetermined—it happens **randomly, a process known as independent assortment.** This **random arrangement ensures** that each new cell will receive a **different mix of chromosomes**, adding another layer to genetic diversity.

Analogy: *Picture two lines of dancers standing opposite each other, awaiting their next move. But unlike a choreographed routine, their order is shuffled at random, ensuring no two dances are ever the same.*

Anaphase I: The Great Separation

As the music swells, the **spindle fibers tighten** and pull the **homologous chromosomes apart**, drawing them toward **opposite sides of the ballroom**. This marks a crucial moment: each **new cell will now have only half the original chromosome number**—preparing for the **next stage of division**.

Analogy: *Imagine the dancers being dramatically pulled apart, each group escorted into separate rooms. They are now in different locations, yet still part of the same grand event.*

Telophase I and Cytokinesis: A New Beginning

As the **curtains close** on this first phase, the ballroom **transforms**. The cell **physically divides** into **two new halls (cells), each with a unique mix of dancers (chromosomes).** A **nuclear membrane reforms** around each set, ensuring that these new cells are ready for the **final act—Meiosis II.**

Analogy: *Picture two smaller but distinct dance halls being set up, each filled with different groups of dancers. Though separated, they are still preparing for the next grand performance—the second division.*

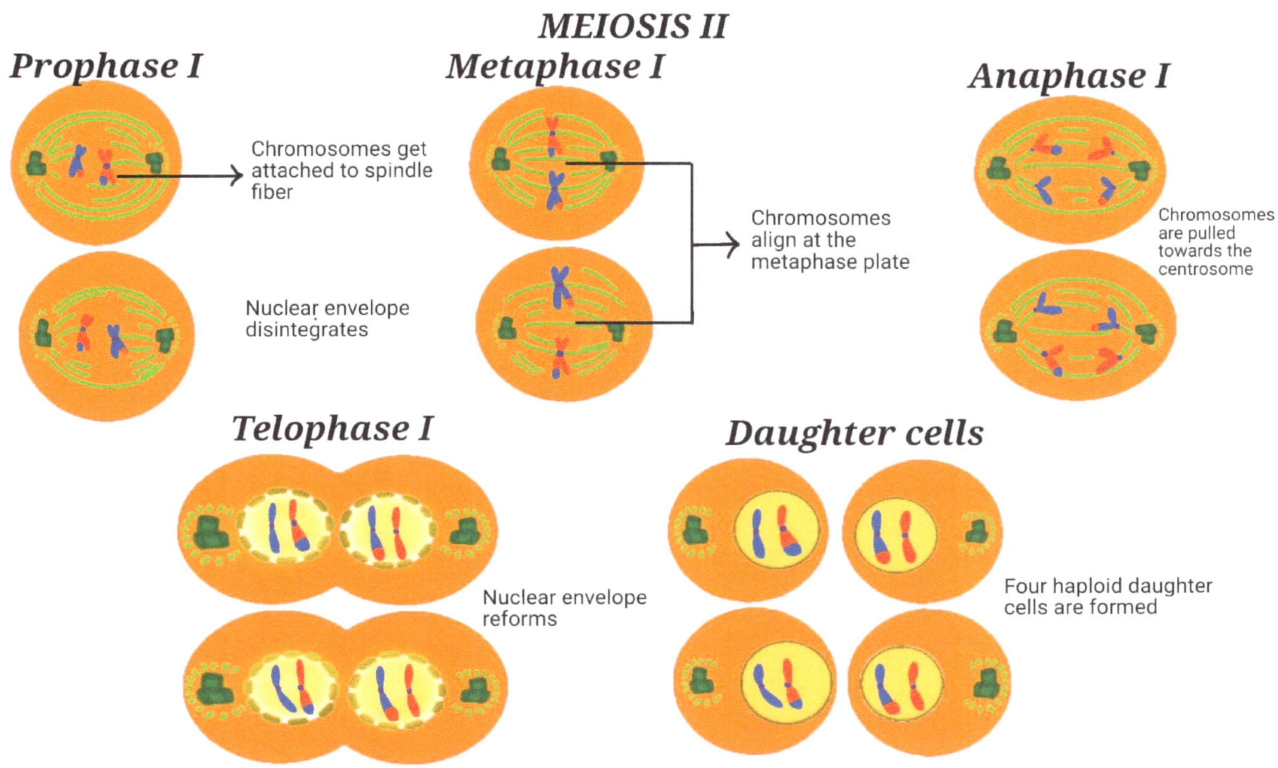

Meiosis II: The Second Division

The second division, **meiosis II**, is like the **final round of a grand performance**. This phase is similar to **mitosis**, but instead of reducing chromosome numbers, it **splits the sister chromatids**, ensuring **each gamete carries only a single copy of each chromosome**.

Prophase II: The Final Preparation

In each of the **two new cells**, the chromosomes **condense once again**, and spindle fibers **begin to form**. Unlike **Meiosis I**, no homologous pairing occurs here—this stage is purely about preparing for **the final act of separation**.

Analogy: *Imagine the dancers returning to the ballroom, preparing for one last performance, but this time, each dancer stands alone, without their previous partners.*

Metaphase II: The Second Lineup

The chromosomes **align at the center** of each cell. The spindle fibers **attach to the centromeres**, ensuring that the **sister chromatids are ready to part ways**.

Analogy: *Picture the dancers standing in a single line in the middle of the ballroom, waiting for the final cue that will send them to opposite sides.*

Anaphase II: The Final Separation

With **a decisive pull**, the spindle fibers **separate the sister chromatids**, dragging them **to opposite poles of the cell**. Each chromatid **is now an independent chromosome**, ensuring that the resulting gametes are **genetically unique**.

Analogy: *Imagine the dancers being split apart one final time, each one moving toward a different exit, ensuring no two groups are the same.*

Telophase II and Cytokinesis: The Birth of Gametes

As the **final curtain falls**, the **two cells divide once more**, resulting in **four genetically distinct gametes**—each with **half the original chromosome number**. These gametes will go on to **create new life**, carrying unique combinations of genes.

Analogy: *Picture four brand-new dance halls, each filled with a unique mix of dancers, ready to embark on their own separate journeys into the world.*

The Importance of Meiosis: The Blueprint of Diversity

Meiosis is **an architect of genetic diversity**. By **halving the chromosome number** and introducing **variation through crossing-over and independent assortment**, meiosis ensures that **no two offspring**

are exactly alike. This genetic diversity fuels **evolution**, allowing species to adapt, survive, and thrive in changing environments.

Analogy: *Imagine a deck of cards. Each time the deck is shuffled (meiosis), the combination of cards (genetic traits) changes, ensuring that every new hand (offspring) is different from the last.*

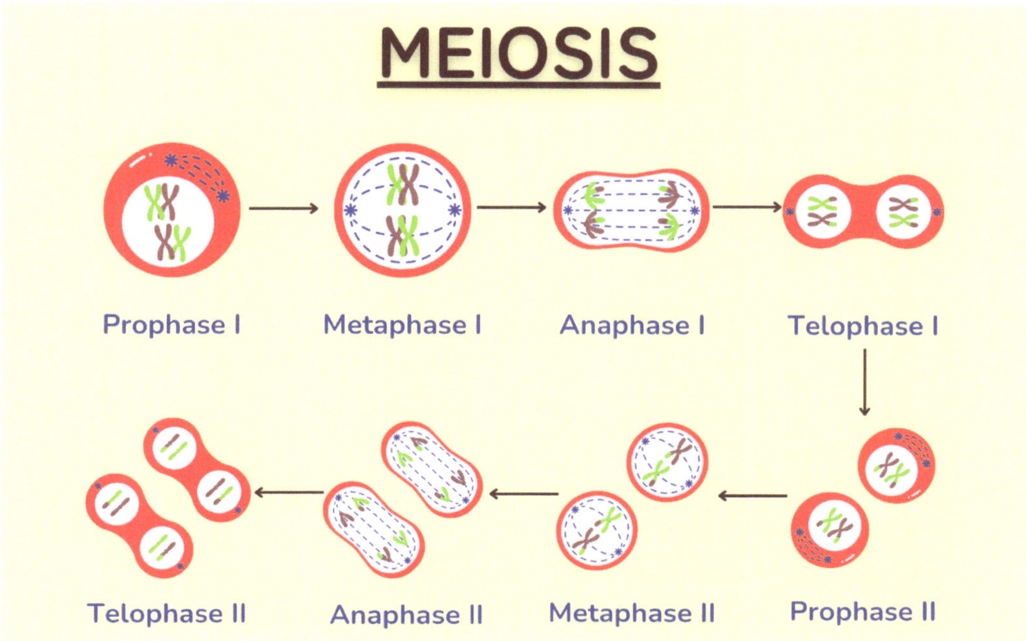

Conclusion: The Endless Dance of Life

The story of meiosis is one of precision, elegance, and purpose—a beautifully choreographed dance of chromosomes that ensures the continuity and diversity of life. From the graceful pairing of homologous chromosomes in prophase I to the final division in telophase II, each step plays a vital role in shaping the future of generations to come.

By understanding meiosis, we unlock the secrets of genetic inheritance, appreciating how variation drives evolution and sustains the incredible diversity of life on Earth.

Simple Questions

1. What is the cell cycle?
2. What happens during the G1 phase of the cell cycle?
3. Why is the G1 phase important for a cell?
4. What is the purpose of the S phase in the cell cycle?
5. How does DNA replication occur during the S phase?
6. What happens during the G2 phase of the cell cycle?
7. Why is the G2 phase considered a final check before mitosis?
8. What is the M phase in the cell cycle?
9. What is the role of prophase in mitosis?
10. What happens during metaphase in mitosis?
11. How does anaphase contribute to cell division?
12. What occurs during telophase?
13. What is cytokinesis, and when does it occur?
14. What are cyclins and CDKs, and how do they regulate the cell cycle?
15. Why is the regulation of the cell cycle important for preventing cancer?
16. What are the key differences between mitosis and meiosis?
17. What is crossing over in meiosis, and why is it important?
18. What happens during prophase I of meiosis?
19. What role does independent assortment play in genetic diversity during meiosis?
20. Why is meiosis essential for sexual reproduction?

Answers

1. The cell cycle is the series of stages a cell goes through to grow, prepare for division, and finally divide into two new cells. It is crucial for growth, development, and repair in all living organisms.
2. During the G1 phase, the cell grows, synthesizes proteins, and produces organelles needed for future tasks. The cell also checks the environment to ensure it is suitable for division.
3. The G1 phase is important because it allows the cell to gather resources, grow, and check its environment for suitable conditions before proceeding with the rest of the cycle.
4. The purpose of the S phase is DNA replication. The cell copies its genetic material to ensure that each daughter cell will receive an exact replica of the genome.
5. During DNA replication in the S phase, helicase unwinds the DNA double helix, and DNA polymerase adds complementary nucleotides to form identical DNA molecules.
6. In the G2 phase, the cell continues to grow, synthesizes proteins, and checks for DNA replication errors. The cell also organizes structures needed for mitosis.
7. The G2 phase acts as a final check before mitosis because the cell ensures DNA replication is error-free and all necessary organelles are prepared for division.
8. The M phase is the mitotic phase where the cell divides its genetic material and cytoplasm to form two identical daughter cells.
9. Prophase is the first step of mitosis where chromosomes condense into visible structures, the nuclear envelope breaks down, and spindle fibers begin to form.
10. During metaphase, chromosomes align at the cell's equator along the metaphase plate, preparing for separation.
11. Anaphase separates sister chromatids by pulling them toward opposite poles of the cell, ensuring that each new cell receives an identical set of chromosomes.
12. During telophase, the chromosomes decondense back into chromatin, a new nuclear envelope forms around each set of chromosomes, and spindle fibers disassemble.
13. Cytokinesis is the final step in cell division where the cytoplasm and cell membrane pinch inward to form two separate daughter cells.
14. Cyclins and CDKs regulate the cell cycle by controlling the timing of cell division. Cyclins activate CDKs, which drive the cell through different stages by phosphorylating target proteins.
15. Regulation of the cell cycle is crucial to prevent cancer because uncontrolled cell division can lead to tumor formation. The checkpoints ensure that the cell only proceeds if it is ready.
16. Mitosis results in two identical daughter cells with the same chromosome number as the parent cell, while meiosis reduces the chromosome number by half and produces four genetically distinct gametes.
17. Crossing over occurs during prophase I of meiosis when homologous chromosomes exchange genetic material. This increases genetic diversity by creating new combinations of genes.

18. During prophase I of meiosis, homologous chromosomes pair up and exchange segments through crossing over, setting the stage for genetic recombination.
19. Independent assortment ensures genetic diversity by randomly distributing maternal and paternal chromosomes into the gametes during metaphase I.
20. Meiosis is essential for sexual reproduction because it reduces the chromosome number by half, ensuring that offspring inherit a complete set of chromosomes when gametes fuse during fertilization.

Problem Based Questions

1. A cell is found to have extra DNA. Which phase of the cell cycle might be affected, and why?
2. A cell is unable to correctly copy its DNA during replication. What consequences would this have during the cell cycle?
3. A mutation causes a spindle fiber defect in a cell. How would this affect cell division?
4. In a certain organism, cells fail to pass the G1 checkpoint. What might be the consequences for this organism?
5. During mitosis, a cell cannot form the nuclear envelope around the chromosomes. What stage of mitosis is affected, and what would happen?
6. A cell is found to skip the S phase. What would happen to the cell's DNA content?
7. In an experiment, cells fail to undergo cytokinesis. What would the result be for the number of daughter cells?
8. A chemical inhibitor is introduced that prevents the activation of cyclin-CDK complexes. What will be the outcome for the cell cycle?
9. A cell has lost the ability to check for DNA errors during the G2 phase. How might this lead to genetic instability?
10. What happens if a cell's checkpoint proteins do not function properly? How might this contribute to cancer?
11. A cell's DNA replication process in the S phase is slower than usual. How might this delay affect cell division?
12. A cell fails to align its chromosomes at the metaphase plate during mitosis. What would happen to the daughter cells?
13. What would happen to the cell if it did not undergo anaphase and the chromosomes did not separate?
14. In a tissue sample, cells are found to have a mix of diploid and haploid chromosome numbers. What part of meiosis may have gone wrong?
15. A cell skips the metaphase stage of meiosis I. What would happen to the chromosome number in the resulting gametes?
16. A cell is unable to form spindle fibers during mitosis. How would this affect chromosome segregation?
17. What would happen if a cell's DNA replication machinery was damaged during the S phase?
18. A cell does not perform independent assortment during meiosis I. How would this affect genetic diversity in the offspring?
19. A cell is missing several key proteins required for the G2 checkpoint. How might this affect the progression of the cell cycle?
20. A cell has an issue where its chromosomes do not condense properly during prophase. What would happen to cell division?

Answers

1. Extra DNA in the cell suggests a problem in the S phase, where DNA replication occurs. The cell might experience issues during mitosis due to the extra chromosomes.
2. A failure to replicate DNA during the S phase would result in incomplete DNA content in the daughter cells, leading to genomic instability or loss of essential genetic information.
3. A spindle fiber defect would affect chromosome alignment and separation during mitosis. This could lead to aneuploidy (incorrect number of chromosomes) in the daughter cells.
4. If a cell fails the G1 checkpoint, it will not progress to the S phase. This could lead to cell cycle arrest, preventing division and halting growth or repair.
5. The inability to form the nuclear envelope during telophase would prevent the formation of two distinct nuclei, possibly leading to incomplete cell division.
6. Skipping the S phase means the cell would not replicate its DNA. This would result in half the normal DNA content in the daughter cells, causing genetic problems.
7. If cytokinesis fails, the result would be a binucleate or multinucleate cell, as the cell's cytoplasm is not divided properly.
8. Preventing the activation of cyclin-CDK complexes would halt the progression of the cell cycle. The cell may become stuck in a specific phase, unable to proceed to the next phase.
9. A failure to check for DNA errors in G2 could lead to the propagation of mutated DNA, causing genetic instability and potentially cancer.
10. Checkpoint proteins that do not function properly can allow unregulated cell division, a hallmark of cancer. This leads to the formation of tumors.
11. A slower DNA replication process would delay the entire cell cycle, leading to delayed mitosis and potentially improper chromosome distribution.
12. If chromosomes do not align at the metaphase plate, it could result in misaligned chromosomes, leading to aneuploidy in daughter cells.
13. Failure to undergo anaphase would result in chromosomes remaining together, and the daughter cells would not receive a complete set of chromosomes.
14. A mix of diploid and haploid chromosome numbers suggests a failure in meiosis I, where homologous chromosomes should separate but instead remain together in some cells.
15. Skipping metaphase in meiosis I would prevent proper alignment of chromosomes, likely resulting in incorrect chromosome distribution to the daughter cells.
16. Without spindle fibers, chromosomes cannot be pulled apart during mitosis, leading to incorrect chromosome segregation.
17. If DNA replication machinery is damaged, it could result in incomplete or inaccurate DNA replication, leading to mutations or genomic instability in daughter cells.
18. Failure of independent assortment would reduce genetic diversity, as chromosomes would not segregate randomly, leading to less variation in offspring.
19. Missing proteins for the G2 checkpoint could result in the cell moving forward to mitosis without correcting any DNA damage, causing genomic instability in the daughter cells.
20. If chromosomes do not condense properly during prophase, the cell may not properly segregate chromosomes during mitosis, leading to misdistribution of chromosomes.

References

1. Uzbekov, R., & Prigent, C. (2022). *A journey through time on the discovery of cell cycle regulation. Cells, 11*(4), Article 704.
2. Alberts, B., Johnson, A., Lewis, J., Raff, M., Roberts, K., & Walter, P. (2015). *Molecular biology of the cell* (6th ed.). Garland Science.

DNA Replication: The Miracle of Life's Blueprint

Introduction: The Heart of Heredity

Imagine opening a treasured family recipe book, filled with detailed instructions for creating your favorite dishes. Just as you can make exact copies of these recipes to pass down to future generations, living organisms have their own way of copying their genetic instructions, ensuring that each new cell has the same set of recipes. This process is known as DNA replication, a fundamental mechanism that preserves life across generations.

This chapter takes you on a journey through DNA replication—breaking down each step in a way that makes this complex process clear and relatable, even for those without a genetics background.

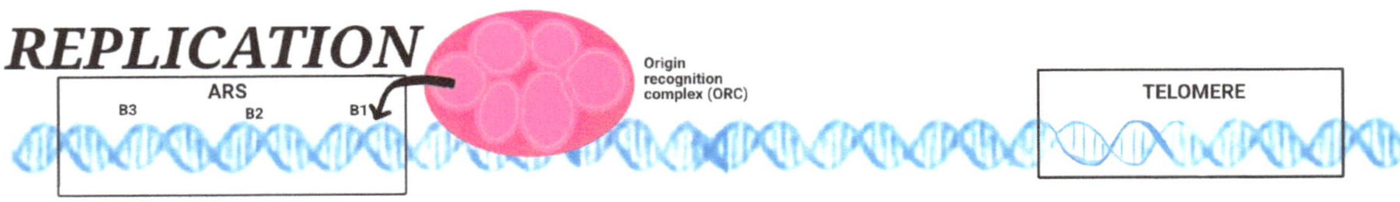

The Role of DNA in Cells

DNA, or deoxyribonucleic acid, is the molecule that carries the genetic blueprint for life. Every cell in an organism contains DNA, which holds instructions for building and maintaining the organism. For a cell to divide and form new cells—whether during growth, repair, or reproduction—it must first make a complete copy of its DNA. This ensures that each new cell inherits the same genetic information, preserving the integrity of life across generations.

The Double Helix: A Perfect Template

The structure of DNA, discovered by James Watson and Francis Crick with crucial contributions from Rosalind Franklin, provides the perfect mechanism for replication. DNA is composed of two strands that form a double helix, with each strand serving as a template for creating a new complementary strand.

The Replication Process: Unzipping the Double Helix

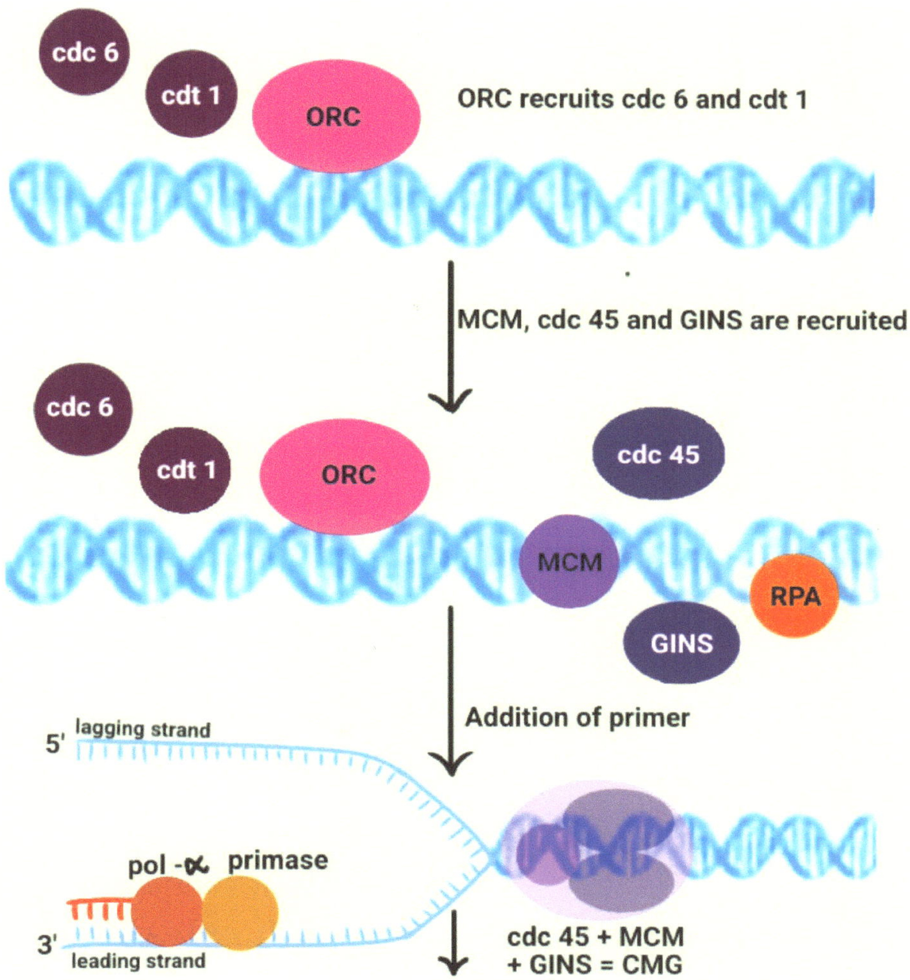

Initiation: The Starting Point

Replication begins at specific locations on the DNA molecule called **origins of replication**. Here, the double helix is unwound, creating two single strands that will serve as templates. Special proteins recognize these origins and recruit the necessary machinery to start the process.

Analogy: *Imagine a zipper—the origin of replication is where you begin unzipping, allowing the two strands to separate.*

The Role of Helicase: The Unzipping Enzyme

The enzyme helicase plays a crucial role in unzipping the DNA double helix. It breaks the hydrogen bonds between the paired bases, separating the two strands and creating a replication fork—a **Y-shaped region** where the DNA is split into two single strands.

Analogy: *Think of helicase as a pair of scissors that carefully cut through the middle of a zipper, separating the two sides so new material can be added.*

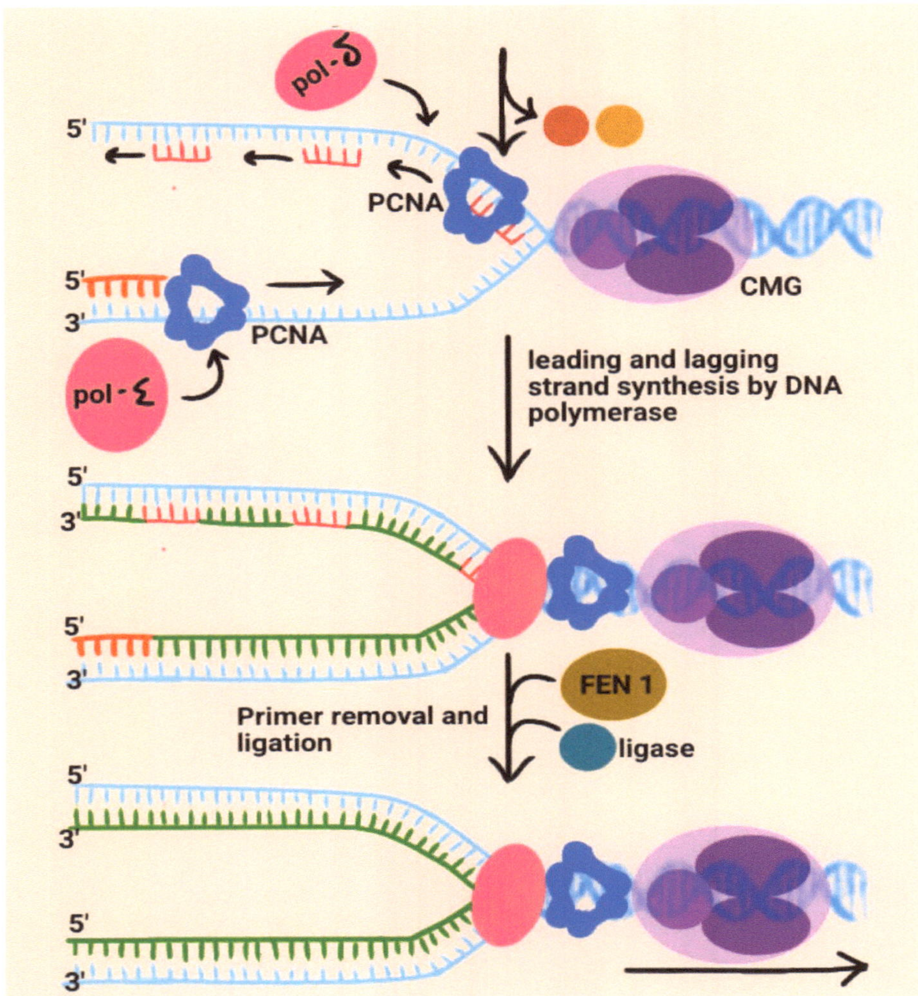

Elongation: Building the New Strands

The Role of DNA Polymerase: The Master Builder

Once the DNA is unzipped, an enzyme called DNA polymerase takes over. **DNA polymerase** is responsible for adding new nucleotides (the building blocks of DNA) to the exposed single strands, creating two new complementary strands.

DNA polymerase reads the exposed template strand and matches each base with its complementary partner:

- Adenine (A) pairs with Thymine (T)
- Guanine (G) pairs with Cytosine (C)

Analogy: *Imagine DNA polymerase as a meticulous chef, carefully following a recipe to ensure each ingredient (nucleotide) is added in the correct order.*

Leading and Lagging Strands: The Challenge

DNA replication isn't as straightforward as copying a simple line of text. The two strands of the DNA double helix run in opposite directions, and DNA polymerase can only add nucleotides in one **direction (5' to 3')**. This creates two different strategies:

The Leading Strand:

- Synthesized continuously as DNA polymerase moves smoothly in the same direction as the replication fork.
- No interruptions, just a seamless extension of the new strand.

The Lagging Strand:

- Moves in the opposite direction of the replication fork, meaning it must be synthesized in small, discontinuous segments called Okazaki fragments.
- Each fragment is later stitched together to form a complete strand.

Analogy: *Think of the leading strand as a smooth highway where cars (nucleotides) travel without stopping, while the lagging strand is like a bumpy road with frequent stop signs, requiring short, start-and-stop movements.*

Primase and RNA Primers: Setting the Starting Line

Before DNA polymerase can begin building, it needs a starting point. That's where primase comes in.

- Primase lays down short RNA primers, which act as launch pads for DNA polymerase.
- On the leading strand, only one primer is needed.
- On the lagging strand, multiple primers are required—one for each **Okazaki fragment**.

Analogy: *Imagine primase as a race official marking the starting lines for runners, ensuring that DNA polymerase knows exactly where to begin.*

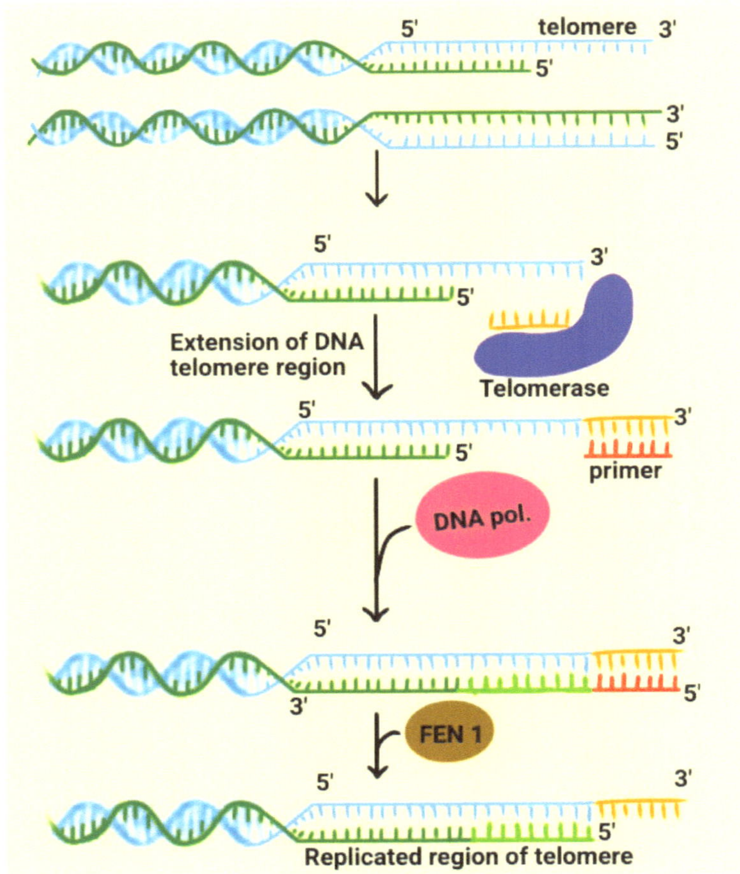

Termination: Finishing the Job

Removing RNA Primers: Swapping Temporary Notes for the Final Copy

Once the new DNA strands are assembled, the **RNA primers** need to be removed and replaced with **DNA nucleotides.** A special type of DNA polymerase performs this task, ensuring that the entire strand is made of pure DNA.

Analogy: *Imagine writing a recipe in pencil (RNA primers) as a draft. Once finalized, you erase the pencil marks and rewrite them in permanent ink (DNA nucleotides) to preserve them forever.*

Ligase: The Molecular Glue – Making It Seamless

While the leading strand is copied continuously, the l**agging strand is synthesized in small Okazaki fragments.** These fragments must be stitched together to form a smooth, continuous strand. This is where DNA ligase comes in—it acts like a molecular glue, sealing the gaps between fragments.

Analogy: *Ligase is like a tape that binds pieces of a torn recipe back together, ensuring it looks as if it was never broken in the first place.*

Proofreading and Error Correction – DNA's Built-in Quality Control

High Fidelity Process: Catching Mistakes on the Go

DNA replication is remarkably accurate, thanks to the proofreading ability of DNA polymerase. As it adds new nucleotides, DNA polymerase checks its work, ensuring that each base is correctly paired. If a mistake is detected, it can remove the incorrect nucleotide and replace it with the correct one.

Analogy: *DNA polymerase works like a meticulous editor carefully reviewing a manuscript, spotting typos, and fixing them before publishing.*

Mismatch Repair: The Final Quality Check

Occasionally, errors slip through the proofreading process. When this happens, a repair mechanism called **mismatch repair** steps in. Specialized proteins recognize and correct these mismatches, maintaining the integrity of the DNA sequence.

Analogy: *Think of mismatch repair as a final team of proofreaders reviewing a book before printing, catching any typos missed by the initial editor.*

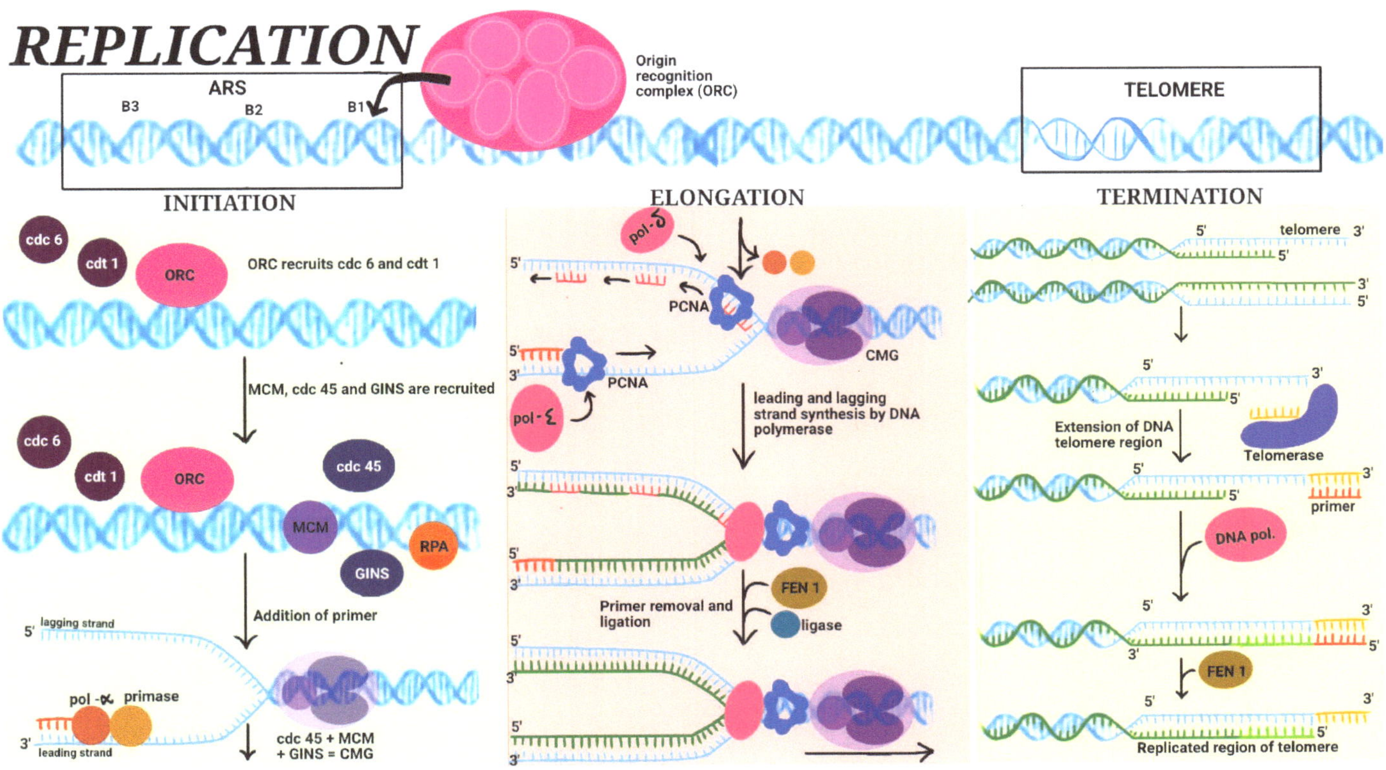

The Significance of DNA Replication

Ensuring Genetic Continuity: Life's Unbreakable Chain

DNA replication is the foundation of life, ensuring that every new cell receives an exact copy of the genetic blueprint. This process preserves the instructions necessary for growth, function, and reproduction. Without precise DNA replication, cells would lose vital information, leading to malfunctions and disease.

Analogy: *DNA replication is like photocopying a master blueprint, ensuring that every new construction project (cell division) follows the correct design, preventing structural failures.*

Implications for Evolution and Medicine: The Power of Tiny Changes

The fidelity of DNA replication has profound implications for evolution and medicine. While the process is highly accurate, occasional errors (mutations) introduce genetic variation, driving evolution.

In medicine, understanding DNA replication has led to groundbreaking advances, including:

- **Cancer research**: Identifying how DNA errors lead to uncontrolled cell growth.
- **Genetic therapies:** Developing treatments for inherited disorders.
- **Antiviral drugs:** Targeting viral replication processes to fight infections.

Analogy: *Just as occasional changes in a recipe can lead to new culinary creations, mutations in DNA contribute to the diversity of life and the potential for adaptation.*

Conclusion: The Marvel of Molecular Machinery

DNA replication is a marvel of molecular machinery, ensuring the faithful transmission of genetic information from one generation to the next. Through a series of well-orchestrated steps involving unwinding, synthesizing, proofreading, and repairing, this process exemplifies the precision and complexity of life at the molecular level.

By understanding DNA replication, we gain insights into the fundamental processes that underlie growth, development, and evolution.

Eukaryotic DNA Replication

Introduction: The Complexity of Eukaryotic Cells

Eukaryotic cells—found in plants, animals, fungi, and protists—are far more complex than their prokaryotic counterparts, like bacteria. This complexity extends to DNA replication, which must efficiently manage larger genomes, multiple chromosomes, and intricate cellular structures.

Unlike prokaryotic replication, which typically begins at a single origin of replication, eukaryotic DNA replication is more coordinated and decentralized, utilizing multiple origins along each chromosome. This chapter explores the intricate mechanisms of eukaryotic DNA replication, while also comparing it to the simpler prokaryotic process.

The Initiation of Eukaryotic DNA Replication

Origins of Replication: Multiple Starting Points

Unlike prokaryotes, which typically have a single origin of replication, eukaryotic chromosomes contain multiple origins of replication. This is necessary to efficiently replicate their larger and more complex genomes.

Analogy: *Imagine trying to transcribe a massive book—instead of starting at just one-page, multiple scribes begin copying at different sections simultaneously to complete the job faster.*

The Role of The Origin Recognition Complex (ORC)

The replication process begins with the formation of the Origin Recognition Complex (ORC) at each origin of replication. The ORC is a protein complex that binds to the DNA, marking the starting point for replication.

Analogy: *The ORC acts like a team of project managers, carefully assigning multiple starting points for a large-scale construction project, ensuring all sections are completed efficiently.*

Loading of MCM Helicase: Unzipping the DNA

Following the binding of the ORC, additional proteins, including **Cdc6 and Cdt1, help load the MCM (Mini-Chromosome Maintenance)** helicase onto the DNA. The **MCM helicase** is responsible for unwinding the double helix to create single-stranded templates for replication.

Licensing the Origins: Ensuring One-Time Use

To prevent uncontrolled re-replication, cells use a careful licensing system. The loading of MCM helicase onto DNA is called **"licensing"** of the origins, ensuring that:

- Each origin is properly prepared for replication.
- Every origin is used only once per cell cycle.

This regulation prevents errors, genome instability, and potential mutations.

Analogy: *Licensing works like a ticketing system at an exclusive event—each guest (replication origin) gets one valid entry pass, preventing duplicate entries and ensuring everything runs smoothly.*

The Elongation Phase: Building the New DNA Strands

Primase and RNA Primers

As in prokaryotic replication, eukaryotic DNA replication requires primase to synthesize short RNA primers. These primers provide starting points for DNA polymerases to begin adding nucleotides.

DNA Polymerase Alpha

Once the **primase** has placed the **RNA primers, DNA polymerase alpha** takes over. This enzyme extends the RNA primer by adding a short stretch of DNA nucleotides. However, **DNA polymerase alpha lacks proofreading ability, meaning it is not highly accurate.** To ensure high-fidelity replication, it is quickly replaced by more specialized polymerases.

Switching to DNA Polymerase Delta and Epsilon

To maintain accuracy and efficiency, the replication machinery switches to:

- **DNA Polymerase Delta** → synthesizes the lagging strand (discontinuous synthesis).
- **DNA Polymerase Epsilon** → synthesizes the leading strand (continuous synthesis).

These polymerases ensure high fidelity, with built-in proofreading mechanisms to correct mistakes, reducing errors in the newly synthesized DNA.

Leading and Lagging Strands

As with prokaryotic replication, eukaryotic DNA replication involves continuous synthesis on the leading strand and discontinuous synthesis on the lagging strand, forming Okazaki fragments.

The Termination Phase: Completing Replication

Telomeres and Telomerase

Eukaryotic chromosomes are linear and have protective ends called telomeres. Replicating the ends of linear chromosomes poses a challenge because DNA polymerase cannot fully replicate the very ends. This issue is resolved by the **enzyme telomerase**, which extends the telomeres, allowing the lagging strand to be completed.

Analogy: *Telomerase acts like a construction crew extending a runway, ensuring that DNA polymerase can land safely and finish replication without cutting off essential parts.*

Sealing the Nicks: DNA Ligase

Once the DNA synthesis is complete, the RNA primers are removed, and the gaps are filled with DNA by DNA polymerase. DNA ligase then seals the nicks, joining the Okazaki fragments on the lagging strand into a continuous strand.

Chromatin Assembly: Organizing the New DNA

After replication, the new DNA strands must be packaged into **chromatin**. This involves the assembly of **nucleosomes**, which are structures of **DNA wrapped around histone proteins**. This packaging is essential for maintaining the structural integrity and regulation of the genome.

Regulation and Checkpoints

Cell Cycle Control: Ensuring Orderly Replication

Eukaryotic DNA replication is carefully coordinated with the cell cycle, which consists of distinct phases:

1. **G1 Phase (Gap 1):** The cell grows and prepares for DNA replication.
2. **S Phase (Synthesis):** DNA replication occurs, ensuring that each chromosome is duplicated.
3. **G2 Phase (Gap 2):** The cell checks for errors and prepares for division.
4. **M Phase (Mitosis):** The cell divides, distributing the replicated DNA into two daughter cells.

To prevent errors, the cell cycle has built-in checkpoints that ensure each phase is properly completed before moving forward.

Analogy: *Cell cycle checkpoints are like quality control inspectors in a factory, ensuring that each step meets the necessary standards before production continues.*

Checkpoint Proteins: The Guardians of Genome Integrity

Checkpoint proteins, such as **ATM and ATR kinases**, detect any DNA damage or replication stress and can halt the cell cycle, allowing time for repairs before replication proceeds. This prevents the propagation of errors to daughter cells.

Analogy: *Checkpoint proteins act like traffic signals, stopping the process when there is a hazard ahead and ensuring safe progression.*

Comparison: Eukaryotic vs. Prokaryotic DNA Replication

To better understand the unique aspects of eukaryotic DNA replication, let's compare it with prokaryotic DNA replication in the following table:

Feature	**Prokaryotic Replication**	**Eukaryotic Replication**
Genome Size	Small, circular chromosomes	Large, linear chromosomes
Origins of Replication	Single origin per chromosome	Multiple origins per chromosome
Initiation Complex	Simple (DnaA initiator protein)	Complex (ORC, Cdc6, Cdt1, MCM helicase)
Primase	Single primase	Primase associated with DNA polymerase alpha
DNA Polymerases	DNA polymerase III	DNA polymerase alpha, delta, epsilon
Okazaki Fragments	Longer fragments	Shorter fragments
Termination	Termination sequences (Ter sites)	Telomeres and telomerase
Replication Rate	Faster (~ 1000 nucleotides/sec)	Slower (~ 50 nucleotides/sec)
Packaging	No histones; supercoiling by gyrase	Chromatin structure with histones
Cell Cycle Regulation	Simple, no distinct cell cycle phases	Complex, tightly regulated with cell cycle phases
Proofreading	High fidelity with DNA polymerase III	High fidelity with DNA polymerase delta and epsilon
Checkpoint Control	Limited	Extensive (ATM, ATR, and other checkpoint proteins)

Conclusion: The Symphony of Eukaryotic DNA Replication

Eukaryotic DNA replication is a finely orchestrated process, ensuring the precise duplication of genetic material essential for life. This intricate dance involves multiple origins of replication, specialized enzymes, and stringent checkpoints that synchronize with the cell cycle. The complexity of this system highlights the elegance of cellular machinery and the importance of maintaining genomic integrity.

Understanding these processes not only sheds light on the fundamental mechanisms of life but also provides insights into the potential for medical advancements in treating genetic diseases and cancers.

DNA Transcription: A Tale of Two Worlds

Introduction: From Blueprint to Messenger

DNA transcription is like converting the blueprint of a building (DNA) into a step-by-step instruction manual (RNA) for construction workers (the cell's machinery). Both **prokaryotic** (bacteria) and **eukaryotic** (animals, plants) cells use this process to pass along genetic information, but they do it in different ways, just like how two artists might paint the same landscape using different techniques. Let's explore these differences.

Prokaryotic Transcription: Simple and Swift

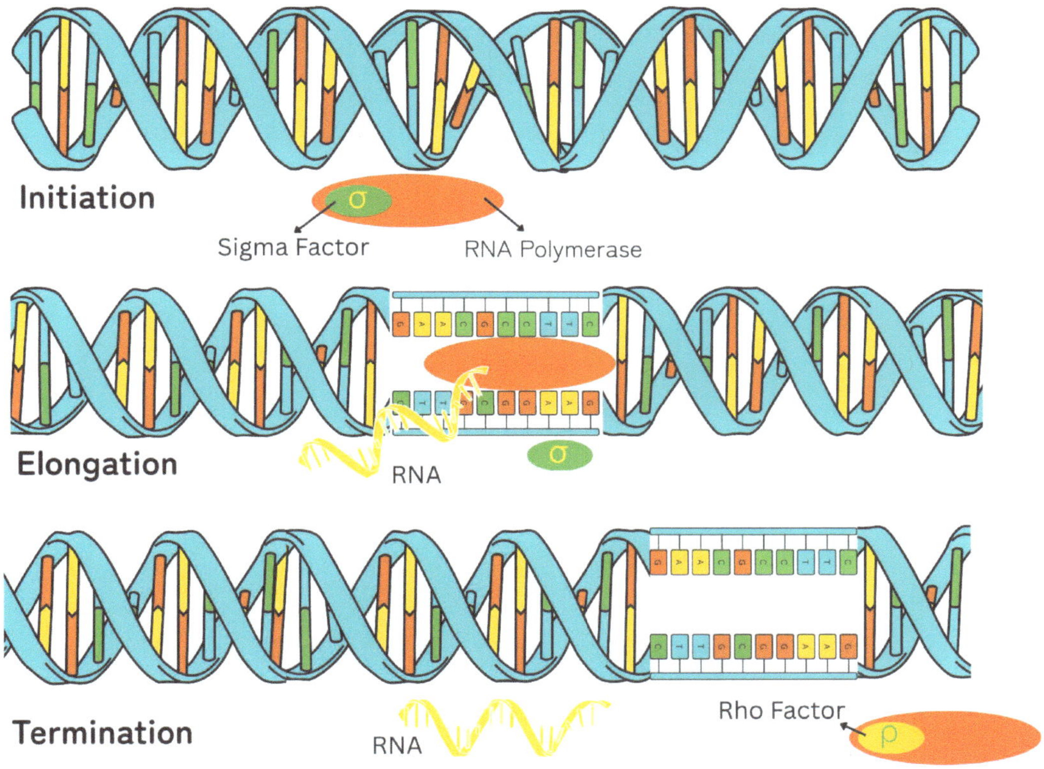

Location and Simplicity

In prokaryotes like bacteria, transcription occurs directly in the cytoplasm, as they lack a nucleus. Imagine a **small bakery** where everything—**mixing the dough, baking, and packaging**—happens in one room. Here, transcription is straightforward, with a **single type of RNA polymerase** acting as the enzyme that transcribes DNA into RNA.

Analogy: Imagine RNA polymerase as a **baker copying a simple recipe** from a wall poster (DNA). The baker writes the instructions on a small piece of paper (RNA), which can immediately be used to start baking (translation).

Promoter Region and Initiation

- **Promoter Region**: Transcription starts at a "green light" on the DNA called the **promoter**. This is where RNA polymerase begins its work.
- **Sigma Factor**: A helper protein called the **sigma factor** guides RNA polymerase to the right starting point, like a navigator telling the baker exactly where to start reading the recipe.

Termination

Transcription continues until RNA polymerase reaches a **termination signal**—similar to a full stop in a sentence—indicating that the RNA transcript is complete and ready for use.

Coupling of Transcription and Translation

In prokaryotes, **transcription and translation occur simultaneously**. As soon as the RNA transcript is written, ribosomes begin translating it into a protein.

Analogy: *Imagine the baker writing down the recipe while another worker simultaneously begins preparing the dough. There's no waiting!*

Eukaryotic Transcription: A Complex Symphony

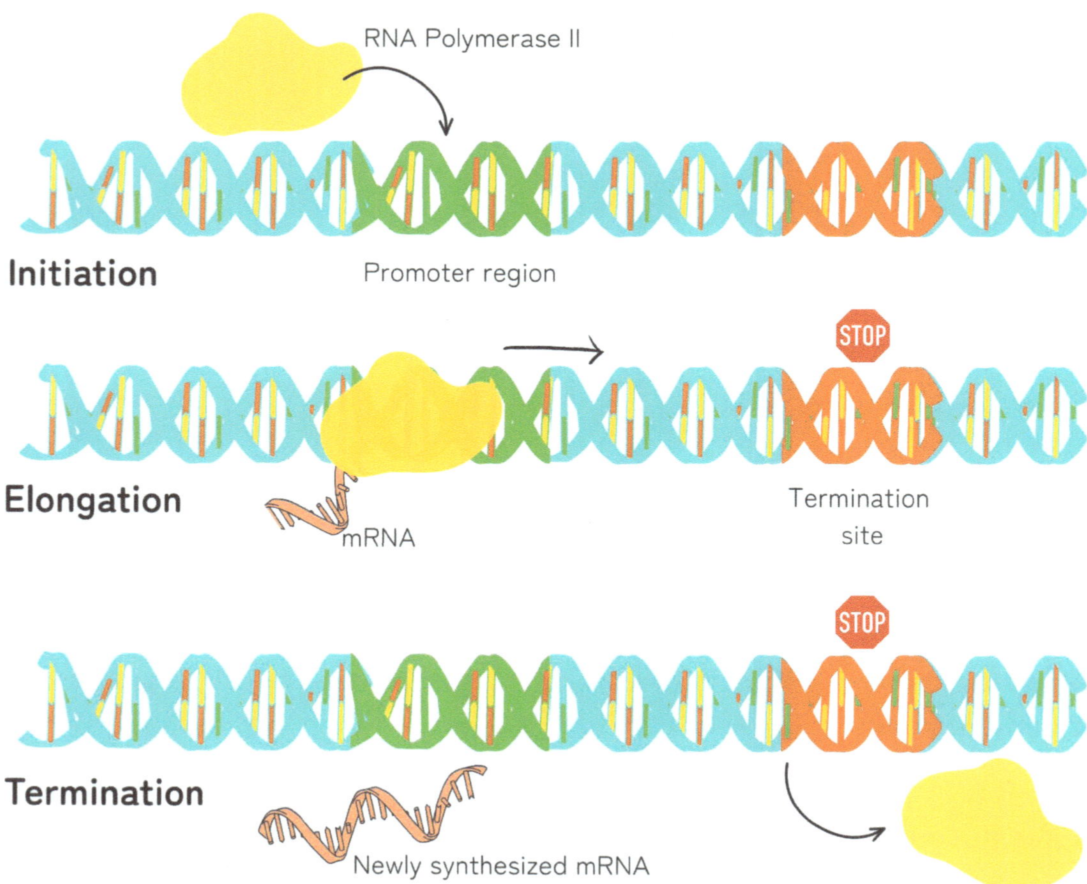

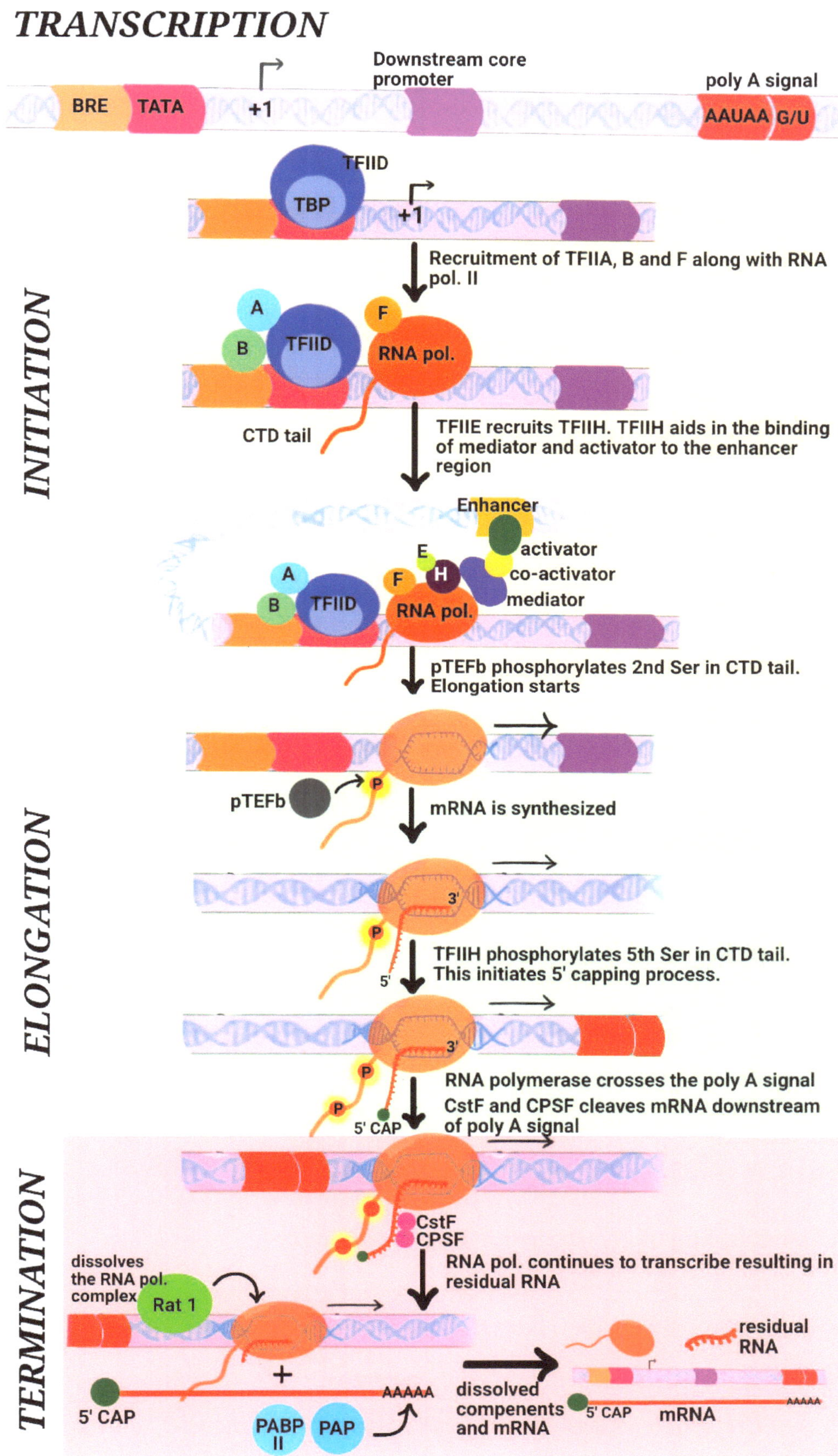
TRANSCRIPTION
Downstream core promoter
poly A signal
BRE
TATA
+1
AAUAA
G/U
TFIID
TBP
+1
Recruitment of TFIIA, B and F along with RNA pol. II
A
F
B
TFIID
RNA pol.
CTD tail
TFIIE recruits TFIIH. TFIIH aids in the binding of mediator and activator to the enhancer region
Enhancer
activator
co-activator
mediator
E
H
A
F
B
TFIID
RNA pol.
pTEFb phosphorylates 2nd Ser in CTD tail. Elongation starts
pTEFb
P
mRNA is synthesized
3'
P
5'
TFIIH phosphorylates 5th Ser in CTD tail. This initiates 5' capping process.
3'
P
P
5' CAP
RNA polymerase crosses the poly A signal
CstF and CPSF cleaves mRNA downstream of poly A signal
CstF
CPSF
RNA pol. continues to transcribe resulting in residual RNA
dissolves the RNA pol. complex
Rat 1
+
AAAAA
5' CAP
PABP II
PAP
dissolved compenents and mRNA
residual RNA
5' CAP
mRNA
AAAAA
INITIATION
ELONGATION
TERMINATION

Location and Complexity

In **eukaryotes**, like humans, transcription happens inside the **nucleus** (a separate room in the cell), and it involves more steps and more types of **RNA polymerase**. This is like a large, professional kitchen where there are specialized chefs for different parts of the recipe.

Analogy: *If DNA is the cookbook in the manager's office (nucleus), only certain authorized workers can access it. These workers carefully write down the instructions (transcription) before handing them off to the kitchen staff (the cytoplasm), where the actual cooking (translation) happens.*

Promoter Region and Transcription Factors

Unlike prokaryotic transcription, which relies on a single sigma factor, eukaryotic RNA polymerase requires multiple **transcription factors** to initiate transcription.

Analogy: *Instead of one chef, a team of sous-chefs gathers ingredients and sets up the kitchen before the head chef (RNA polymerase II) starts cooking.*

Elongation and Processing

As RNA polymerase II moves along the DNA strand, the RNA recipe is written but needs several changes before it's fully ready. These extra steps don't happen in prokaryotes.

1. **5' Capping**: The mRNA gets a protective "cap" on one end.
   - **Analogy**: A plastic lid on a coffee cup prevents spills, just as the 5' cap protects mRNA from degradation while it travels through the cell.
2. **Splicing**: The RNA has unnecessary sections called **introns**, which are cut out. Only the useful parts, called **exons**, are kept.
   - **Analogy**: It's like removing unwanted paragraphs from a recipe to make it easier to follow.
3. **Polyadenylation**: A "tail" of extra nucleotides is added to the RNA's end, keeping it stable and easy to handle, like tying up a stack of papers with a ribbon so they don't scatter.

Analogy: *Imagine a chef who edits the recipe by cutting out irrelevant steps and putting a cover on it for protection before sending it to the kitchen.*

Termination and Uncoupling of Transcription and Translation

Once transcription is done, the mRNA must leave the nucleus and travel to the cytoplasm (the cell's kitchen), where translation happens. Unlike in prokaryotes, this is a **separate step**, adding more control and regulation.

Analogy: *The chef in the office (nucleus) completes the recipe, covers it, and passes it down to the kitchen staff. They cannot start cooking until the recipe is in their hands.*

Comparison: Prokaryotic vs. Eukaryotic Transcription

Feature	Prokaryotic Transcription	Eukaryotic Transcription
Location	Cytoplasm	Nucleus
RNA Polymerases	Single RNA polymerase	Three RNA polymerases (I, II, III)
Promoter	Simple, requires sigma factor	Complex, includes TATA box and other elements
Transcription Factors	Minimal involvement of transcription factors	Requires multiple general transcription factors
mRNA Processing	Minimal (no capping, splicing, or tailing)	Extensive (5′ cap, splicing, poly-A tail)
Transcription & Translation	Coupled (occur simultaneously)	Uncoupled (transcription in nucleus, translation in cytoplasm)
Termination	Simple, uses rho-dependent or rho-independent mechanisms	Complex, involves multiple signals

Conclusion: Two Paths to the Same Goal

Despite their differences, both **prokaryotic and eukaryotic transcription serve the same fundamental purpose**—to convert DNA instructions into RNA for protein synthesis. **Prokaryotic transcription** is like a **small, fast-paced bakery** where everything happens simultaneously, maximizing efficiency. In contrast, **eukaryotic transcription** resembles a **large, professional kitchen**, where each step is carefully regulated to ensure precision and quality. This added complexity allows eukaryotic cells to **fine-tune gene expression**, ensuring that the right proteins are produced at the right time, in the right amounts, and under the right conditions.

The Translation Process: From mRNA to Protein

Introduction: Decoding the Message

Translation is the process of converting the genetic code in mRNA into a specific sequence of amino acids to build proteins. It's like taking a written recipe (mRNA) and using it in the kitchen (ribosome) to create a dish (protein). This process happens in both **prokaryotes** (bacteria) and **eukaryotes** (animals and plants), but they each follow different steps in their respective "kitchens."

Prokaryotic Translation: Simple and Efficient

Location and Overview

In **prokaryotic cells**, like bacteria, translation happens directly in the **cytoplasm** because there's no nucleus. Transcription and translation take place in the same space, allowing protein synthesis to begin immediately after mRNA is produced.

Analogy: *Imagine a small café where the chef writes down the recipe and cooks the meal all in one space without any waiting time.*

Step-by-Step Translation in Prokaryotes

1. **Ribosomes: The Workbench**

   Prokaryotic ribosomes are made of two parts: the **30S (small)** and **50S (large)** subunits, which together form a **70S ribosome**. This is the site where translation occurs.

   Analogy: *Think of the ribosome as a workbench in a kitchen, where ingredients are assembled to make a meal (protein).*

2. **mRNA: The Blueprint**

   In prokaryotes, the mRNA is often **polycistronic**, meaning it contains instructions for several proteins on one molecule. This allows for simultaneous translation of multiple proteins.

   Analogy: *It's like a recipe book with multiple recipes on a single page, allowing the chef to make different dishes at once.*

3. **Shine-Dalgarno Sequence: The Starting Signal**

   The **Shine-Dalgarno sequence** is a specific section on the mRNA that tells the ribosome where to begin translation.

   Analogy: *This sequence is like a bold, underlined note in a recipe that says, "Start Here!"*

4. **Initiation Factors: The Organizers**

   Initiation factors (IF-1, IF-2, IF-3) help assemble the ribosome, mRNA, and initiator tRNA, which carries the first amino acid (**formyl-methionine**).

   Analogy: *Think of initiation factors as event planners who ensure everything is in place before the cooking begins.*

5. **Elongation: Building the Protein Chain**

   During elongation, **tRNA molecules** bring amino acids to the ribosome, matching their anticodons with the codons on the mRNA.

   Analogy: *tRNAs are like sous-chefs who bring specific ingredients (amino acids) to the head chef (ribosome), following the recipe.*

6. **Termination: Completing the Protein**

   Translation continues until the ribosome hits a **stop codon** (UAA, UAG, UGA), which signals the end of translation.

   Analogy: *Stop codons are like the final step in a recipe, signaling that no more ingredients are needed and the dish is complete.*

7. **Release Factors**

   Release factors (**RF1, RF2, RF3**) recognize the stop codon and help disassemble the ribosome, releasing the newly formed protein.

   Analogy: *Release factors are like waiters signaling that the dish is ready to be plated and served.*

Eukaryotic Translation: A Sophisticated Process

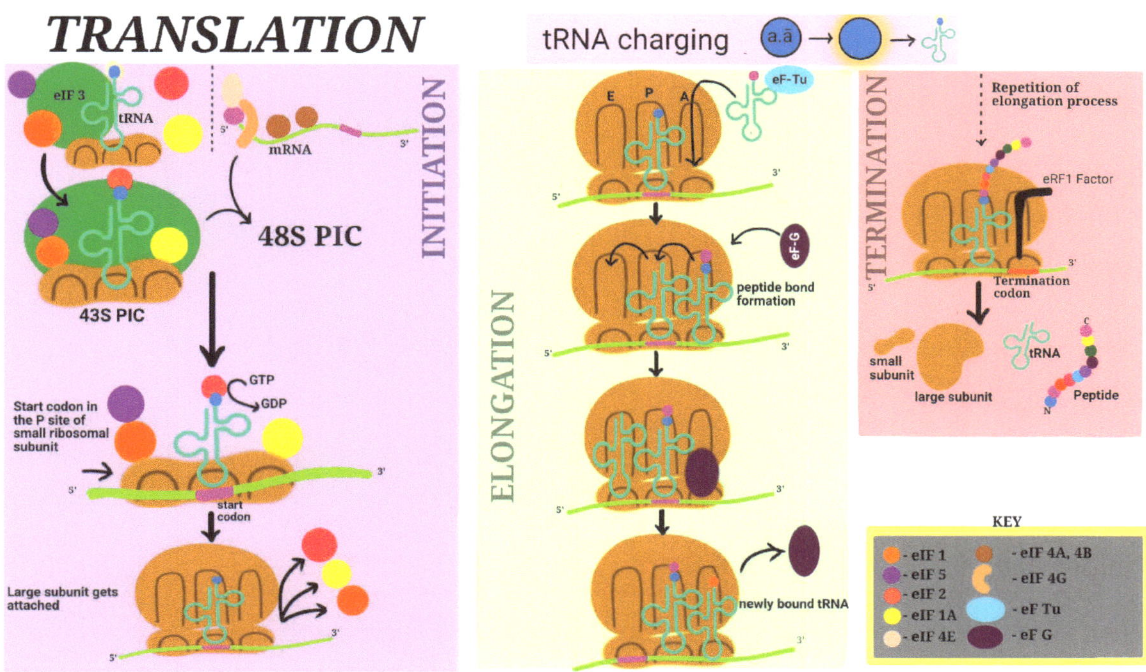

Location and Overview

In **eukaryotic cells**, translation is more complex and takes place in the **cytoplasm**, but only after the mRNA has been prepared in the nucleus. Since transcription and translation are separated by space and time, this adds additional layers of regulation and control.

Analogy: *Imagine a large, gourmet restaurant where the recipe (mRNA) is prepared in the manager's office (nucleus) before being sent to the kitchen (cytoplasm) for cooking.*

Step-by-Step Translation in Eukaryotes

1. **Ribosomes: The Workbench**

   Eukaryotic ribosomes consist of two subunits: the **40S (small)** and **60S (large)** subunits, forming an **80S ribosome** when assembled.

   Analogy: *The ribosome is the workbench in a high-end kitchen, where ingredients (mRNA and amino acids) are assembled to make an exquisite meal (protein).*

2. **mRNA: The Blueprint**

   Eukaryotic mRNA is typically **monocistronic**, meaning it codes for a single protein. The mRNA undergoes modifications like adding a **5' cap** and a **poly-A tail**, and introns are spliced out.

   Analogy: *A monocistronic mRNA is like a single, detailed recipe for one dish, carefully edited and proofread before it reaches the kitchen.*

3. **5' Cap and Poly-A Tail: Protective Covers**

   The **5' cap** and **poly-A tail** protect the mRNA and help it leave the nucleus and bind to the ribosome.

   Analogy: *These modifications are like wrapping the recipe in a protective cover so it doesn't get damaged on its way to the kitchen.*

4. **Initiation Factors: The Organizers**

   In eukaryotes, **eukaryotic initiation factors (eIFs)** help bring together the ribosome, mRNA, and the first tRNA (which carries **methionine**).

   Analogy: *eIFs are like expert chefs who ensure that the kitchen is properly set up before cooking begins.*

5. **Scanning Mechanism: Finding the Start**

   The small ribosomal subunit binds to the 5' cap of the mRNA and **scans** along the mRNA until it finds the start codon (AUG).

   Analogy: *This is like a chef scanning through a long recipe to find the right place to start cooking.*

6. **Elongation: Building the Protein Chain**

   Similar to prokaryotic translation, **tRNA molecules** bring specific amino acids to the ribosome, which links them together via **peptide bonds**, forming a growing protein chain.

   Analogy: *tRNAs function like sous-chefs, bringing in the right ingredients (amino acids) as the head chef (ribosome) assembles the dish.*

7. **Termination: Completing the Protein**

   Translation ends when the ribosome encounters a **stop codon**. **Release factors (eRF1 and eRF3)** cause the ribosome to release the finished protein.

   Analogy: *The stop codon marks the end of the recipe, just like the final step in cooking, where no more ingredients are needed, and the dish is ready to be served.*

Comparison: Prokaryotic vs. Eukaryotic Translation

Feature	Prokaryotic Translation	Eukaryotic Translation
Location	Cytoplasm (no nucleus)	Cytoplasm (after mRNA is processed in nucleus)
Ribosome	70S ribosome (30S and 50S subunits)	80S ribosome (40S and 60S subunits)
mRNA	Polycistronic (can code for multiple proteins)	Monocistronic (codes for one protein)
Initiation Sequence	Shine-Dalgarno sequence	Scanning from 5′ cap to start codon (AUG)
Initiation Factors	IF-1, IF-2, IF-3	eIFs (many more factors involved)
mRNA Modifications	None	5′ cap, poly-A tail, splicing
Coupling of Transcription & Translation	Yes, occurs simultaneously	No, separated by nuclear membrane

Conclusion: Two Ways to Make the Same Dish

Both prokaryotic and eukaryotic translation serve the same purpose—building proteins—but they follow different approaches. Prokaryotic translation is like a small, fast-paced café where everything happens quickly in one space. In contrast, eukaryotic translation resembles a high-end restaurant, with specialized steps and extra quality control to ensure precision and efficiency.

Questions

1. A DNA molecule is exposed to high heat and begins to denature. What phase of DNA replication might be affected, and why?
2. What happens if helicase is unable to unwind the DNA during the initiation phase?
3. A cell has a defect in its DNA polymerase enzyme, preventing it from adding nucleotides. What would be the result of this issue in DNA replication?
4. During DNA replication, a mutation causes the primer to be incorrectly placed. How would this affect the elongation process?
5. If the enzyme primase were not functional, what part of DNA replication would be disrupted?
6. What would happen if DNA polymerase added nucleotides in the wrong order during replication?
7. A cell has a malfunctioning ligase enzyme. What would be the impact on the lagging strand during DNA replication?
8. How would a mutation in the 3′ to 5′ exonuclease proofreading ability of DNA polymerase affect replication fidelity?
9. What would happen if a cell's mismatch repair system was defective during DNA replication?
10. During DNA replication, a segment of the lagging strand has incomplete Okazaki fragments. What would the cell do to fix this?
11. How would a defect in telomerase affect the replication of the ends of eukaryotic chromosomes?
12. If the origin of replication in a eukaryotic cell failed to form, what would happen to the replication process?
13. What would be the result if the cell's checkpoint proteins did not function properly during DNA replication?
14. If the leading strand were synthesized in fragments, what would this indicate about the DNA replication machinery?
15. What would happen if RNA primers were not removed during DNA replication?
16. A mutation causes the replication fork to move in the opposite direction. How would this impact DNA synthesis on the lagging strand?
17. What happens if DNA polymerase is unable to extend the RNA primer on the leading strand?
18. If a eukaryotic cell's replication machinery failed to recruit the necessary transcription factors, how would DNA replication be affected?
19. A DNA strand has a mismatched base pair after replication. How would the cell correct this error?
20. What would happen if DNA ligase could not seal the nicks between Okazaki fragments?

Answers

1. Denaturation of the DNA would impact the initiation phase because the double-stranded DNA would not be properly unwound into single strands, preventing proper template access for replication.
2. Without helicase unwinding the DNA, the replication fork would not form, and DNA replication would not start properly, blocking the process.
3. If DNA polymerase cannot add nucleotides, elongation would be halted. The DNA strand would remain incomplete, and no new DNA strands would be synthesized.
4. If primers are incorrectly placed, DNA polymerase would not have the correct starting point, leading to errors in strand elongation or a failure to initiate replication.
5. Without primase, RNA primers could not be laid down to start DNA synthesis. This would prevent DNA polymerase from beginning replication.
6. If DNA polymerase adds nucleotides incorrectly, mismatched base pairs would occur, leading to mutations in the replicated DNA.
7. A malfunctioning ligase would prevent the Okazaki fragments on the lagging strand from being joined together, leading to gaps in the lagging strand.
8. A loss of proofreading activity in DNA polymerase would increase the number of errors (mutations) in the newly synthesized DNA, reducing the fidelity of replication.
9. If the mismatch repair system is defective, errors introduced during DNA replication would not be corrected, leading to permanent mutations in the genome.
10. If Okazaki fragments are incomplete, ligase and DNA polymerase would fill in the gaps, and the fragments would be joined to form a continuous strand.
11. A defect in telomerase would prevent the full replication of chromosome ends, leading to progressive loss of genetic material over successive cell divisions, potentially causing cell death.
12. If the origin of replication fails to form, the DNA would not be properly unwound, and replication would not proceed in that region of the genome, leading to incomplete DNA synthesis.
13. If checkpoint proteins malfunction, the cell might proceed through the cell cycle without proper replication, potentially leading to genetic instability and tumors.
14. If the leading strand is synthesized in fragments, it indicates a defect in DNA polymerase or helicase, as the leading strand should be synthesized continuously.
15. If RNA primers are not removed, the newly synthesized DNA would contain RNA sequences instead of DNA, potentially affecting the integrity of the genome.
16. If the replication fork moves in the opposite direction, the lagging strand would not be synthesized properly in the correct orientation, disrupting the replication process.
17. If DNA polymerase cannot extend the RNA primer on the leading strand, DNA replication would halt, and the replication fork would be stalled.

18. If the necessary transcription factors are not recruited, DNA polymerase cannot begin replication properly, leading to delayed or failed DNA synthesis.
19. If a mismatched base pair occurs, mismatch repair proteins would recognize and correct the error by replacing the incorrect base with the correct one.
20. If ligase cannot seal the nicks between Okazaki fragments, the lagging strand would be incomplete, resulting in broken DNA strands.

Reference

Alberts, B., Johnson, A., Lewis, J., Raff, M., Roberts, K., & Walter, P. (2015). *Molecular biology of the cell* (6th ed.). Garland Science.

The Genesis of Nutritional Genetics

In the late 20th century, a scientific revolution was quietly brewing—one that would forever change our understanding of biology, health, and nutrition. This was the dawn of the **Human Genome Project (HGP)**, an ambitious international endeavor aimed at mapping the entire human genetic code. The completion of this monumental task in 2003 marked the beginning of a new era in science, laying the groundwork for the fields of nutrigenetics and nutrigenomics.

Let's delve into this scientific saga, exploring how the **Human Genome Project** gave rise to personalized nutrition and the transformative potential it holds for our health.

The Human Genome Project: A Leap into the Genetic Frontier

Imagine a vast library—one meticulously organized into sections, each containing numerous books. Every book is filled with detailed chapters and pages, providing comprehensive information on a particular topic.

Now, think of the **human genome** as this vast library. The entire library represents the genome—the complete set of genetic material in an organism. Each section corresponds to a set of genes, which are segments of DNA encoding specific functions or traits. Within these sections, individual books symbolize specific genes, and just as books contain chapters and pages, each gene consists of DNA sequences that provide precise instructions for building and maintaining the human body.

The Human Genome Project faced the enormous task of cataloging and understanding every section, book, and page in this genetic library. By mapping the entire human genome, scientists aimed to unlock the complex instructions encoded in our genes—paving the way for advancements in personalized nutrition, medicine, and health.

To fully grasp the development and discovery of various genomics fields such as nutrigenetics, nutrigenomics, pharmacogenomics, and beyond, it is essential to have a comprehensive understanding of the Human Genome Project (HGP). The HGP's completion marked a pivotal moment in scientific history, providing the foundational knowledge necessary to explore how our genetic makeup influences health, disease, and treatment responses. Furthermore, understanding the HGP is crucial for recognizing advancements in personalized medicine, targeted therapies, improved diagnostic tools, and the deeper insights gained into human evolution and genetic diversity.

The Human Genome Project (HGP) is an international research initiative with the primary goal of decoding the entire human genetic material, known as the genome. This involves identifying all 50,000 to 100,000 genes within the genome and developing tools to analyze this extensive genetic information.

The fundamental premise of the HGP was that by isolating and studying DNA, scientists could gain critical insights into disease development and devise innovative prevention and treatment strategies. Nearly all human medical conditions—except for physical injuries—are linked to changes (mutations) in DNA structure and function. These conditions include:

- Approximately 4,000 inherited "Mendelian" diseases, caused by mutations in a single gene.
- Complex, multifactorial disorders, arising from alterations in multiple genes.
- Cancers and other acquired diseases, which result from DNA mutations accumulated over a person's lifetime.

The Role of Recombinant DNA Technology

Recombinant DNA technology laid the critical foundation for the Human Genome Project, providing scientists with the tools to manipulate and understand the vast complexity of genetic information. By the late 1970s and early 1980s, the ability to recombine DNA from different sources revolutionized genetic research, enabling detailed mapping and sequencing of genes. This technological advancement was pivotal, demonstrating that it was possible to systematically decode and catalog the entire human genome, an ambitious endeavor that would ultimately transform our understanding of biology and medicine.

Breakthroughs in Genetic Disease Research

Recombinant DNA technology has been revolutionary, allowing scientists to identify genes responsible for various genetic disorders. Some key discoveries include:

- Cystic fibrosis gene (*CFTR*): This breakthrough helped uncover the gene responsible for cystic fibrosis, a condition characterized by thick mucus production, affecting the lungs and digestive system.
- *BRCA1* and *BRCA2* genes: Mutations in these genes significantly increase the risk of breast and ovarian cancers.
- Huntington's disease gene (*HTT*): This discovery pinpointed the gene responsible for Huntington's disease, a neurodegenerative disorder that leads to progressive brain cell death.

Ethical Implications and Public Applications

"**Seeing is believing with GloFish**. They are absolutely stunning!" proclaims the marketing material on the **GloFish website**. Beauty may be subjective, but almost everyone would agree that these first—and currently only—transgenic animals available to the general public in the United States (excluding California, where their environmental impact is under review) are fascinating conversation starters.

A transgenic (genetically modified) organism is one that has been altered using recombinant DNA technology, a process that involves combining DNA from different genomes or inserting foreign DNA into an existing genome. GloFish, a type of **transgenic zebrafish** have been modified by inserting a **green fluorescent protein (GFP)** gene that was originally extracted from a **jellyfish** (***Aequorea victoria***), or the **red fluorescent protein (RFP)** originated from **Discosoma sp.**, an Indo-Pacific ocean relative of sea anemones and coral. However, not all GloFish are green; **different *GFP* gene constructs create a variety of fluorescent colors, from yellow to red.**

Currently, GloFish is the only **recombinant-DNA animal approved for human use by the U.S. Food and Drug Administration (FDA).** Their approval raises important ethical and regulatory questions about the extent to which genetically modified animals should be made available to consumers.

Finding Disease Genes: Functional vs. Positional Cloning

Since the advent of recombinant DNA technology 46 years ago, scientists have identified and studied hundreds of disease-related genes. Most of these discoveries were possible because researchers had prior knowledge of the underlying biochemical problem. Often, they could identify the normal protein involved, analyze part of its amino acid sequence, or use antibodies to locate the protein. In some cases, they directly identified genes based on their function—a technique known as functional cloning.

However, when the biological defect behind a disease is unknown, functional cloning is not an option. To address this, scientists developed positional cloning, a breakthrough method that has revolutionized human genetics and modern medicine.

Positional Cloning: Mapping Genes Without Knowing Their Function

Positional cloning allows scientists to identify the precise location of a disease-causing gene on a chromosome without prior knowledge of its function. Researchers study families affected by the disease, analyzing which DNA markers are consistently inherited alongside the condition. By tracking these markers, they pinpoint the chromosome region where the gene is likely located. They then narrow down the search until they identify the specific gene responsible for the disorder.

This technique has been instrumental in discovering many disease-causing genes, advancing our understanding of genetics, and paving the way for targeted treatments and personalized medicine.

Analogy: *Positional cloning can be understood using the analogy of finding a faulty house in a large city. In this analogy, the city represents the chromosome, and the houses represent genes. Scientists do not know which house is faulty, just as they do not know the function of the disease-causing gene. Families affected by the disease are like people who keep getting sick in the same area. The landmarks near the house (such as schools or parks) represent DNA markers, which are inherited along with the disease. By tracking these landmarks across families, researchers narrow the search* *to a specific neighborhood, representing a chromosomal region, and then inspect each house until they find the exact faulty house, which represents the disease-causing gene.*

Diseases Identified with Positional Cloning

Disease	Gene Name	Protein	Gene Mutation	Gene Defect	Disease Characteristics	Reference
Chronic Granulomatous Disease (CGD)	*CYBB*	gp91^phox	Various mutations	Immune system dysfunction	Frequent bacterial and fungal infections	Royer-Pokora B et al., 1986
Duchenne Muscular Dystrophy (DMD)	*DMD*	Dystrophin	Deletions, duplications, point mutations	Progressive muscle degeneration	Muscle weakness, loss of mobility	Monaco et al., 1986
Retinoblastoma	*RB1*	Retinoblastoma protein (pRB)	Various mutations	Tumor suppressor gene defect	Eye cancer, primarily in children	Friend et al., 1986
Cystic Fibrosis	*CFTR*	CFTR protein	ΔF508 and other mutations	Defective chloride ion transport	Thick mucus affecting lungs & digestive system	Riordan et al., 1989
Huntington's Disease	*HTT*	Huntingtin	CAG trinucleotide repeat expansion	Neurodegenerative disorder	Progressive motor, cognitive, and psychiatric decline	Huntington's Disease Collaborative Research Group, 1993
Fragile X Syndrome	*FMR1*	FMRP	CGG trinucleotide repeat expansion	Loss of FMRP function	Intellectual disability, autism, elongated face	Fu, Y.-H., Kuhl et al., 1991
Wilms Tumor	*WT1*	Wilms tumor protein	Various mutations	Tumor suppressor gene defect	Kidney cancer, primarily in children	Gessler et al., 1990
Neurofibromatosis Type 1	*NF1*	Neurofibromin	Various mutations	Defective cell growth regulation	Tumors on nerves, skin changes, bone deformities	Marchuk, D. A et al., 1990
Testis Determining Factor	*SRY*	Testis-determining factor	Mutations affecting sex determination	Disruption in male sex development	Sex reversal, gonadal dysgenesis	Harley, V.R et al., 1994

Familial Polyposis Coli	*APC*	APC protein	Various mutations	Tumor suppressor gene defect	Colon polyps, high colorectal cancer risk	Fredrich, A et al., 2003
Choroideremia	*CHM*	Rab escort protein-1	Various mutations	X-linked retinal degeneration	Progressive vision loss	van Bokhoven et al., 1994
Kallmann Syndrome	*KAL1*	Anosmin-1	Various mutations	Defective neural migration	Delayed puberty, impaired sense of smell	Petit C et al., 1993
Aniridia	*PAX6*	Paired box protein Pax-6	Various mutations	Eye development disorder	Absence of the iris, vision problems	Ton C. C et al., 1991
Myotonic Dystrophy	*DMPK*	Myotonin-protein kinase	CTG trinucleotide repeat expansion	Defective RNA processing	Muscle weakness, myotonia, cataracts, heart issues	Brook et al., 1992

Positional Cloning and Its Role in the Human Genome Project

The Human Genome Project revolutionized genetics by mapping the entire human genome, enabling scientists to pinpoint genes linked to various traits and diseases. One of the most powerful techniques developed during this effort was positional cloning, a method used to identify disease-causing genes without prior knowledge of their function.

To achieve this, researchers relied on three key approaches:

1. **Gene Mapping** – Identifying the approximate locations of genes on chromosomes.
2. **Physical Mapping** – Determining the actual distances between genetic markers.
3. **Complete Sequence Mapping** – Deciphering the precise DNA sequence of a gene.

Each of these tools played a crucial role in uncovering the genetic basis of inherited disorders. Let's go ahead and break down each of these.

Gene Mapping

What It Is?

Gene mapping is like creating a roadmap that shows the approximate locations of genes on the chromosomes.

Description: Scientists use genetic markers—specific DNA sequences that vary among individuals—to track the inheritance of genes through families. By analyzing how these markers are passed down, they can determine the general location of a gene on a chromosome. This process is also called linkage mapping.

How It's Done?

1. **Identify Traits or Markers**

   Think of gene mapping like a treasure hunt. Scientists first identify specific traits (like eye color) or markers (unique DNA sequences) they want to locate on the genome.

2. **Study Families or Populations**

   Just as explorers rely on clues from past adventurers, geneticists study families or populations to observe how traits or markers are inherited.

3. **Look for Linkage**

   If two treasures are always found close together on an island, they must be in the same area. Similarly, if two genetic markers are frequently inherited together, they are likely located near each other on a chromosome. This is called linkage.

4. **Calculate Distances**

   To make the map more precise, scientists measure how often markers appear together in individuals. The closer two markers are, the less likely they are to be separated by recombination during inheritance.

5. **Create the Map**

   Using this information, scientists draw a genetic map that shows the relative positions of genes and markers along chromosomes—just like plotting treasure locations on an island map.

6. **Use the Map for Discovery**

   Once the map is complete, it guides scientists to find specific genes related to diseases, traits, and biological functions—just like a treasure map leads to hidden gold!

Analogy: *Gene mapping is like drawing a simple city map that shows where major buildings are located in relation to one another. In this analogy, the chromosome represents the city and* ***genes*** *represent buildings. This type of map helps identify the approximate location of genes and which genes are close together, but it does not show the exact distances between them.*

Physical Mapping

What It Is?

Physical mapping is a more detailed version of gene mapping that looks at the physical distance between genes.

Description: Think of physical mapping as creating a more precise and detailed version of the roadmap. It involves breaking down the chromosome into smaller pieces and determining the order and distance between these pieces. Techniques like restriction mapping, yeast artificial chromosomes (YACs), and bacterial artificial chromosomes (BACs) are used to place markers more accurately along the DNA.

How It's Done?

1. **Collecting the DNA:**

   Imagine having a book but it's all shredded into tiny pieces. Scientists start by collecting these tiny pieces of DNA from an organism, just like picking up all the shreds of paper from the floor.

2. **Cutting DNA into Smaller Pieces:**

   These DNA pieces are still too big to work with, so they cut them into even smaller, more manageable fragments. Think of this as cutting the shreds into even smaller bits so they are easier to handle and analyze.

3. **Arranging the Pieces:**

   Next, they need to figure out how these small fragments fit together. They do this by looking for overlapping sequences, much like solving a puzzle by finding pieces that match up. For example, if one fragment ends with the sentence "...was a great day," and another starts with "It was a great day...," you can tell these two fragments go next to each other.

4. **Creating Contigs:**

   By identifying overlapping sequences, scientists' piece together longer stretches of DNA called contigs. This process is like assembling enough puzzle pieces to form a complete paragraph or page in our book analogy.

5. **Mapping the DNA Fragments:**

   To make the map more precise, they use landmarks on the DNA called "markers" or "tags." These markers are like specific words or phrases that you know are in certain parts of the book, helping to orient where you are. Techniques like restriction mapping or using known genes as reference points help in placing these landmarks correctly.

6. **Building the Complete Map:**

   Once all the fragments are pieced together and markers are placed correctly, scientists create a comprehensive map showing the order and spacing of DNA segments. This is equivalent to having a book's table of contents and index, allowing easy navigation through the genetic material.

Why It's Useful?

Just as a detailed book index helps you find key topics in a complex novel, a physical map of DNA helps scientists understand the layout of genes and other critical regions. This information is invaluable for:

- Identifying genes associated with diseases
- Understanding gene interactions
- Developing targeted treatments and therapies

Analogy: *Physical mapping is similar to using a detailed city map or GPS to measure the exact distance between buildings. Here, genetic markers act as landmarks, and distances are measured precisely, like kilometers or meters. This approach reveals how far apart genes or markers truly are on the chromosome.*

Complete Sequence Mapping

What It Is?

Complete sequence mapping in genetics involves determining the exact order of all the DNA letters (A, T, C, G) in an organism's genome. Scientists do this by breaking the DNA into small pieces, reading these pieces using sequencing machines, and then assembling them back together to create the entire sequence. This map reveals the full genetic code, helping us understand genes, genetic variations, and how they influence traits and diseases.

How is it done?

1. **Collect the DNA:**

   Scientists begin by extracting the complete set of DNA from the organism they're studying. Imagine this DNA as an enormous book filled with billions of letters—like picking up a massive encyclopedia from a library.

2. **Break DNA into Small Pieces:**

   Since the book is too big to read all at once, scientists break the DNA into smaller, more manageable fragments. Think of this as dividing a book into chapters or individual pages to make it easier to read.

3. **Read the DNA Fragments:**

   Scientists then read these smaller pieces using machines called DNA sequencers. These machines determine the order of the letters (A, T, C, G) in each fragment. It's like scanning each page of the book to get the exact text.

4. **Assemble the Fragments**:

   After reading the small fragments, scientists need to put them back together in the right order. They look for overlapping parts of the fragments to fit them together, much like piecing together a shredded letter where each piece has a bit of text that matches the next piece.

5. **Build the Complete Sequence:**

   Once all fragments are correctly arranged, the entire DNA sequence is reconstructed. This is similar to reassembling all the pages and chapters of a book, ensuring every sentence is in the right place.

6. **Annotate the Sequence:**

   After assembling the genome, scientists annotate it—marking important regions, such as genes, regulatory elements, and genetic markers. This step is like adding footnotes and chapter headings to a book, helping researchers identify key sections and understand their functions.

Analogy: *Complete sequence mapping is like reading every street name, house number, and address in the city. In this analogy, the DNA bases (A, T, C, and G) are comparable to individual letters and numbers, allowing scientists to determine the exact DNA sequence of a gene with complete accuracy.*

Conclusion

Gene mapping, physical mapping, and complete sequence mapping are three essential tools that have transformed genetic research. Gene mapping provides a roadmap of gene locations, physical mapping offers a more detailed layout by arranging DNA fragments, and complete sequence mapping reveals the exact genetic code. Together, these techniques have advanced our understanding of genetics, enabling breakthroughs in disease research, diagnostics, and personalized medicine.

Unveiling the Biology of Genetic Variations

Imagine building a car. Each model follows a standard blueprint, but minor modifications—like a new paint color, an upgraded engine, or a sunroof—make each car unique while maintaining the same fundamental structure. Genetic variations in our DNA work in a similar way: small changes in the genetic code make each person distinct while preserving the essential blueprint of human life.

Genetic variation refers to the differences in DNA sequences between individuals. These variations account for why some people have curly hair while others have straight hair, why some are tall while others are short, and even why individuals respond differently to various diets or medications. In simple terms, genetic variation explains what makes each of us unique—just as small modifications make each car distinct.

Types of Genetic Variation

Just like cars can be customized in different ways, DNA variations come in different forms. Scientists have categorized these variations based on the specific changes they cause in the DNA sequence. The most common types of genetic variation include:

- **Mutations**
- **Single Nucleotide Polymorphisms (SNPs)**
- **Insertion/Deletion Polymorphisms (Indels)**
- **Copy Number Variations (CNVs)**
- **Structural Variants**

Each type of variation has unique characteristics and can influence how our bodies function. Let's explore these variations with simple examples.

1. Mutations: The Blueprint Errors

A mutation is like an error in the car's blueprint. Imagine if the blueprint mistakenly instructed the manufacturer to use square wheels instead of round ones—this would drastically affect how the car functions. Similarly, in DNA, a mutation is a permanent change in the genetic sequence, ranging from a single base change to large structural alterations.

Example: In humans, **sickle cell anemia** is caused by a mutation that changes a single DNA base, resulting in red blood cells that are sickle-shaped instead of round. This alteration affects the cells' ability to transport oxygen, leading to health complications.

Some mutations are inherited, while others occur spontaneously due to environmental factors like radiation or chemicals. While some mutations cause diseases, others may be beneficial or have no significant impact.

2. Single Nucleotide Polymorphisms (SNPs): The Minor Tweaks

If a mutation is an error, an SNP (pronounced "snip") is more like a minor tweak—such as choosing between two slightly different shades of paint for a car. An SNP is a single-letter change in the DNA sequence, but it usually doesn't drastically alter function.

Example: An SNP might change an adenine (A) to a cytosine (C) in the DNA. These changes are very common and typically have no major effect. However, certain SNPs can influence traits like drug metabolism, disease risk, or even how individuals respond to specific nutrients.

SNPs play a key role in **nutrigenetics**, the study of how genes affect nutrient metabolism. For example, some SNPs determine whether a person can metabolize caffeine quickly or if they are more sensitive to its effects.

3. Insertion/Deletion Polymorphisms (Indels): Adding or Removing Parts

An indel is like modifying a car by adding or removing a feature—such as removing the radio or installing a new spoiler. In DNA, an indel refers to the insertion or deletion of one or more DNA bases.

Example: An insertion could add an extra base to the DNA sequence, while a deletion removes one. If these changes occur within a crucial gene, they can disrupt its function, sometimes leading to genetic disorders.

4. Copy Number Variations (CNVs): Doubling Up on Features

A CNV is like deciding to install two engines in the car instead of one. In genetics, CNVs involve duplicating or deleting large segments of DNA, affecting the number of copies of certain genes.

Example: CNVs can be associated with conditions such as **autism** or **schizophrenia**. In some cases, having extra copies of certain genes can contribute to disease, while in others, it may provide an advantage.

5. Structural Variants: Major Overhauls

Structural variants are large-scale changes in the DNA that can be likened to flipping a section of the car's blueprint upside down or swapping parts between two car models. These include:

- **Inversions** – flipping DNA segments
- **Translocations** – moving DNA segments between chromosomes

Example: Structural variants can disrupt entire genes or regulatory regions, sometimes leading to significant effects. **Chronic myeloid leukemia (CML)**, for instance, is caused by a **translocation** between chromosomes, creating an abnormal DNA sequence that drives uncontrolled cell growth.

The Importance of SNPs in Nutrigenetics

Among all these variations, **SNPs** are the most common and hold special importance in **nutrigenetics**, which explores how genes interact with nutrients. Nutrigenetics helps explain why one person might thrive on a low-fat diet while another gains weight on the same regimen.

In nutrigenetics, specific SNPs are studied to understand how they affect nutrient absorption, metabolism, and utilization. For example:

- **Caffeine Sensitivity**: Certain SNPs in the ***CYP1A2*** gene determine whether someone is a fast or slow metabolizer of caffeine, affecting how they respond to coffee or tea.
- **Lactose Intolerance**: A well-known SNP in the **LCT** gene influences the ability to digest lactose. People with certain versions of this SNP may experience discomfort after consuming dairy.
- **Folate Metabolism**: The **MTHFR** gene contains SNPs that impact folate processing. Those with certain variations may require higher folate intake to support normal bodily functions.

Genetic Variation and Phenylketonuria (PKU)

One of the earliest examples of how genetic variation influences diet is **Phenylketonuria (PKU)**, a metabolic disorder caused by mutations in the **PAH** gene. Individuals with PKU **lack the ability to break down phenylalanine**, an amino acid found in many protein-rich foods. If left untreated, phenylalanine builds up in the body, leading to **brain damage and developmental issues**.

By identifying this genetic variation early, doctors can recommend a **phenylalanine-free diet**, preventing harmful effects and allowing individuals with PKU to lead healthy lives. This highlights how understanding genetic variations can lead to **personalized dietary recommendations** that improve health outcomes.

Genetic Variations and Their Role in Health

Nutrigenetics helps us understand how specific genetic variations influence our responses to nutrients. Some key examples include:

- **Metabolism & Disease Risk:** Certain genes influence a person's risk for obesity, diabetes, or cardiovascular diseases by affecting how they metabolize fats and sugars.
- **Vitamin & Mineral Absorption:** Genetic testing can reveal variations that impact the body's ability to absorb essential nutrients like vitamin D, iron, or folate.
- **Personalized Diet Plans:** Customized diets, such as low-carb, Mediterranean, or plant-based diets, can be tailored based on a person's unique genetic profile for optimal health.

Conclusion

By studying genetic variations, particularly **SNPs**, nutrigenetics provides valuable insights into **personalized nutrition**. Instead of a one-size-fits-all approach, this field leverages genetic information to create **tailored dietary recommendations** that align with an individual's DNA. As research advances, we move closer to a future where nutrition is not just **generalized advice**, but a **customized plan** designed to optimize health and prevent disease.

Questions

1. What was the main goal of the Human Genome Project (HGP)?
2. When was the Human Genome Project completed?
3. What role did recombinant DNA technology play in the Human Genome Project?
4. What is a gene, and how is it related to the human genome?
5. How did the Human Genome Project contribute to personalized nutrition?
6. How are mutations in DNA linked to inherited diseases?
7. What is recombinant DNA technology, and how does it work?
8. What breakthroughs in genetic disease research were made possible by recombinant DNA technology?
9. What is a transgenic organism?
10. What is the significance of GloFish, and how does recombinant DNA technology relate to them?
11. What is the difference between functional cloning and positional cloning in genetics?
12. How does positional cloning work to identify disease-causing genes?
13. What role did the Human Genome Project play in the development of positional cloning?
14. How does gene mapping contribute to understanding genetic diseases?
15. What is physical mapping in genetics, and how does it differ from gene mapping?
16. Why is complete sequence mapping important for understanding genetic diseases?
17. What are the steps involved in complete sequence mapping?
18. What are the common types of genetic variation?
19. How do mutations impact DNA function?
20. What are Single Nucleotide Polymorphisms (SNPs), and how do they influence traits?
21. How do insertions and deletions (Indels) affect genetic sequences?
22. What are Copy Number Variations (CNVs), and how do they influence genetic diseases?
23. What are structural variants in DNA, and what effects can they have?
24. How do SNPs play a role in nutrigenetics?
25. What is Phenylketonuria (PKU), and how is it related to genetic variation?
26. How can understanding genetic variation help personalize diets?
27. What is the relationship between genetic variation and metabolism?
28. How can genetic testing help in understanding the body's absorption of vitamins and minerals?
29. How can SNPs influence an individual's risk for diseases like obesity and diabetes?
30. What are the benefits of personalized diet plans based on genetic profiles?
31. How does the understanding of SNPs influence the development of personalized nutrition strategies?
32. How does the human genome relate to disease prevention?
33. Why is the study of genetic variation important for advancing medical treatments?
34. What are the implications of genetic research on future cancer therapies?
35. How do mutations in the CFTR gene cause cystic fibrosis?
36. What is the role of the BRCA1 and BRCA2 genes in breast and ovarian cancer risk?

37. How do positional cloning techniques contribute to the discovery of disease-related genes?
38. What is the significance of understanding gene function in genetic disease research?
39. How does recombinant DNA technology impact the field of gene therapy?
40. How does personalized nutrition benefit individuals with metabolic disorders like PKU?

Answers

1. The main goal of the Human Genome Project was to map the entire human genetic code and identify all the genes within the genome.
2. The Human Genome Project was completed in 2003.
3. Recombinant DNA technology allowed scientists to manipulate and study DNA in ways that enabled mapping and sequencing of the human genome.
4. A gene is a segment of DNA that encodes instructions for making proteins, which carry out the functions necessary for life.
5. The Human Genome Project contributed to personalized nutrition by identifying genetic variations that affect nutrient metabolism, leading to individualized dietary recommendations.
6. Mutations in DNA can lead to inherited diseases by disrupting the normal function of genes.
7. Recombinant DNA technology involves combining DNA from different organisms, enabling scientists to study genes and create transgenic organisms.
8. Breakthroughs include identifying genes responsible for cystic fibrosis, breast cancer, Huntington's disease, and more, all made possible by recombinant DNA technology.
9. A transgenic organism is one that has been genetically modified by incorporating DNA from another organism.
10. GloFish are transgenic zebrafish modified with fluorescent proteins, demonstrating the application of recombinant DNA technology.
11. Functional cloning identifies genes based on their function, while positional cloning identifies genes based on their location on a chromosome.
12. Positional cloning uses DNA markers to track the inheritance of genes and pinpoint disease-causing genes without knowing their function.
13. The Human Genome Project provided the genetic map necessary for positional cloning, helping scientists identify disease-causing genes.
14. Gene mapping involves identifying the locations of genes on chromosomes, which helps in understanding how genes are inherited and associated with diseases.
15. Physical mapping is more precise than gene mapping and involves determining the actual distances between genes and markers.
16. Complete sequence mapping reveals the exact DNA sequence, helping scientists understand genetic variations, genes, and their roles in diseases.
17. Complete sequence mapping involves collecting DNA, breaking it into fragments, sequencing the fragments, assembling them, and annotating the sequence.
18. The most common types of genetic variation include mutations, SNPs, insertions/deletions, CNVs, and structural variants.
19. Mutations in DNA can cause genetic disorders by altering the function of proteins, leading to diseases.
20. SNPs are minor variations in DNA sequence that can influence traits like disease susceptibility and drug metabolism.

21. Indels are insertions or deletions of DNA bases that can disrupt gene function, leading to disease.
22. CNVs involve changes in the number of copies of a gene or DNA segment, influencing genetic disorders like autism or schizophrenia.
23. Structural variants include large-scale changes like inversions and translocations, which can disrupt gene function or regulation.
24. SNPs affect how genes interact with nutrients, influencing how an individual metabolizes food and absorbs nutrients.
25. PKU is caused by mutations in the PAH gene, which prevents the breakdown of phenylalanine, leading to brain damage if untreated.
26. Understanding genetic variation helps tailor diets to individual genetic needs, improving health outcomes.
27. Genetic variation affects metabolism by altering how the body processes fats, proteins, and carbohydrates, impacting disease risk.
28. Genetic testing can identify variations in genes that affect nutrient absorption, allowing for optimized vitamin and mineral intake.
29. SNPs in genes like *FTO* and PPAR can influence an individual's risk for diseases like obesity and diabetes by affecting metabolism.
30. Personalized diet plans based on genetic profiles can optimize health by targeting individual metabolic needs.
31. Understanding SNPs enables personalized nutrition strategies by identifying how an individual processes specific nutrients.
32. The human genome plays a crucial role in disease prevention by providing insights into genetic predispositions to conditions like cancer, diabetes, and heart disease.
33. Studying genetic variation enables the development of targeted medical treatments based on a person's unique genetic makeup.
34. Genetic research on mutations in genes like BRCA1 and BRCA2 has paved the way for targeted cancer therapies, improving patient outcomes.
35. Mutations in the CFTR gene cause cystic fibrosis by disrupting chloride ion transport, leading to mucus buildup in the lungs and digestive system.
36. BRCA1 and BRCA2 mutations significantly increase the risk of breast and ovarian cancer by disrupting the repair of DNA damage.
37. Positional cloning enables the discovery of disease-related genes by identifying the location of genes associated with genetic disorders.
38. Gene function is crucial in genetic disease research because understanding the role of a gene helps develop effective treatments and therapies.
39. Recombinant DNA technology has enabled gene therapy by allowing the modification of genes to treat genetic disorders.
40. PKU is a prime example of how genetic variation influences diet, where individuals must avoid phenylalanine-rich foods to prevent brain damage.

References

1. Moraes, F., & Góes, A. (2016). A decade of Human Genome Project conclusion: Scientific diffusion about our genome knowledge. *Biochemistry and Molecular Biology Education, 44*(3), 215–223. https://doi.org/10.1002/bmb.20952.
2. Gannett, L. (n.d.). *The human genome project*. In E. N. Zalta (Ed.), *The Stanford encyclopedia of philosophy* (Spring 2025 ed.). Stanford University. Retrieved July 13, 2025, from https://plato.stanford.edu/entries/human-genome/.
3. Bose, K. (Ed.). (2022). *Textbook on cloning, expression and purification of recombinant proteins*. Springer Nature. https://doi.org/10.1007/978-981-16-4987-5.
4. Yi, D., & Mertz, J. E. (2024). Paul Berg and the origins of recombinant DNA. *Cell, 187*(5), 1019–1023. https://doi.org/10.1016/j.cell.2024.01.007.
5. Brookes, A. J. (1999). The essence of SNPs. *Gene, 234*(2), 177–186. https://doi.org/10.1016/S0378-1119(99)00219-X
6. Feero, W. G., Guttmacher, A. E., & Collins, F. S. (2010). Genomic medicine—an updated primer. *New England Journal of Medicine, 362*(21), 2001–2011. https://doi.org/10.1056/NEJMra0907175
7. Guttmacher, A. E., & Collins, F. S. (2002). Genomic medicine—a primer. *New England Journal of Medicine, 347*(19), 1512–1520. https://doi.org/10.1056/NEJMra012240
8. Venter, J. C., Adams, M. D., Myers, E. W., Li, P. W., Mural, R. J., Sutton, G. G., Smith, H. O., Yandell, M., Evans, C. A., *et al.* (2001). The sequence of the human genome. *Science, 291*(5507), 1304–1351. https://doi.org/10.1126/science.1058040.
9. Monaco, A. P., Neve, R. L., Colletti-Feener, C., Bertelson, C. J., Kurnit, D. M., & Kunkel, L. M. (1986). Isolation of candidate cDNAs for portions of the Duchenne muscular dystrophy gene. *Nature, 323*(6089), 646–650. https://doi.org/10.1038/323646a0
10. Friend, S. H., Bernards, R., Rogelj, S., Weinberg, R. A., Rapaport, J. M., Albert, D. M., Dryja, T. P., … Dryja, T. P. (1986). A human DNA segment with properties of the gene that predisposes to retinoblastoma and osteosarcoma. *Nature, 323*(6089), 643–646. https://doi.org/10.1038/323643a0
11. Huntington's Disease Collaborative Research Group. (1993). A novel gene containing a trinucleotide repeat that is expanded and unstable on Huntington's disease chromosomes. *Cell, 72*(6), 971–983. https://doi.org/10.1016/0092-8674(93)90585-E
12. Fu, Y.-H., Kuhl, D. P., Pizzuti, A., Pieretti, M., Sutcliffe, J. S., Richards, S., Verkerk, A. J., Holden, J. J., Fenwick, R. G., Jr., & Warren, S. T. (1991). Variation of the CGG repeat at the fragile X site results in genetic instability: Resolution of the Sherman paradox. *Cell, 67*(6), 1047–1058. https://doi.org/10.1016/0092-8674(91)90283-5
13. Gessler, M., Poustka, A., Cavenee, W., Neve, R. L., Orkin, S. H., & Bruns, G. A. (1990). Homozygous deletion in Wilms tumours of a zinc-finger gene identified by chromosome jumping. *Nature, 343*(6260), 774–778. https://doi.org/10.1038/343774a0

14. Marchuk, D. A., Andersen, L. B., Buchberg, A. M., Viskochil, D., & Collins, F. S. (1990). Type 1 neurofibromatosis gene: Identification of a large transcript disrupted in three NF1 patients. *Science, 249*(4965), 181–186. https://doi.org/10.1126/science.2134734
15. Riordan, J. R., Rommens, J. M., Kerem, B., Alon, N., Rozmahel, R., Grzelczak, Z., & Tsui, L.-C. (1989). Identification of the cystic fibrosis gene: Cloning and characterization of complementary DNA. *Science, 245*(4922), 1066–1073. https://doi.org/10.1126/science.2475911
16. van Bokhoven, H., van den Hurk, J. A., Bogerd, L., Philippe, C., Gilgenkrantz, S., de Jong, P., ... Khattabi, A. (1994). Cloning and characterization of the human choroideremia gene. *Human Molecular Genetics, 3*(7), 1041–1046. https://doi.org/10.1093/hmg/3.7.1041 molvis.org+13UpToDate+13PNAS+13
17. Brook, J. D., McCurrach, M. E., Harley, H. G., Buckler, A. J., Church, D., Aburatani, H., ... Muntoni, F. (1992). Molecular basis of myotonic dystrophy: expansion of a trinucleotide (CTG) repeat at the 3′ end of a transcript encoding a protein kinase family member. *Cell, 68*(4), 799–808. https://doi.org/10.1016/0092-8674(92)90154-5
18. Glaser, T., Walton, D. S., & Maas, R. L. (1992). Genomic structure, evolutionary conservation and aniridia mutations in the human PAX6 gene. *Nature Genetics, 2*(4), 232–239. https://doi.org/10.1038/ng0492-232
19. Huntington's Disease Collaborative Research Group. (1993). A novel gene containing a trinucleotide repeat that is expanded and unstable on Huntington's disease chromosomes. *Cell, 72*(6), 971–983. https://doi.org/10.1016/0092-8674(93)90585-E
20. Harley, V. R., & Goodfellow, P. N. (1994). The biochemical role of SRY in sex determination. *Molecular Reproduction and Development, 39*(2), 184–193. https://doi.org/10.1002/mrd.1080390211
21. Friedrich, A., & Kullmann, F. (2003). *Familial adenomatous polyposis syndrome (FAP): pathogenesis and molecular mechanisms*. *Medizinische Klinik, 98*(12), 776–782. https://doi.org/10.1007/S00063-003-1325-2
22. Petit, C. (1993). Molecular basis of the X-chromosome-linked Kallmann's syndrome. *Trends in Endocrinology and Metabolism, 4*(1), 8–13. https://doi.org/10.1016/1043-2760(93)90057-I
23. Royer-Pokora, B., Kunkel, L. M., Monaco, A. P., Goff, S. C., Newburger, P. E., Baehner, R. L., Cole, F. S., Curnutte, J. T., & Orkin, S. H. (1986). Cloning the gene for an inherited human disorder—chronic granulomatous disease—on the basis of its chromosomal location. *Nature, 322*(6074), 32–38. https://doi.org/10.1038/322032a0
24. Ton, C. C., Hirvonen, H., Miwa, H., Weil, M. M., Monaghan, P., Jordan, T., van Heyningen, V., Hastie, N. D., Meijers-Heijboer, H., Drechsler, M., et al. (1991). Positional cloning and characterization of a paired box- and homeobox-containing gene from the aniridia region. *Cell, 67*(6), 1059–1074. https://doi.org/10.1016/0092-8674(91)90284-6

INTRODUCTION TO NUTRIGENETICS AND NUTRIGENOMICS

The fields of **nutrigenetics** and **nutrigenomics** have revolutionized our understanding of how diet and genes interact to influence health and disease. *Nutrigenetics focuses on how genetic variations influence an individual's response to specific nutrients, while nutrigenomics explores how nutrients and dietary components affect gene expression and biological pathways.* **In simple terms, nutrigenetics asks, "How do my genes respond to food?" while nutrigenomics asks, "How does food influence my genes?"** As scientists continue to uncover the intricate relationship between our genetic makeup and nutrition, the potential for personalized nutrition becomes increasingly evident. This chapter aims to provide a clear and accessible introduction to these emerging disciplines, focusing on epigenomics, molecular mechanisms, gene–environment interactions, and their implications for health and disease prevention.

Introduction to Epigenomics

Epigenomics is the study of changes in gene expression that **do not alter the DNA sequence itself**. Instead, these modifications regulate how genes are turned **on or off** in response to **environmental factors, including diet**. Unlike genetic mutations, epigenetic changes are reversible and can be influenced by lifestyle choices, making them a key focus in personalized nutrition.

Example:

Think of DNA as a book containing instructions for building a person. Epigenetics acts like a bookmark, highlighting certain sections to be read more often while skipping others. What we eat and how we live can influence where these bookmarks are placed, affecting which genes are active at any given time.

Molecular Mechanisms of Epigenomics

Epigenetic regulation involves several key molecular mechanisms that control gene expression without altering the DNA sequence itself. These mechanisms include **DNA methylation, histone modification, chromatin remodeling, non-coding RNAs, and RNA methylation**, all of which can be influenced by dietary factors.

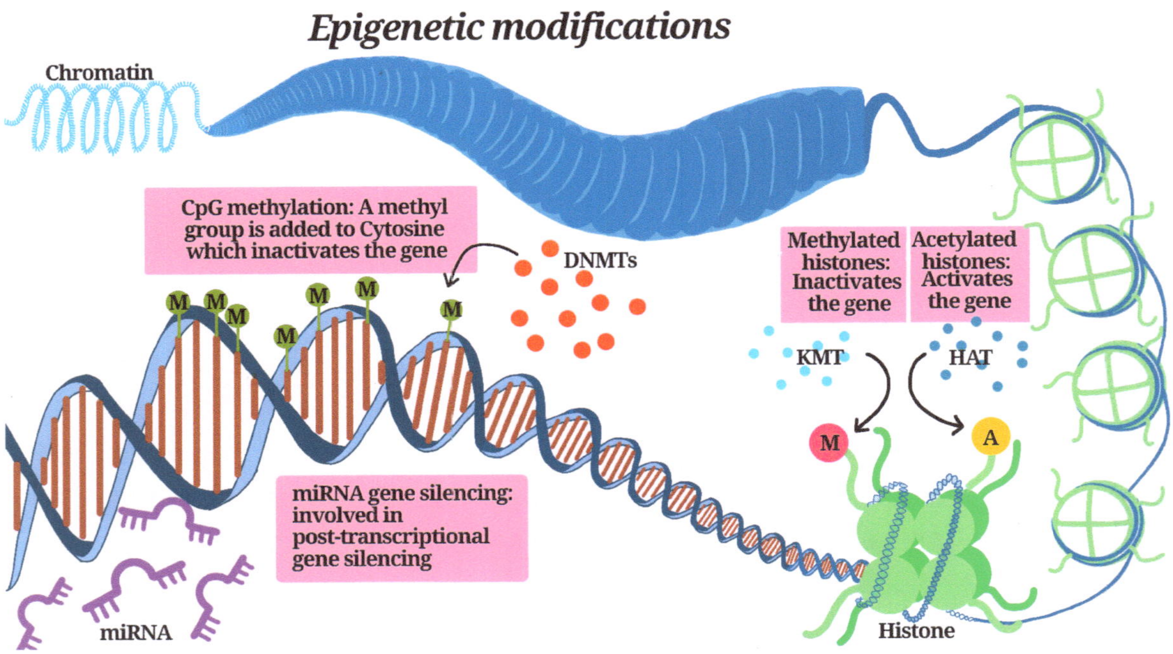

1. DNA Methylation: Silencing Gene Expression

The addition of methyl groups to cytosine bases in the DNA sequence can silence gene expression by preventing transcription factors from binding to DNA. This mechanism is crucial in regulating developmental processes and maintaining cell differentiation. DNA methylation is influenced by dietary components such as folate, vitamin B12, and choline, which serve as methyl donors.

Example: *Research has shown that folate-rich diets contribute to proper DNA methylation patterns, reducing the risk of cardiovascular diseases and neural tube defects. In contrast, deficiency in folate can lead to hypomethylation, resulting in aberrant gene expression and increased disease susceptibility.*

2. Histone Modification: Controlling DNA Accessibility

Histones are proteins around which DNA is wrapped to form chromatin. Post-translational modifications such as acetylation, methylation, and phosphorylation alter histone interactions with DNA, making genes more or less accessible for transcription. Histone acetylation is commonly associated with gene activation, whereas histone methylation can either activate or repress genes depending on the specific histone residue involved.

Example: *Polyphenols such as epigallocatechin-3-gallate (EGCG) from green tea have been shown to modulate histone modifications, particularly by inhibiting histone deacetylases (HDACs) and increasing histone acetylation marks like H3K9 and H3K14. These epigenetic alterations lead to loosening of chromatin structure and activation of genes involved in antioxidant defenses, while suppressing pro-inflammatory signaling pathways including NF-κB and COX-2. Through this mechanism, green tea polyphenols help reduce oxidative stress and chronic inflammation, thereby contributing to healthier aging and metabolic resilience.*

3. Non-Coding RNA (ncRNA): Regulating Gene Expression

Non-coding RNAs (ncRNAs), including microRNAs (miRNAs) and long non-coding RNAs (lncRNAs), regulate gene expression at transcriptional and post-transcriptional levels. They can bind to messenger RNA (mRNA), preventing its translation or promoting its degradation.

Example: *Omega-3 polyunsaturated fatty acids (PUFAs) found in fish and flaxseed have been shown to regulate non-coding RNA activity—particularly microRNAs that control lipid metabolism. In animal and human omics studies, omega-3 PUFAs such as EPA and DHA enhance expression of miRNAs that suppress lipogenesis and promote fatty acid oxidation, thereby reducing adiposity, improving insulin sensitivity, and decreasing inflammation. This regulatory effect on miRNA expression provides a mechanistic pathway through which omega-3 intake lowers the risk of obesity and metabolic disorders.*

4. Chromatin Remodeling: Restructuring Gene Accessibility

Chromatin remodeling refers to the dynamic restructuring of chromatin architecture, making DNA more or less accessible for transcription. Chromatin remodeling complexes modify how tightly DNA is wrapped around histones, influencing gene activation or repression.

Example: *Dietary selenium has been shown to influence chromatin remodeling by modulating both DNA methylation and histone modification pathways, particularly in genes involved in oxidative stress response and immune regulation. Adequate selenium intake enhances the expression and activity of selenoproteins such as glutathione peroxidases and thioredoxin reductases, which support antioxidant defense and stimulate DNA repair mechanisms. Supplementation with selenium has been associated with reduced DNA damage, improved immune cell function, and potentially lower risk of certain cancers and inflammatory disorders. These epigenetic and genomic actions of selenium underpin its role in maintaining genomic stability and supporting immune homeostasis.*

5. RNA Methylation (m6A Modification): Regulating Protein Synthesis

RNA methylation, specifically N6-methyladenosine (m6A) modification, is an emerging area in epigenetics where methyl groups are added to messenger RNA (mRNA). This modification influences RNA stability, translation efficiency, and degradation, ultimately impacting protein production and metabolic pathways.

Example: *High-fat diets have been shown to disrupt N6-methyladenosine (m^6A) RNA methylation, leading to dysregulation of genes involved in lipid metabolism, inflammation, and insulin signaling. Increased expression of the m^6A demethylase FTO and altered activity of the methyltransferase METTL3 have been observed in liver and adipose tissues of high-fat diet-fed models, contributing to insulin resistance and metabolic dysfunction. Conversely, modulation of dietary fat intake or targeting m^6A pathway components, such as METTL14 in brown adipose tissue, has been linked to restored RNA methylation profiles and improved insulin sensitivity, independent of changes in body weight. These findings underscore the epigenetic influence of dietary fat on metabolic health through m^6A-dependent gene regulation.*

Why Do These Mechanisms Matter in Nutrition?

Each of these epigenetic mechanisms demonstrates how **diet influences gene regulation**, highlighting the potential for **personalized nutrition**. By understanding these interactions, researchers can develop dietary strategies tailored to an individual's genetic and epigenetic profile, promoting **optimal health and disease prevention**.

Nutrients Driven Epigenetics Modulation

We have explored various mechanisms of epigenetic regulation. Now, let's delve into how **nutrients act as dynamic modulators of the epigenome**, influencing gene expression in ways that can be **both beneficial and detrimental** to health.

Nutrients play a **pivotal role in shaping epigenetic landscapes** by providing essential cofactors and substrates for biochemical reactions such as **DNA methylation, histone modification, and non-coding RNA regulation**. Certain dietary components can **enhance protective gene expression**, reducing the risk of chronic diseases, while others may **trigger harmful epigenetic changes**, potentially leading to disease development. Let's explore how different nutrients influence and modify epigenetic mechanisms.

Folate and DNA Methylation: An Essential Connection

Folate (vitamin B9) is a **crucial nutrient** that regulates **DNA methylation**, a fundamental process that controls **gene activation and silencing** without altering the DNA sequence itself. This regulatory mechanism plays a key role in **development, disease prevention, and overall cellular function**.

How Does Folate Influence DNA Methylation?

Folate is required for a biochemical pathway called **one-carbon metabolism**, which provides **methyl groups** (chemical tags) necessary for DNA methylation. These methyl groups are transferred to **cytosine bases in DNA** by **DNA methyltransferases (DNMTs)**, helping regulate **gene expression, genomic stability, and cellular differentiation**. This process primarily occurs at **CpG sites** (regions in DNA where cytosine and guanine are linked).

For methylation to occur efficiently, the body needs enough **S-adenosylmethionine (SAM)**, a universal methyl donor. SAM is produced in a cycle that depends on folate. **5-methyltetrahydrofolate (5-methylTHF)**, the active form of folate, helps convert **homocysteine to methionine**, which is then used to produce SAM.

A key enzyme in this pathway, **methylenetetrahydrofolate reductase (MTHFR)**, regulates this conversion. **Genetic variations in the MTHFR gene**, such as the **C677T polymorphism**, can **reduce folate metabolism efficiency**, leading to **lower SAM levels and disrupted DNA methylation**. This can affect **gene activity and disease risk**, making folate intake particularly important for individuals with this genetic variation.

Example 1: Neural Tube Defects and Pregnancy

One of the most well-documented examples of **folate's role in DNA methylation** is its importance during **pregnancy and fetal development**. In the early stages of pregnancy, the **baby's brain and spinal cord** develop rapidly, relying on **proper DNA methylation** for **cell division and tissue formation**.

If a mother has insufficient folate intake, it can lead to errors in DNA methylation, increasing the risk of **neural tube defects (NTDs)**, serious birth defects affecting the spinal cord and brain. A common NTD is **spina bifida**, where the baby's spinal cord fails to develop properly, potentially leading to lifelong disability.

To prevent this, many countries **fortify grains and cereals with folic acid** (a synthetic form of folate), and doctors recommend **folic acid supplements for pregnant women**. This has **significantly reduced birth defects worldwide**.

Example 2: Cancer Risk – The Balance of Folate

Folate's role in DNA methylation is a **double-edged sword** when it comes to **cancer risk**:

- **Too little folate** can lead to **DNA hypomethylation** (insufficient methylation), causing **genetic instability**. This may **activate oncogenes** (cancer-causing genes), increasing the risk of **uncontrolled cell growth and tumor formation**.
- **Too much folate**, however, may lead to **DNA hypermethylation** (excessive methylation), which can **silence tumor suppressor genes**—the body's natural defense against cancer. When these protective genes are turned off, cancer cells may **proliferate unchecked**.

This delicate balance highlights the importance of optimal folate intake for good health. Achieving the right amount—not too little and not too much—is key to reducing cancer risk.

Example 3: Folate, Brain Health, and Aging

Folate also plays a major role in **brain function, memory, and cognitive health**, playing a crucial role in **DNA methylation and neurotransmitter synthesis**. Research has shown that **low folate levels** are linked to **Alzheimer's disease and dementia**.

This happens because low folate levels lead to a **buildup of homocysteine**, a compound that can cause brain cell damage and interfere with DNA methylation, impairing cognitive function.

In simple terms:

- **Sufficient folate = Supports healthy brain cells, enhances memory, and reduces the risk of cognitive decline.**
- **Low folate = Increases the risk of memory loss, accelerated brain aging, and neurodegenerative diseases.**

This is why older adults are encouraged to eat **leafy green vegetables, beans, and fortified grains,** which are rich in folate, to **support brain health**.

Polyphenols and Histone Modifications

Polyphenols are **naturally occurring compounds** found in various plant-based foods and beverages, renowned for their **antioxidant properties** and potential health benefits. Among these, **resveratrol**, a polyphenol predominantly found in **red grapes, berries, and peanuts**, has garnered significant attention for its role in **modulating epigenetic mechanisms**, particularly **histone modifications**.

How Do Polyphenols Influence Histone Modifications?

Histones are proteins around which DNA is wrapped, forming a structure called **chromatin**. Their chemical modifications such as **acetylation and methylation**, control gene activity by making DNA **more or less accessible** for transcription.

- **Histone Acetylation**: Resveratrol **promotes histone acetylation**, leading to **the activation of tumor suppressor genes** such as **BRCA1, p53, and p21(CIP1)**.
- **Histone Methylation**: Resveratrol **modulates histone methylation patterns**, helping restore the expression of genes **silenced in cancer cells**.

Example: Resveratrol and Cancer Prevention

Studies have shown that **resveratrol can slow cancer progression** by promoting **histone acetylation**, which reactivates **tumor suppressor genes** and enhances **DNA repair mechanisms**. This highlights the potential of **dietary polyphenols in cancer prevention.**

Note: Polyphenols like **resveratrol** can influence **both histone modifications and DNA methylation**, making them powerful dietary components in **disease prevention and health promotion**.

Curcumin and Epigenetic Modifications

Curcumin, the active compound in **turmeric (Curcuma longa)**, is a powerful **polyphenol** known for its **anti-inflammatory, antioxidant, and anti-cancer** properties. Emerging research shows that **curcumin acts as an epigenetic modulator**, influencing both **DNA methylation and histone modifications**, which play a crucial role in gene regulation and disease prevention.

How Does Curcumin Influence Epigenetics?

Curcumin regulates gene expression through multiple **epigenetic mechanisms**:

- **DNA Methylation**: Curcumin **inhibits DNA methyltransferases (DNMTs)**, leading to **DNA demethylation** and **reactivation of silenced tumor suppressor genes**.
- **Histone Modifications**: Curcumin acts as a **histone deacetylase (HDAC) inhibitor**, increasing **histone acetylation**, which promotes gene activation and reduces cancer cell proliferation.
- **MicroRNA (miRNA) Regulation**: Curcumin **modulates microRNAs (miRNAs)**, which control gene silencing and activation, particularly in **cancer progression and inflammatory diseases**.

Example: Curcumin and Cancer Therapy

Studies have shown that curcumin inhibits DNMT activity, leading to hypomethylation of tumor suppressor genes, thereby slowing cancer progression. Additionally, as an HDAC inhibitor, curcumin enhances histone acetylation, promoting the expression of protective genes that prevent tumor growth.

Curcumin in Chronic Disease Prevention

Beyond cancer, curcumin's ability to modulate **DNA methylation and histone modifications** suggests **therapeutic potential** in:

- **Neurodegenerative diseases** (e.g., Alzheimer's, Parkinson's)
- **Cardiovascular diseases**
- **Inflammatory disorders** (e.g., arthritis, inflammatory bowel disease)

Selenium and Epigenetic Modifications

Selenium is an essential **trace element** that plays a critical role in **DNA methylation, histone modifications, and microRNA regulation**. It influences **gene expression and cellular processes** by integrating into selenoproteins, which are involved in **antioxidant defense, immune function, and cancer prevention**.

How Does Selenium Influence Epigenetics?

Selenium affects epigenetic regulation through several mechanisms:

- **DNA Methylation:** Selenium influences **one-carbon metabolism**, which provides **methyl groups for DNA methylation**. It has been shown to regulate **DNA methyltransferase (DNMT) activity**, leading to either **gene activation or repression** depending on cellular needs.

- **Histone Modifications:** Selenium has been found to **modulate histone acetylation and methylation**, thereby influencing chromatin structure and gene accessibility.
- **MicroRNA Regulation:** Selenium regulates **microRNAs (miRNAs)**, small RNA molecules that control gene expression by targeting mRNA for degradation or translational repression.

Example: Selenium and Cancer Prevention

Research indicates that **selenium prevents hypermethylation of tumor suppressor genes, reactivating key cancer-fighting genes**. For instance, selenium has been shown to restore the expression of the **GSTP1 gene;** a tumor suppressor frequently **silenced by DNA hypermethylation in prostate cancer**.

Furthermore, selenium enhances **histone acetylation**, promoting a **chromatin structure that facilitates tumor suppressor gene activation**. This dual action on **DNA methylation and histone modifications** suggests selenium's **potential in cancer prevention and therapy.**

Selenium and Inflammation-Related Diseases

Beyond cancer, selenium plays a key role in **modulating inflammatory gene expression**, making it beneficial for:

- Autoimmune diseases (e.g., rheumatoid arthritis, Hashimoto's thyroiditis)
- Cardiovascular health (by reducing oxidative stress and regulating lipid metabolism)
- Neuroprotection (by supporting antioxidant defenses in the brain)

Maintaining Optimal Selenium Levels

Both selenium deficiency and excess can be harmful:

- **Deficiency →** Impaired immune response and increased oxidative stress
- **Excess →** Toxicity leading to DNA damage and metabolic disturbances

Overall, Selenium's ability to modulate DNA methylation, histone modifications, and miRNA expression highlights its potential as a dietary component in disease prevention and health optimization.

Omega-3 Fatty Acids and Epigenetic Modifications

Omega-3 polyunsaturated fatty acids (n-3 PUFAs), particularly **eicosapentaenoic acid (EPA) and docosahexaenoic acid (DHA)**, play a crucial role in **epigenetic regulation**, influencing **DNA methylation, histone modifications, and inflammation-related gene expression**.

How Do Omega-3 Fatty Acids Influence Epigenetics?

- **DNA Methylation:** Omega-3 fatty acids are known to regulate **DNA methylation patterns** by altering the activity of **DNA methyltransferases (DNMTs)**. This can influence inflammatory genes and metabolic pathways.

- **Histone Modifications:** Omega-3s can modulate **histone acetylation and methylation**, impacting genes involved in **inflammation, lipid metabolism, and cardiovascular health**.
- **Regulation of Inflammatory Pathways:** Omega-3s interact with key transcription factors, such as:
  - **NF-κB (nuclear factor kappa B)** → a master regulator of inflammation. Omega-3s **reduce NF-κB activation**, suppressing pro-inflammatory gene expression.
  - **PPARγ (peroxisome proliferator-activated receptor gamma)** → a regulator of lipid metabolism. Omega-3s **activate PPARγ**, promoting beneficial metabolic effects.

Example: Omega-3 Fatty Acids and Inflammation Regulation

A study on the **Yup'ik population in Alaska**, who consume a diet rich in omega-3 fatty acids, found that higher omega-3 intake was associated with **increased DNA methylation at key inflammation-related genes**. This suggests a protective role of omega-3 fatty acids in reducing **chronic inflammation**, a factor linked to cardiovascular diseases, obesity, and autoimmune disorders.

Another study demonstrated that **EPA and DHA supplementation reduced pro-inflammatory cytokine expression** by altering **DNA methylation patterns** in immune cells, highlighting their potential for managing inflammatory conditions.

Omega-3s, Metabolism, and Obesity Risk

Omega-3 fatty acids also regulate *Leptin* gene expression (a hormone involved in hunger and metabolism) through histone modifications, influencing:

- Appetite control
- Energy balance
- Obesity risk

Additionally, omega-3 fatty acids exert **anti-inflammatory and metabolic benefits** by modulating **DNA methylation and histone modifications**, making them a key dietary component in **preventing chronic diseases** such as cardiovascular disease, obesity, and neurodegenerative disorders.

Butyrate and Epigenetic Modifications

Butyrate is a **short-chain fatty acid (SCFA)** produced through the microbial fermentation of **dietary fiber** in the colon. It serves as a critical **epigenetic regulator**, influencing **DNA methylation, histone modifications, and non-coding RNA regulation**, which in turn impact **gene expression, inflammation, and metabolic processes**.

How Does Butyrate Influence Epigenetics?

1. **Histone Deacetylase (HDAC) Inhibition:**
    - Butyrate is a **histone deacetylase inhibitor (HDACi)**, meaning it prevents the removal of acetyl groups from histone proteins.
    - This **promotes histone acetylation**, resulting in a **relaxed chromatin structure** that enhances gene transcription.
    - By increasing histone acetylation, butyrate can **reactivate tumor suppressor genes**, which are often silenced in cancers.
2. **DNA Methylation Modulation:**
    - Butyrate **modulates DNA methylation** by affecting **DNA methyltransferase (DNMT) activity**.
    - It can promote **DNA demethylation of tumor suppressor genes**, preventing the silencing of genes that regulate cell growth and apoptosis.
    - Butyrate also regulates **one-carbon metabolism**, which supplies methyl groups for proper DNA methylation patterns.
3. **Regulation of Non-Coding RNAs:**
    - Butyrate influences **microRNAs (miRNAs)** that control gene silencing by targeting messenger RNA (mRNA) for degradation.
    - Specific miRNAs regulated by butyrate are involved in **inflammation control, metabolic pathways, and immune response**.
4. **Anti-Inflammatory Effects:**
    - By modulating histone acetylation and DNA methylation, butyrate downregulates **pro-inflammatory cytokines** such as **IL-6 and TNF-α**, while upregulating **anti-inflammatory genes**.
    - This **reduces inflammation**, helping to maintain **gut homeostasis** and **lowering the risk of inflammatory bowel diseases (IBD)**, such as **Crohn's disease and ulcerative colitis**.

Example: Butyrate and Colorectal Cancer Prevention

Research suggests that butyrate **induces apoptosis (programmed cell death) in colorectal cancer cells** while supporting **healthy colon cells** through epigenetic modulation. A diet rich in fiber leads to **increased butyrate production**, which has been associated with a **lower risk of colorectal cancer** by:

- **Reactivating tumor suppressor genes** that are silenced due to aberrant DNA methylation.
- **Enhancing histone acetylation**, making chromatin more accessible for gene expression.
- **Regulating immune response genes**, reducing chronic inflammation linked to cancer progression.

In populations with **high-fiber diets**, butyrate production is enhanced, demonstrating **protective effects against colorectal cancer, metabolic syndrome, and inflammatory disorders**.

Butyrate's ability to **modulate histone modifications, regulate DNA methylation, and influence non-coding RNAs** highlights its critical role in **gut health, metabolic regulation, and disease prevention**. Regular consumption of **fiber-rich foods** like whole grains, vegetables, and legumes promotes butyrate production, emphasizing its importance in **epigenetic health and chronic disease prevention.**

Vitamin D and Epigenetic Modifications

Vitamin D is a **steroid hormone** that plays a crucial role in **calcium homeostasis, immune function, and various metabolic processes**. Beyond its classical roles, vitamin D acts as an epigenetic regulator, influencing DNA methylation, histone modifications, and gene expression patterns.

How Does Vitamin D Influence Epigenetics?

1. **DNA Methylation Regulation:**
    - Vitamin D influences DNA methylation patterns by altering the expression of DNA methyltransferases (*DNMT*s).
    - Studies suggest that hypomethylation of the Vitamin D Receptor (*VDR*) gene enhances vitamin D signaling, improving immune responses, and cancer prevention.
    - Methylation patterns of vitamin D metabolism genes can influence vitamin D bioavailability and individual susceptibility to disease.
2. **Histone Modifications:**
    - Vitamin D can modify histone acetylation and methylation, affecting chromatin accessibility and gene transcription.
    - It enhances histone acetylation, leading to the activation of genes related to bone metabolism, immune function, and cancer prevention.
    - By promoting histone deacetylase (HDAC) inhibition, vitamin D facilitates a more open chromatin structure, enhancing gene expression.
3. **Regulation of Vitamin D Metabolism Genes:**
    - Vitamin D affects the expression of key metabolic genes such as CYP2R1, CYP27B1, and CYP24A1, which regulate vitamin D activation and breakdown.
    - Increased methylation of CYP24A1 leads to its silencing, reducing vitamin D breakdown and increasing its bioavailability.
    - Methylation changes in CYP2R1 have been linked to variations in vitamin D levels among different populations.

4. **Immune System Modulation:**
    - Vitamin D regulates immune cell differentiation and function by altering DNA methylation patterns in T cells and macrophages.
    - It downregulates pro-inflammatory cytokines such as IL-6 and TNF-α, reducing inflammation-associated diseases.
    - Vitamin D deficiency is associated with aberrant epigenetic modifications, leading to an increased risk of autoimmune conditions.

Example: Vitamin D and Cancer Prevention

Studies have shown that vitamin D supplementation can restore proper DNA methylation patterns, leading to the reactivation of tumor suppressor genes such as *VDR* and p53. In cancers where *VDR* is silenced due to hypermethylation, vitamin D can reduce methylation levels, restoring gene function and inhibiting tumor growth.

Additionally, vitamin D inhibits histone deacetylases (HDACs), which helps in reducing the growth of cancer cells by promoting a more accessible chromatin state for tumor suppressor gene activation.

The Dual Role of Vitamin D in Epigenetic Regulation

Vitamin D plays a **crucial role in both DNA methylation and histone modifications**, impacting multiple biological processes, including:

- **Immune Regulation** – Reduces inflammation and autoimmune risks.
- **Metabolic Health** – Regulates genes involved in calcium balance, energy metabolism, and insulin sensitivity.
- **Cancer Prevention** – Reactivates tumor suppressor genes through DNA demethylation and histone acetylation.

Limitations

While nutrition plays a powerful role in shaping gene expression through epigenetic mechanisms, it is important to understand that dietary influence is only one part of a broader biological landscape. Epigenetic patterns are shaped by multiple factors—including age, early-life programming, microbiome composition, physical activity, stress exposure, sleep patterns, medications, and environmental pollutants such as heavy metals and endocrine disruptors. Additionally, epigenetic responses can be tissue-specific, time-dependent, and may vary significantly between individuals due to genetic background and biological context. Therefore, while dietary interventions can meaningfully modify gene expression, they should be viewed within a holistic framework of lifestyle, environment, and individual variability rather than as isolated determinants. Recognizing these limitations helps ensure realistic expectations and reinforces the need for personalized, evidence-based nutritional strategies.

Conclusion

The emerging field of nutrigenomics underscores how dietary choices shape epigenetic landscapes, influencing gene expression without altering DNA sequences. Various nutrients—including folate, polyphenols (resveratrol, curcumin), selenium, omega-3 fatty acids, butyrate, and vitamin D—serve as epigenetic modulators, influencing DNA methylation, histone modifications, and microRNA regulation.

Incorporating epigenetically active nutrients—through whole foods, healthy fats, plant-based polyphenols, and adequate vitamin D levels—can optimize genetic potential, promote longevity, and reduce disease susceptibility. Understanding and harnessing nutrition's role in epigenetics paves the way for personalized medicine, precision nutrition, and holistic health strategies for future generations.

Diet–Epigenome–Health Pathway

Dietary Component	Epigenetic Mark	Cellular Response	Health Outcome
Folate, B12, Choline	↑ DNA methylation	Silencing of unnecessary or harmful gene expression	Reduced neural tube defect risk; genomic stability
Polyphenols (Resveratrol, Curcumin, EGCG)	Histone acetylation/ HDAC inhibition	Activation of antioxidant and anti-inflammatory genes	Reduced oxidative stress, lower cancer risk
Omega-3 Fatty Acids (EPA/DHA)	miRNA modulation, altered DNA methylation	Reduced inflammatory gene expression	Lower cardiovascular and metabolic disease risk
Fiber → Butyrate	Histone acetylation (HDAC inhibition)	Apoptosis of damaged cells; improved gut barrier	Reduced colorectal cancer risk; improved gut health
Vitamin D	Histone modification + altered methylation of immune genes	Enhanced immune regulation and cell differentiation	Reduced autoimmunity and inflammation
High-fat/ultra-processed diet	Dysregulated RNA methylation (m^6A)	Increased lipogenesis, impaired insulin signaling	Increased risk of metabolic disease

Questions

1. What is the primary focus of nutrigenetics?
2. How do nutrigenetics and nutrigenomics differ from each other?
3. What role does epigenomics play in personalized nutrition?
4. What is the definition of epigenetics?
5. How do lifestyle and diet influence epigenetic modifications?
6. What is DNA methylation, and how does it affect gene expression?
7. How does folate influence DNA methylation?
8. What are histones, and how do they affect gene expression?
9. What is the role of histone acetylation in gene activation?
10. How do polyphenols influence histone modifications?
11. What are non-coding RNAs (ncRNAs), and how do they regulate gene expression?
12. How do omega-3 fatty acids influence non-coding RNA activity?
13. What is chromatin remodeling, and why is it important for gene expression?
14. How does selenium impact chromatin remodeling?
15. What is RNA methylation (m6A modification), and how does it affect gene expression?
16. How do high-fat diets influence RNA methylation?
17. How can DNA methylation patterns influence disease risk?
18. What is the role of vitamin B12 in DNA methylation?
19. How does genetic variation influence the response to nutrients?
20. What is the importance of the MTHFR gene in folate metabolism?
21. How does folate intake affect neural tube defects during pregnancy?
22. What is the relationship between folate and cancer risk?
23. How does curcumin influence DNA methylation and histone modifications?
24. What role does curcumin play in cancer therapy?
25. How do polyphenols like resveratrol influence cancer prevention?
26. How does curcumin affect microRNA regulation in cancer progression?
27. What is the significance of selenium in DNA methylation and cancer prevention?
28. How does selenium influence inflammation-related diseases?
29. What is the impact of omega-3 fatty acids on inflammatory pathways?
30. How do omega-3 fatty acids regulate DNA methylation and histone modifications?
31. What is butyrate, and how does it influence epigenetic modifications?
32. How does butyrate impact inflammation and metabolic pathways?
33. What role does butyrate play in colorectal cancer prevention?
34. How does vitamin D influence gene expression through epigenetic mechanisms?
35. What is the impact of vitamin D deficiency on epigenetic modifications?
36. How does vitamin D regulate immune function through epigenetic mechanisms?
37. How does vitamin D supplementation affect tumor suppressor genes?
38. What are the epigenetic effects of vitamin D on metabolic health?
39. How do nutrients like folate, polyphenols, and selenium work together to optimize health?
40. How can personalized nutrition based on epigenetic regulation improve health outcomes?

Answers

1. Nutrigenetics focuses on how individual genetic variations affect a person's response to nutrients, influencing metabolism, health, and disease susceptibility.
2. Nutrigenetics studies the genetic factors that influence how individuals respond to food, while nutrigenomics focuses on how nutrients and diet influence gene expression and function.
3. Epigenomics is key in personalized nutrition because it explains how environmental factors, including diet, can alter gene expression without changing the DNA sequence.
4. Epigenetics refers to changes in gene expression that do not involve changes to the underlying DNA sequence but are influenced by environmental factors.
5. Lifestyle choices such as diet, physical activity, and stress levels can lead to epigenetic modifications that influence gene expression, impacting health outcomes.
6. DNA methylation involves adding methyl groups to DNA, typically silencing gene expression by preventing transcription factors from binding to the DNA.
7. Folate influences DNA methylation by donating methyl groups that are essential for the proper regulation of gene expression.
8. Histones are proteins around which DNA is wrapped. Their modifications affect how accessible the DNA is for transcription, thereby influencing gene expression.
9. Histone acetylation makes DNA more accessible for transcription, generally associated with gene activation.
10. Polyphenols, such as those found in green tea and berries, can promote histone acetylation, activating genes involved in antioxidant defense and reducing inflammation.
11. Non-coding RNAs (ncRNAs) regulate gene expression by binding to mRNA, blocking translation, or promoting mRNA degradation.
12. Omega-3 fatty acids can influence ncRNA activity to regulate genes involved in inflammation, lipid metabolism, and other metabolic pathways.
13. Chromatin remodeling refers to the alteration of chromatin structure, making DNA more or less accessible for transcription, which regulates gene expression.
14. Selenium influences chromatin remodeling by modifying histone acetylation and affecting genes associated with oxidative stress and immune response.
15. RNA methylation (m6A modification) regulates RNA stability, translation efficiency, and degradation, affecting protein production and metabolic processes.
16. High-fat diets can disrupt RNA methylation patterns, influencing genes involved in obesity and insulin resistance, impairing metabolic health.
17. Changes in DNA methylation patterns can lead to genetic instability, increasing the risk of diseases such as cancer, cardiovascular conditions, and neurological disorders.
18. Vitamin B12 is essential for DNA methylation because it helps produce SAM, the primary methyl donor involved in the process.
19. Genetic variations influence how individuals metabolize nutrients, which can affect their health and response to dietary interventions.
20. MTHFR gene variations (like the C677T polymorphism) can reduce folate metabolism efficiency, affecting DNA methylation and disease risk.

21. Folate intake is crucial during pregnancy as it influences DNA methylation patterns that ensure proper neural tube development, reducing the risk of defects like spina bifida.
22. Low folate intake can lead to DNA hypomethylation, activating oncogenes and increasing cancer risk, while excess folate can silence tumor suppressor genes.
23. Curcumin promotes DNA demethylation and histone acetylation, reactivating tumor suppressor genes and preventing cancer cell proliferation.
24. Curcumin has been shown to inhibit DNA methyltransferase (DNMT), restoring the expression of tumor suppressor genes and slowing cancer progression.
25. Polyphenols, like resveratrol, activate tumor suppressor genes by promoting histone acetylation, reducing cancer cell proliferation.
26. Curcumin regulates microRNAs that control gene silencing, particularly in cancer progression, helping to block cancer cell growth.
27. Selenium affects DNA methylation, preventing hypermethylation of tumor suppressor genes, and plays a role in cancer prevention.
28. Selenium modulates inflammatory gene expression, which is beneficial in conditions like autoimmune diseases, cardiovascular health, and neuroprotection.
29. Omega-3 fatty acids reduce NF-κB activation, suppressing pro-inflammatory gene expression, which is beneficial for inflammation-related diseases.
30. Omega-3s influence DNA methylation and histone modifications, regulating genes involved in inflammation and cardiovascular health.
31. Butyrate is a histone deacetylase inhibitor, promoting histone acetylation and enhancing gene expression related to tumor suppression and cancer prevention.
32. Butyrate also modulates DNA methylation, reactivating tumor suppressor genes and preventing colorectal cancer progression.
33. A diet rich in fiber increases butyrate production, enhancing tumor suppression through histone acetylation and DNA methylation changes.
34. Vitamin D influences DNA methylation patterns, enhancing immune responses and helping in cancer prevention through epigenetic modifications.
35. Vitamin D deficiency leads to hypomethylation, impairing immune function and increasing autoimmune diseases risk.
36. Vitamin D regulates immune responses by altering DNA methylation patterns in immune cells, which reduces inflammation.
37. Vitamin D supplementation restores tumor suppressor genes such as *VDR* and p53, reducing cancer growth.
38. Vitamin D influences histone modifications, activating genes involved in bone metabolism, immune function, and cancer prevention.
39. Folate, polyphenols, and selenium work together to modulate epigenetic mechanisms, improving health outcomes and disease prevention.
40. Personalized nutrition based on epigenetic regulation can improve longevity, prevent disease, and optimize health by aligning dietary recommendations with individual genetic profiles.

References

1. Anderson, O. S., Sant, K. E., & Dolinoy, D. C. (2012). Nutrition and epigenetics: An interplay of dietary methyl donors, one-carbon metabolism and DNA methylation. *Journal of Nutritional Biochemistry, 23*(8), 853–859. https://doi.org/10.1016/j.jnutbio.2012.03.003
2. Choi, S.-W., & Friso, S. (2010). Epigenetics: A new bridge between nutrition and health. *Advances in Nutrition, 1*(1), 8–16. https://doi.org/10.3945/an.110.1004
3. Fang, M., Chen, D., & Yang, C. S. (2007). Dietary polyphenols may affect DNA methylation. *The Journal of Nutritional Biochemistry, 18*(5), 287–296. https://doi.org/10.1016/j.jnutbio.2006.10.007
4. Smithells, R. W., Sheppard, S., Schorah, C. J., & Harris, R. (1981). Neural tube defects and folic acid: prevention with folic acid. *The Lancet*, *317*(8226), 339–340. https://doi.org/10.1016/S0140-6736(81)92400-1
5. Glier, M. B., Green, T. J., & Devlin, A. M. (2014). Methyl nutrients, DNA methylation, and cardiovascular disease. *Molecular Nutrition & Food Research*, *58*(1), 172–182. https://doi.org/10.1002/mnfr.201200636.
6. Li, X., Xie, F., Huang, W., Hu, Y., & Zhou, S. (2020). METTL3 modulates lipid metabolism and insulin resistance via m6A-dependent regulation of mTORC1–NF-κB signaling in high-fat diet–induced obesity. *Frontiers in Endocrinology*, *11*, 577566. https://doi.org/10.3389/fendo.2020.577566
7. Wu, R., Liu, Y., Yao, Y., Zhao, Y., Bi, Z., Jiang, Q.,... & Wang, Y. (2019). *FTO* regulates adipogenesis by controlling cell cycle progression via m6A-YTHDF2-dependent mechanism. *Biochimica et Biophysica Acta (BBA) - Molecular and Cell Biology of Lipids*, *1864*(9), 1323–1330. https://doi.org/10.1016/j.bbalip.2019.06.011
8. Xiao, Y., Wang, L., Wang, Q., Liu, L., Tan, H., & Lin, Q. (2024). METTL14 deletion in brown adipose tissue improves systemic insulin sensitivity through m6A-regulated prostaglandin signaling. *Nature Metabolism*, *6*(1), 33–46. https://doi.org/10.1038/s42255-023-00853-3.
9. Li, J., Wang, H., Guo, Y., Wu, J., & Zhao, Y. (2024). Natural flavonoid dihydromyricetin ameliorates obesity by regulating gut microbiota and N6-methyladenosine RNA methylation. *Phytotherapy Research, 38*(7), 3437–3452. https://doi.org/10.1002/ptr.8176.
10. Ciesielski, O., Biesiekierska, M., & Balcerczyk, A. (2020). Epigallocatechin-3-gallate alters histone acetylation and methylation and impacts chromatin architecture profile in human endothelial cells. *Molecules, 25*(10), 2326. https://doi.org/10.3390/molecules25102326 mdpi.com+9sciencedirect.com+9pmc.ncbi.nlm.nih.gov+9pmc.ncbi.nlm.nih.gov+2pubmed.ncbi.nlm.nih.gov+2researchgate.net+2
11. Lorente-Cebrián, S. (2025). Phenolic compounds and epigenetic mechanisms: Polyphenols promote histone acetylation, leading to gene expression activation. *Journal of Physiological Biochemistry*. link.springer.com
12. Pereira, Q. C., et al. (2023). The molecular mechanism of polyphenols in inflammation and aging: Modulation of epigenetic enzymes including HATs and HDACs. *International Journal of Molecular Sciences, 24*(6), 5508. mdpi.com

13. Karbowska, J., & Kochan, Z. (2025). *Crosstalk between dietary fatty acids and microRNAs in the regulation of hepatic ApoB-containing lipoprotein synthesis in humans*. International Journal of Molecular Sciences, 26(10), 4817. https://doi.org/10.3390/ijms26104817 pmc.ncbi.nlm.nih.gov+1jomes.org+1mdpi.com
14. Li, J., Zhang, et al. (2025). *Dietary omega-3 polyunsaturated fatty acids improve metabolic health and regulate miRNA expression linked to adipogenesis and inflammation*. Nutrients, 17(11), 1836. https://doi.org/10.3390/nu17111836 mdpi.com
15. MacDonald-Ramos, K., et al. (2021). *Effect of dietary fatty acids on microRNA expression in models of metabolic disease and inflammation*. PMC. https://pubmed.ncbi.nlm.nih.gov/PMC8226960
16. Avery, J. C., & Hoffmann, P. R. (2018). Selenium, selenoproteins, and immunity. *Nutrients, 10*(9), 1203. https://doi.org/10.3390/nu10091203 researchgate.net+9pmc.ncbi.nlm.nih.gov+9mdpi.com+9mdpi.com
17. Speckmann, B., & Grune, T. (2015). Epigenetic effects of selenium and their implications for health. *Environmental and Molecular Mutagenesis, 56*(7), 477–492. https://doi.org/10.1002/em.22039 tandfonline.com+1researchgate.net+1
18. Barchielli, G., & Maleczek, M. (2022). The role of selenium in pathologies: an updated review. *Antioxidants, 11*(2), 251. https://doi.org/10.3390/antiox11020251

CHAPTER 4

KEY DATABASES FOR SEARCHING SNPS AND TRAIT ASSOCIATIONS

The study of single nucleotide polymorphisms (SNPs) and their association with human traits has become a cornerstone of modern genetics, personalized nutrition, and precision medicine. Advances in genomic research have led to the development of specialized databases that store, organize, and provide access to vast amounts of genetic variation data.

This chapter provides an overview of key online databases essential for SNP research and trait association studies. Each database offers unique features, data types, and search functionalities, enabling users to explore the genetic landscape and its relevance to health, nutrition, and personalized interventions.

dbSNP (Database of Single Nucleotide Polymorphisms)

Who Created It

- Developed and maintained by the **National Center for Biotechnology Information (NCBI)**, part of the **U.S. National Library of Medicine**.

History and Purpose

- Launched in **1998** as a central repository for genetic variation.
- Created to store information on **single nucleotide polymorphisms (SNPs)** and other small genetic variants such as insertions and deletions (indels).
- Aimed to support research in genetics, genomics, and personalized medicine.

What You Can Discover

- SNP IDs (rs numbers), their genomic location, alleles, reference sequences.
- Population-specific allele frequencies.
- Clinical significance and validation status of SNPs.
- Links to publications and genomic annotations.

Benefits

- A foundational resource for SNP identification.
- Crucial for linking genetic variants with health outcomes, drug responses, and trait predispositions.
- Frequently used in bioinformatics pipelines and annotation tools.

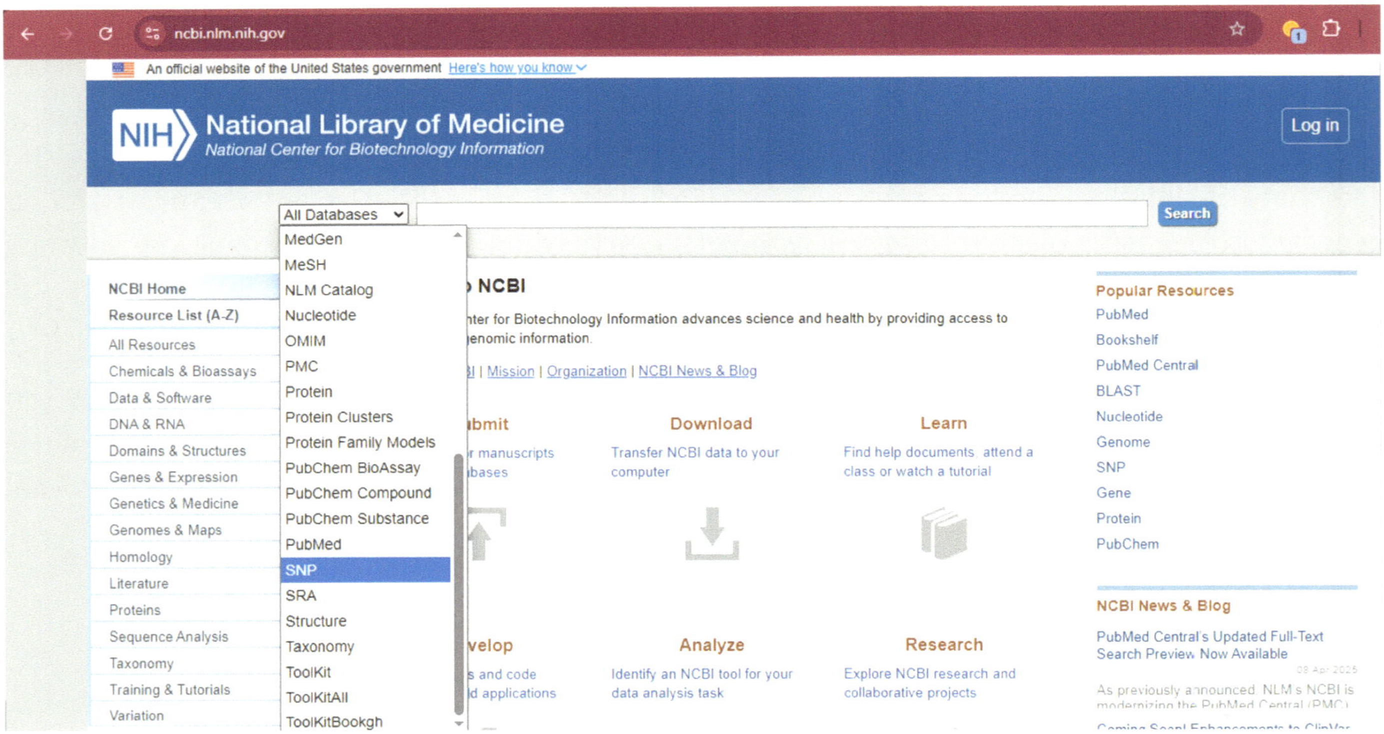

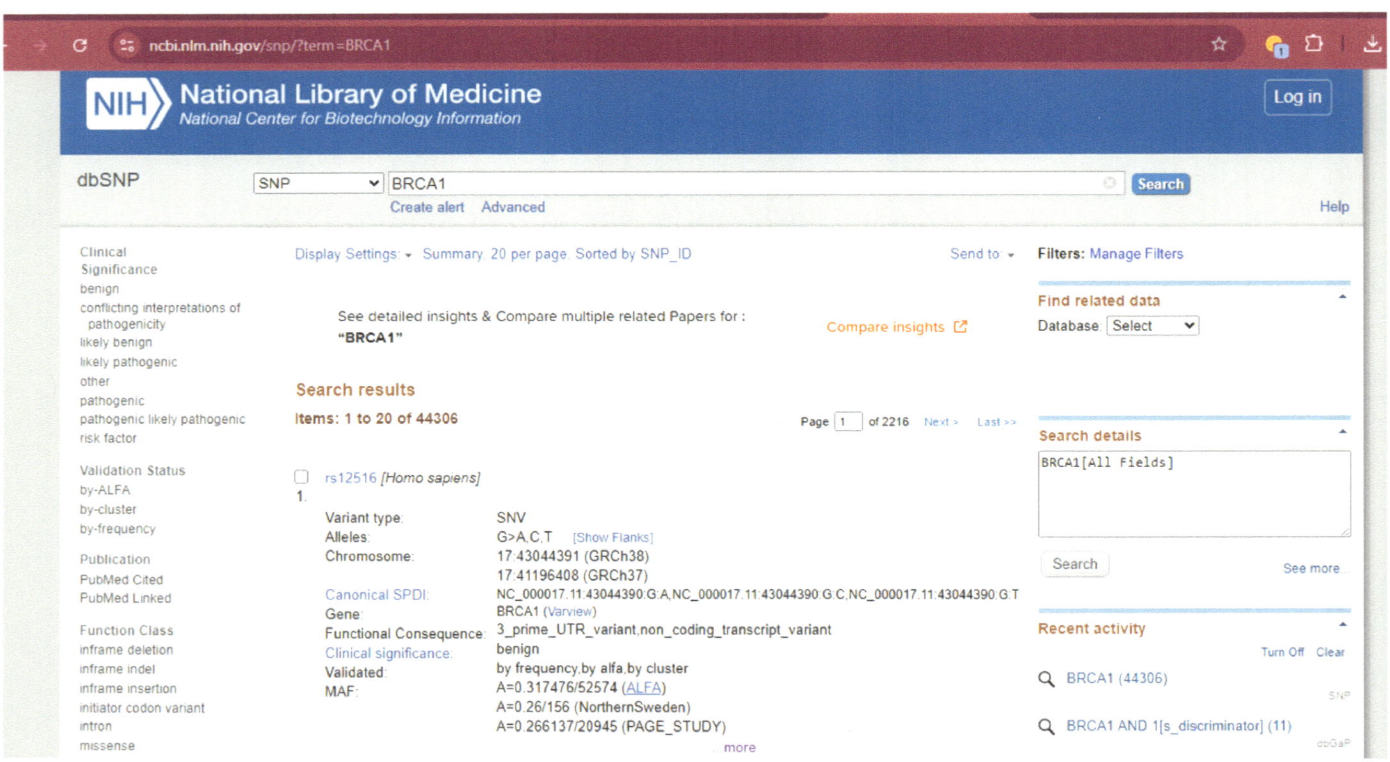

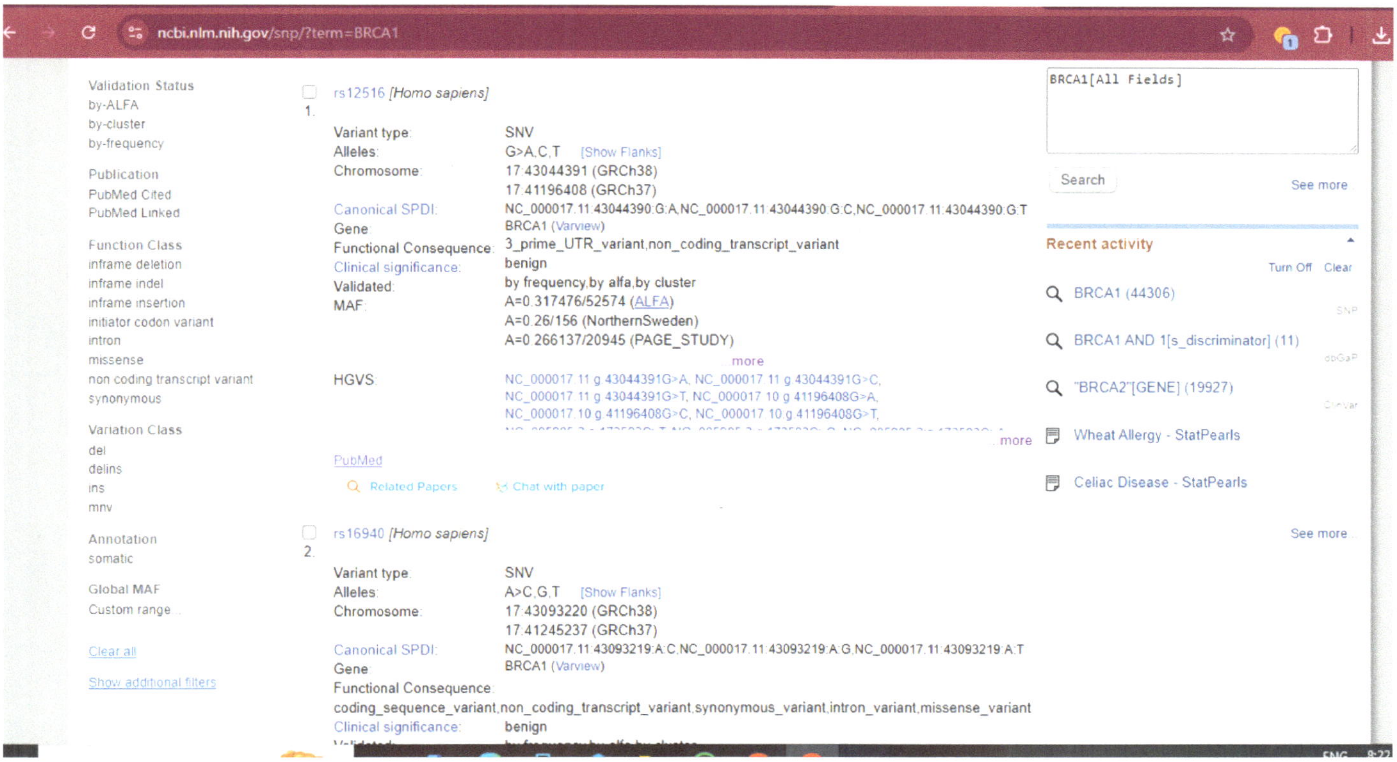

GWAS Catalog

Who Created It

- Jointly maintained by the **European Bioinformatics Institute (EMBL-EBI)** and the **National Human Genome Research Institute (NHGRI)**.

History and Purpose

- Initiated in **2008** to catalog published **Genome-Wide Association Studies (GWAS)**.
- Tracks SNP-trait associations based on statistical significance across multiple human populations.

What You Can Discover

- SNPs associated with diseases and traits like BMI, blood pressure, metabolic disorders and vitamin levels.
- Effect size of SNP-trait associations.
- P-values indicating statistical significance.
- Allele information and risk allele identification.
- Sample sizes, population ancestry, and study characteristics.
- Direct links to peer-reviewed publications for in-depth study details.

Benefits

- A key resource for nutrigenomics and personalized nutrition research.
- Helps identify SNPs associated with metabolism, nutrient absorption, obesity, and chronic diseases.
- Enables filtering of data based on trait type, population, study design, or chromosomal region.

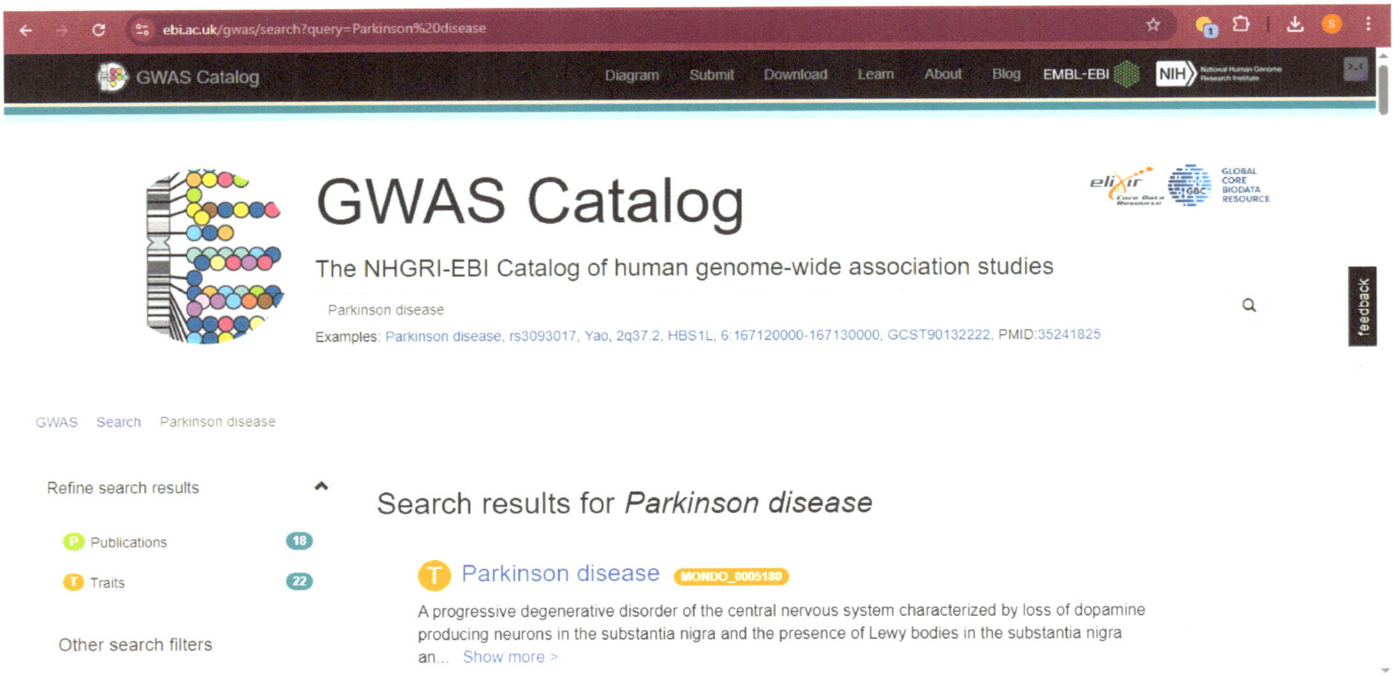

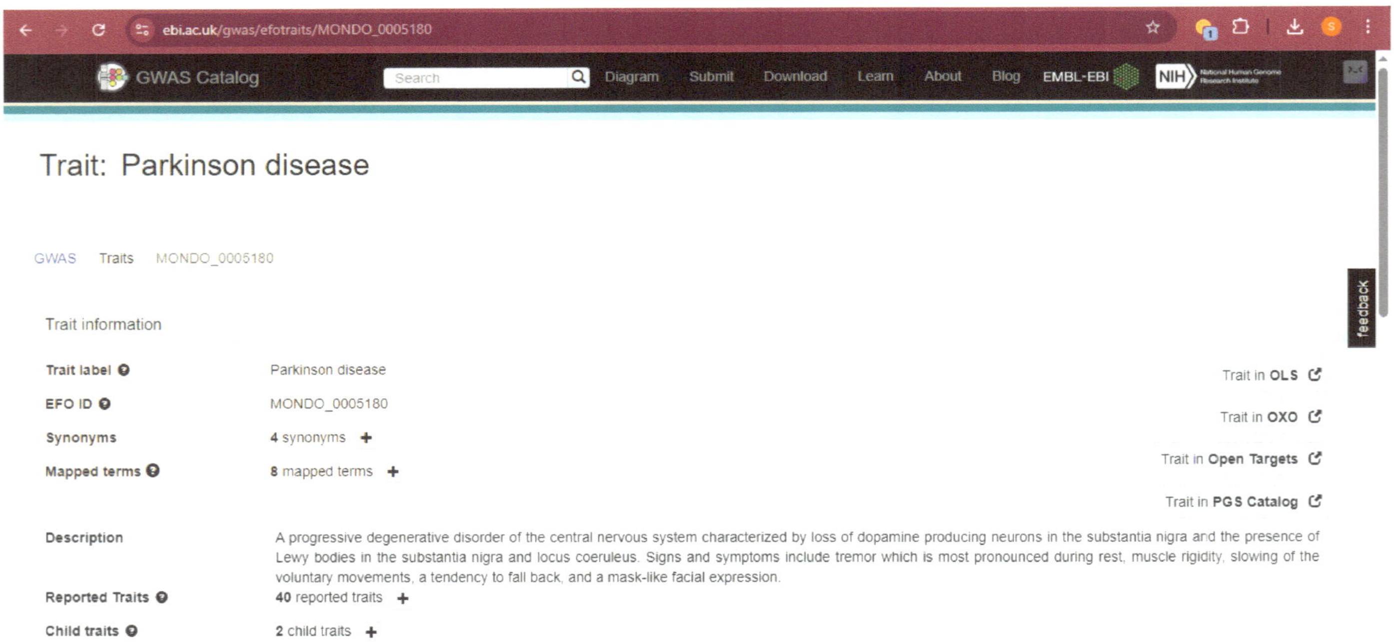

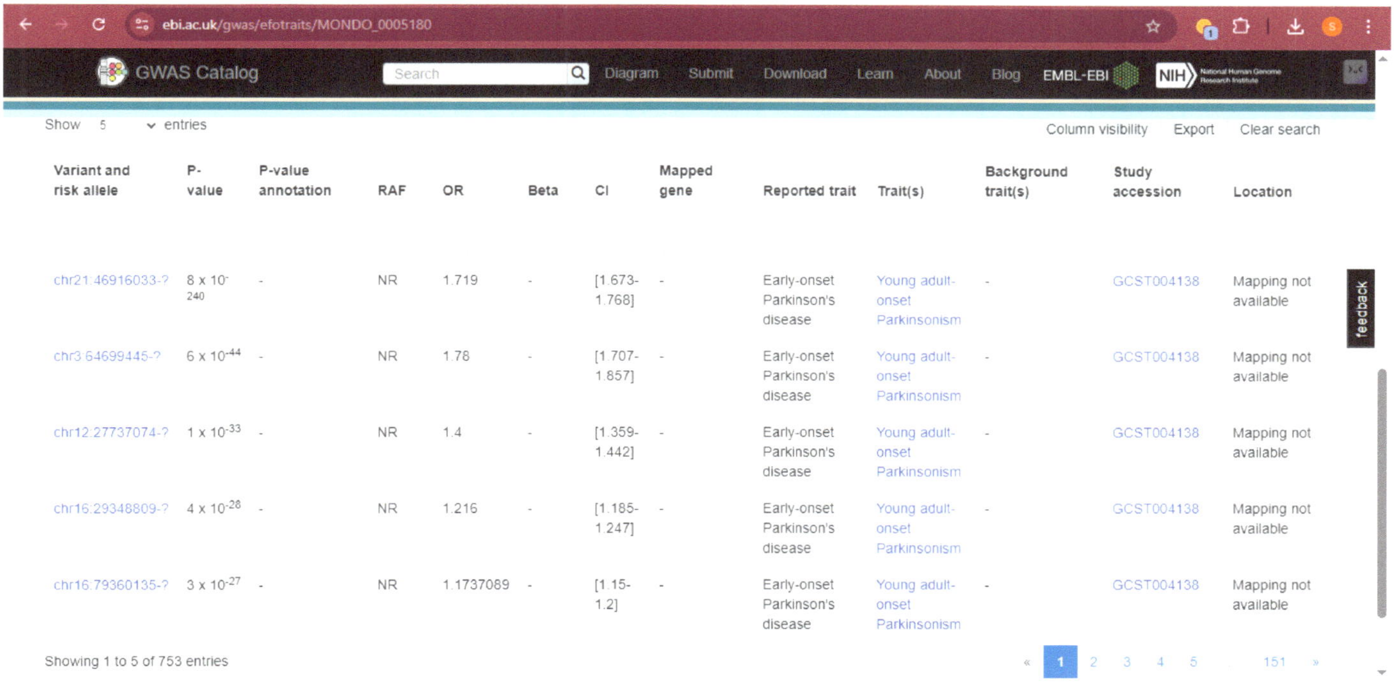

Variant and risk allele	P-value	P-value annotation	RAF	OR	Beta	CI	Mapped gene	Reported trait	Trait(s)	Background trait(s)	Study accession	Location
chr21:46916033-?	8×10^{-240}	-	NR	1.719	-	[1.673-1.768]	-	Early-onset Parkinson's disease	Young adult-onset Parkinsonism	-	GCST004138	Mapping not available
chr3:64699445-?	6×10^{-44}	-	NR	1.78	-	[1.707-1.857]	-	Early-onset Parkinson's disease	Young adult-onset Parkinsonism	-	GCST004138	Mapping not available
chr12:27737074-?	1×10^{-33}	-	NR	1.4	-	[1.359-1.442]	-	Early-onset Parkinson's disease	Young adult-onset Parkinsonism	-	GCST004138	Mapping not available
chr16:29348809-?	4×10^{-28}	-	NR	1.216	-	[1.185-1.247]	-	Early-onset Parkinson's disease	Young adult-onset Parkinsonism	-	GCST004138	Mapping not available
chr16:79360135-?	3×10^{-27}	-	NR	1.1737089	-	[1.15-1.2]	-	Early-onset Parkinson's disease	Young adult-onset Parkinsonism	-	GCST004138	Mapping not available

Ensembl Genome Browser

Who Created It

- Developed by the **European Bioinformatics Institute (EMBL-EBI)** and the **Wellcome Sanger Institute**.

History and Purpose

- First launched in **1999** to visualize the human genome.
- Offers a browser-based interface to explore multiple genome annotations.

What You Can Discover

- Gene structures, transcript isoforms, and regulatory regions.
- SNPs and their annotations, evolutionary conservation, and linkage disequilibrium.
- Comparative genomics and orthologs in other species.

Benefits

- Excellent visualization and filtering tools.
- Integration with multiple genomic databases, such as GTEx (gene expression), dbSNP (variant data), and ClinVar (clinical significance).
- Supports batch queries, variant effect prediction, and genome builds.

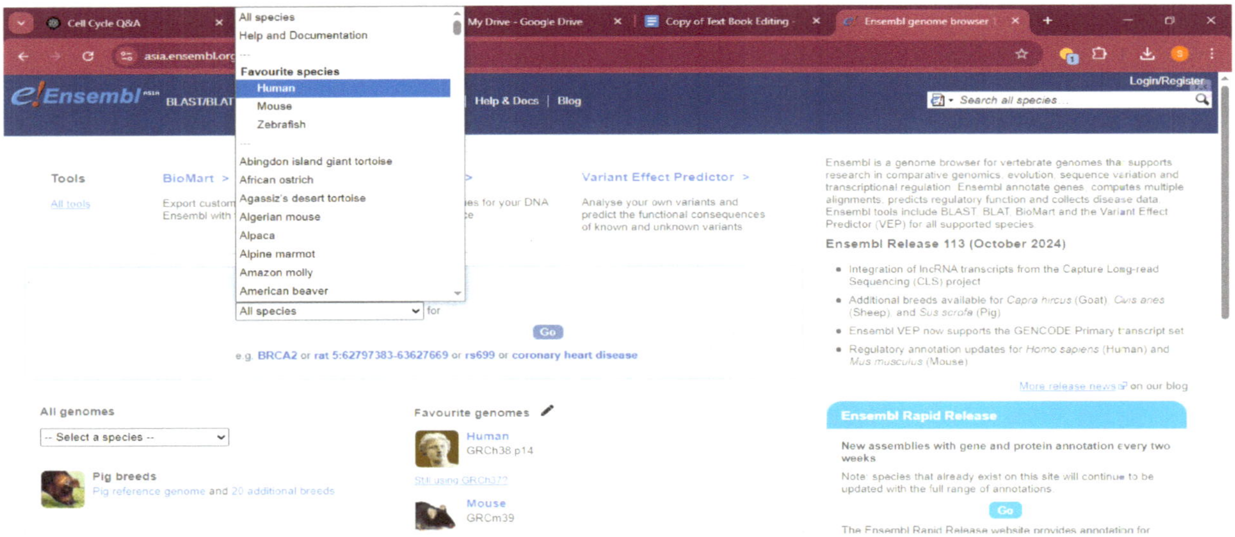
All species
Help and Documentation
Favourite species
Human
Mouse
Zebrafish
Abingdon island giant tortoise
African ostrich
Agassiz's desert tortoise
Algerian mouse
Alpaca
Alpine marmot
Amazon molly
American beaver
All species
Go
e.g. BRCA2 or rat 5:62797383-63627669 or rs699 or coronary heart disease
Tools
BioMart
Variant Effect Predictor
Analyse your own variants and predict the functional consequences of known and unknown variants
Ensembl Release 113 (October 2024)
All genomes
-- Select a species --
Pig breeds
Favourite genomes
Human
GRCh38.p14
Mouse
GRCm39
Ensembl Rapid Release
New assemblies with gene and protein annotation every two weeks

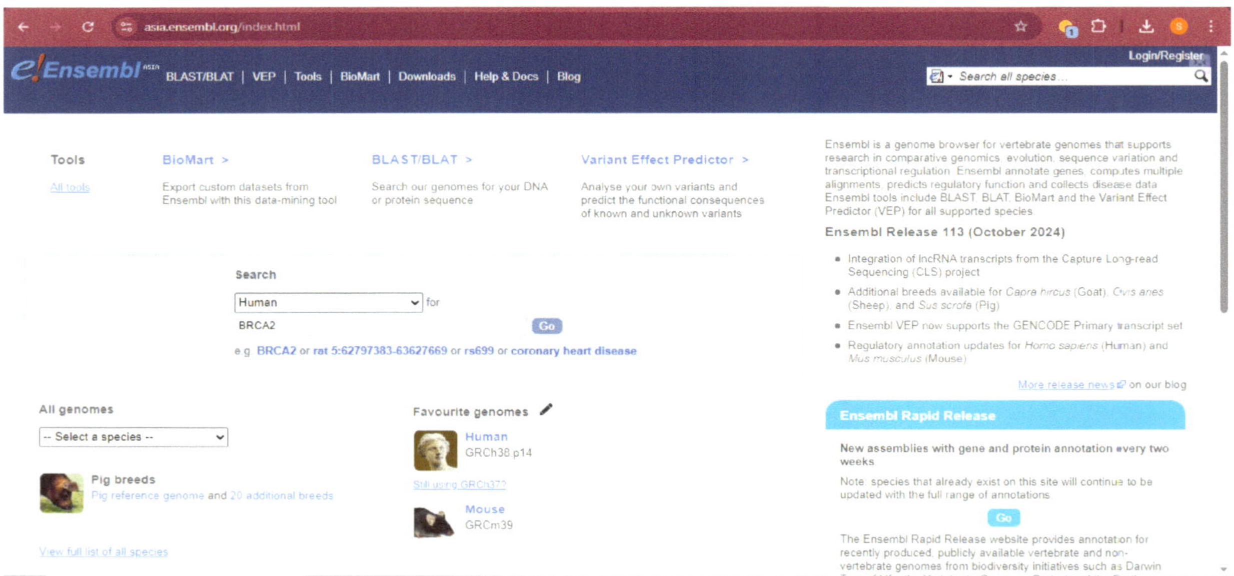
asia.ensembl.org/index.html
Ensembl
BLAST/BLAT | VEP | Tools | BioMart | Downloads | Help & Docs | Blog
Login/Register
Search all species...
Tools
BioMart
Export custom datasets from Ensembl with this data-mining tool
BLAST/BLAT
Search our genomes for your DNA or protein sequence
Variant Effect Predictor
Analyse your own variants and predict the functional consequences of known and unknown variants
Ensembl Release 113 (October 2024)
Search
Human
BRCA2
Go
e.g. BRCA2 or rat 5:62797383-63627669 or rs699 or coronary heart disease
All genomes
-- Select a species --
Pig breeds
Favourite genomes
Human
GRCh38.p14
Mouse
GRCm39
Ensembl Rapid Release
New assemblies with gene and protein annotation every two weeks

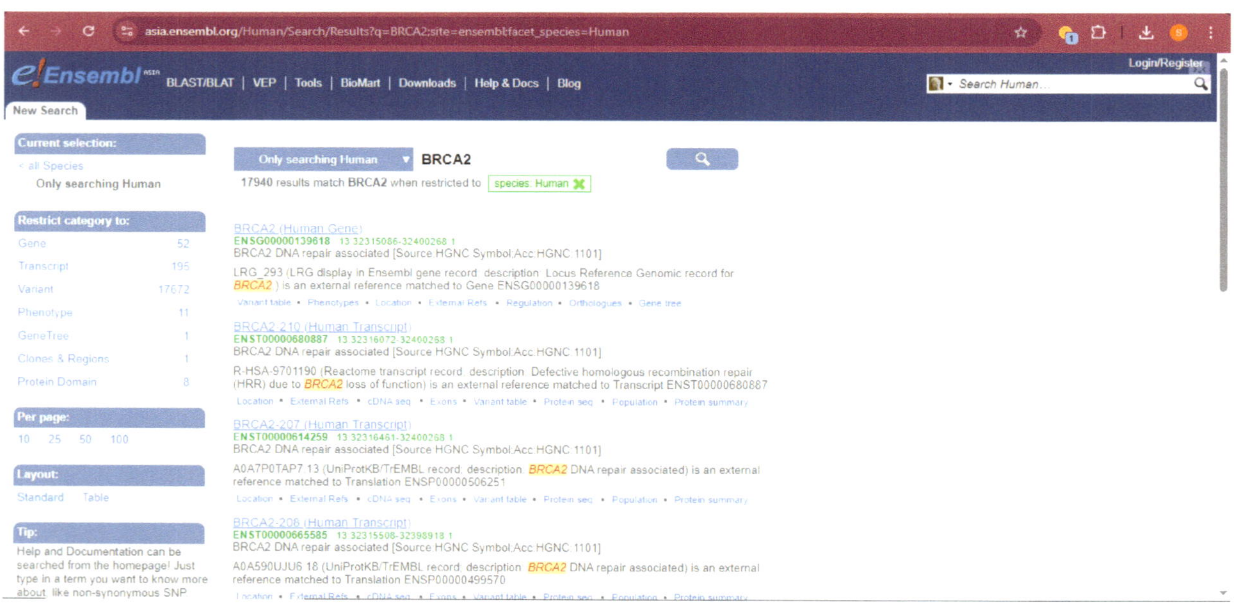
asia.ensembl.org/Human/Search/Results?q=BRCA2;site=ensembl;facet_species=Human
Ensembl
BLAST/BLAT | VEP | Tools | BioMart | Downloads | Help & Docs | Blog
New Search
Current selection:
Only searching Human
Restrict category to:
Per page:
Layout:
Tip:
Only searching Human
BRCA2
17940 results match BRCA2 when restricted to species: Human
BRCA2 (Human Gene)
ENSG00000139618
BRCA2 DNA repair associated [Source:HGNC Symbol;Acc:HGNC:1101]
BRCA2-210 (Human Transcript)
ENST00000680887
BRCA2-207 (Human Transcript)
ENST00000614259
BRCA2-206 (Human Transcript)
ENST00000665585

ClinVar

Who Created It

- Maintained by the **NCBI** and supported by the **National Institutes of Health (NIH)**.

History and Purpose

- Launched in **2013** to serve as a public archive of reports linking genetic variants to human health.

What You Can Discover

- Clinical interpretations of SNPs and variants (e.g., pathogenic, benign, uncertain).
- Associations of specific variants with diseases, conditions, and phenotypic traits.
- Supporting evidence from labs, researchers, and health providers.

Benefits

- Highly relevant for medical genetics and clinical nutrigenomics.
- Aids in identifying variants of clinical concern.
- Incorporates data from genetic testing companies, research institutions, and clinical laboratories.

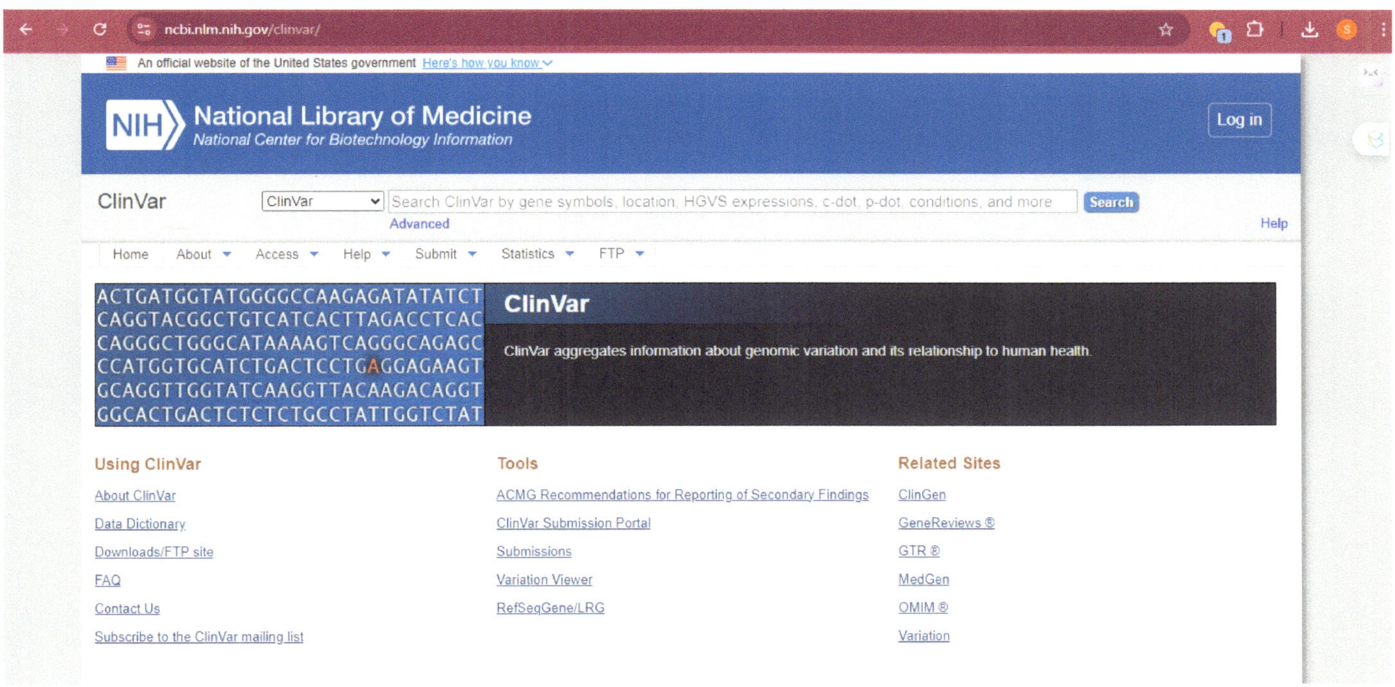

SNPedia

Who Created It

- Created by **Greg Lennon** and **Mike Cariaso**, co-founders of the personal genome analysis tool **Promethease**.

History and Purpose

- Started in **2006** as a wiki-based resource.
- Intended to crowdsource knowledge of SNP-trait associations from literature and public sources.

What You Can Discover

- Descriptions of SNP effects on health, nutrition, and ancestry.
- Traits like caffeine sensitivity, folate metabolism, or lactose intolerance.
- Links to supporting articles and scientific evidence.

Benefits

- Highly user-friendly and educational, suitable for both professionals and non-specialists.
- A valuable starting point for students and early-stage researchers in nutrigenomics.
- Supports interpretation of personal genomic data from consumer genetic testing services like 23andMe and AncestryDNA.

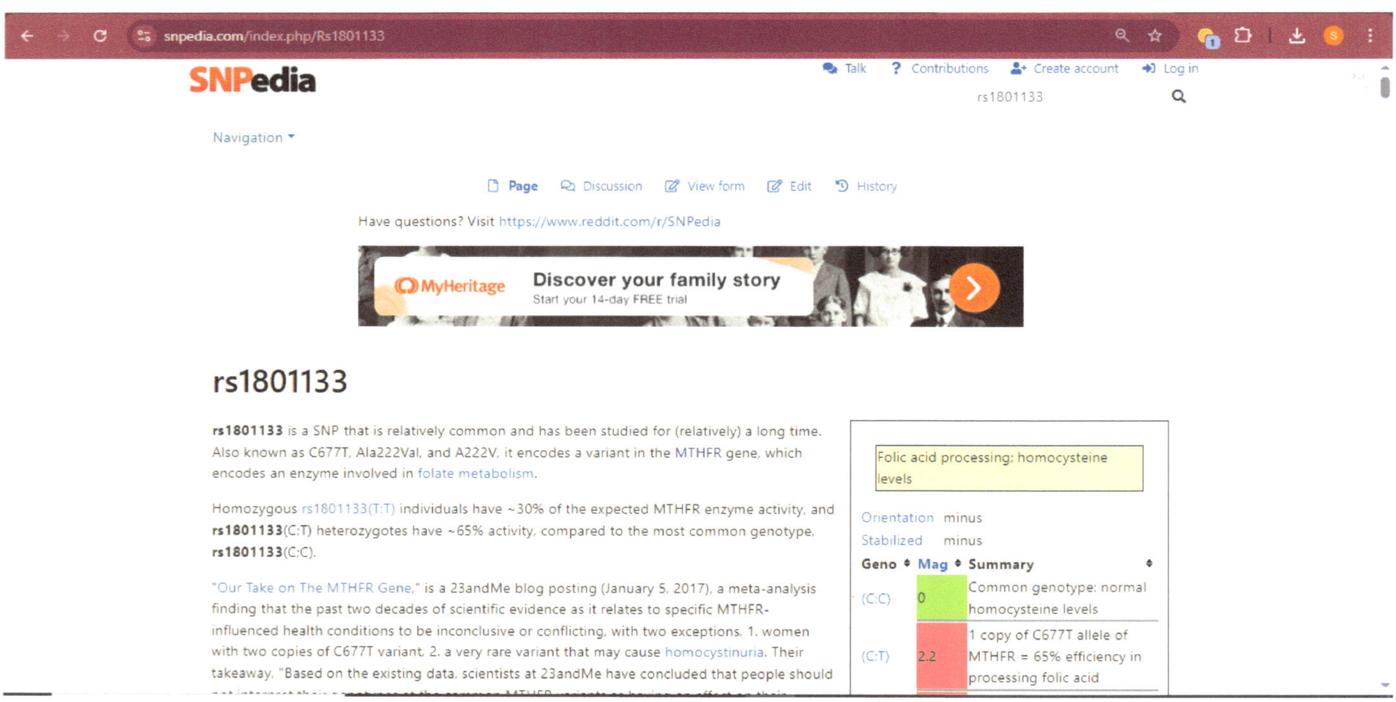

PhenoScanner

Who Created It

- Developed by researchers at the **University of Cambridge** and other academic collaborators.

History and Purpose

- Released in **2016** to enable a lookup of **genotype-to-phenotype associations** across traits and studies.

What You Can Discover

- SNP associations with traits, gene expression (eQTL), methylation (mQTL), and protein levels (pQTL).
- Filtering options by tissue type, population group, and study design.

Benefits

- Provides multidimensional data beyond traditional trait associations.
- Facilitates functional interpretation of genetic variants.
- Essential for integrative nutrigenomics research.

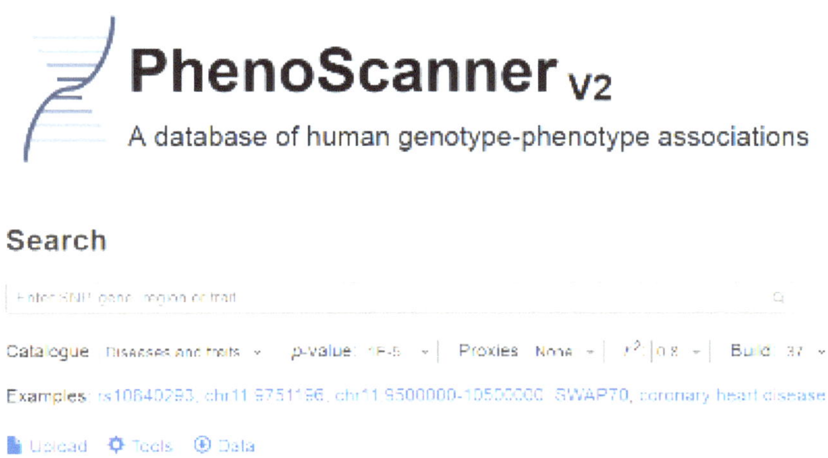

LDlink

Who Created It

- Developed by the **National Cancer Institute (NCI)**, NIH.

History and Purpose

- Created to analyze **linkage disequilibrium (LD)** among SNPs across diverse human populations.

What You Can Discover

- LD patterns between SNPs within specific populations.
- Identification of proxy SNPs (tagSNPs) that represent regions of the genome.
- Haplotype structures and LD heatmaps for visualizing SNP correlations.
- Chromosome browsing tools to locate variants within specific genomic regions.

Benefits

- Vital for designing genotyping assays and understanding SNP interactions.
- Facilitates the selection of representative SNPs for association studies.
- Valuable in ancestry-specific trait analysis, particularly in diverse or underrepresented populations.

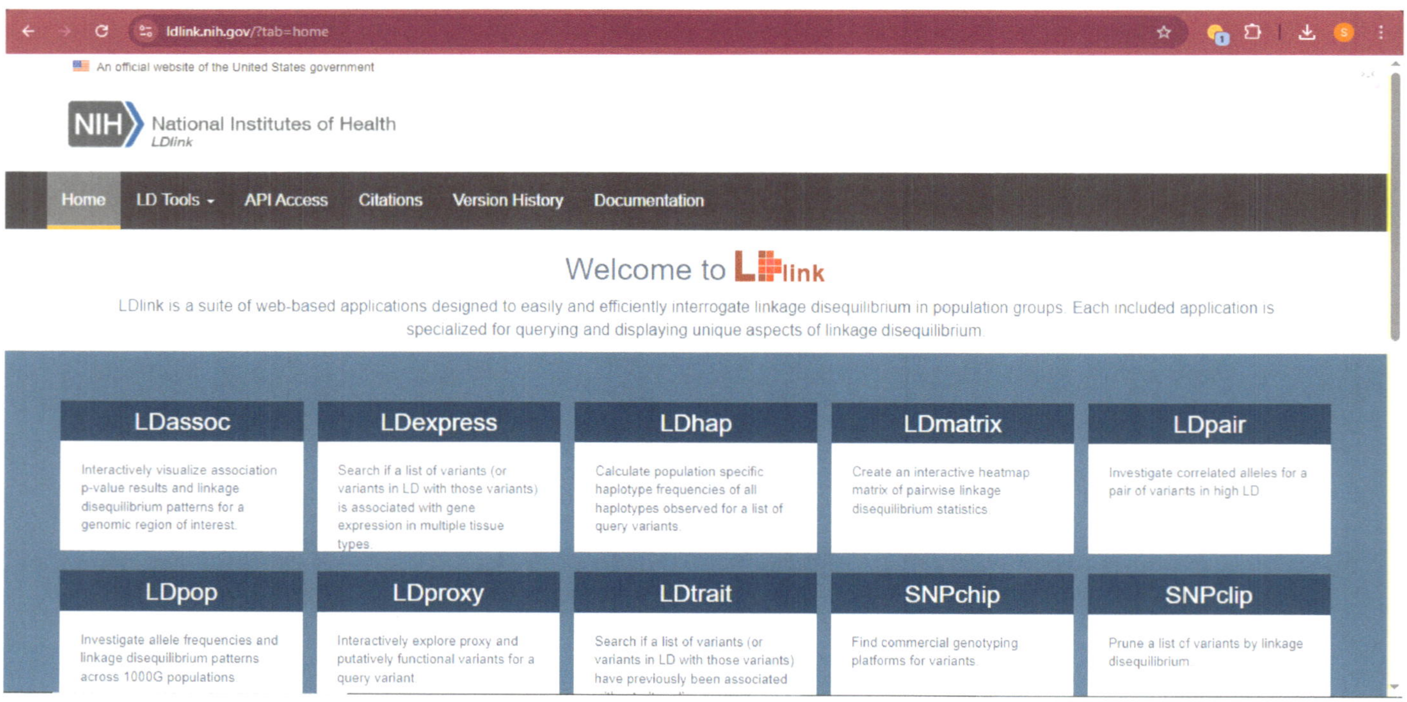

Key Databases for Searching SNPS and Trait Associations

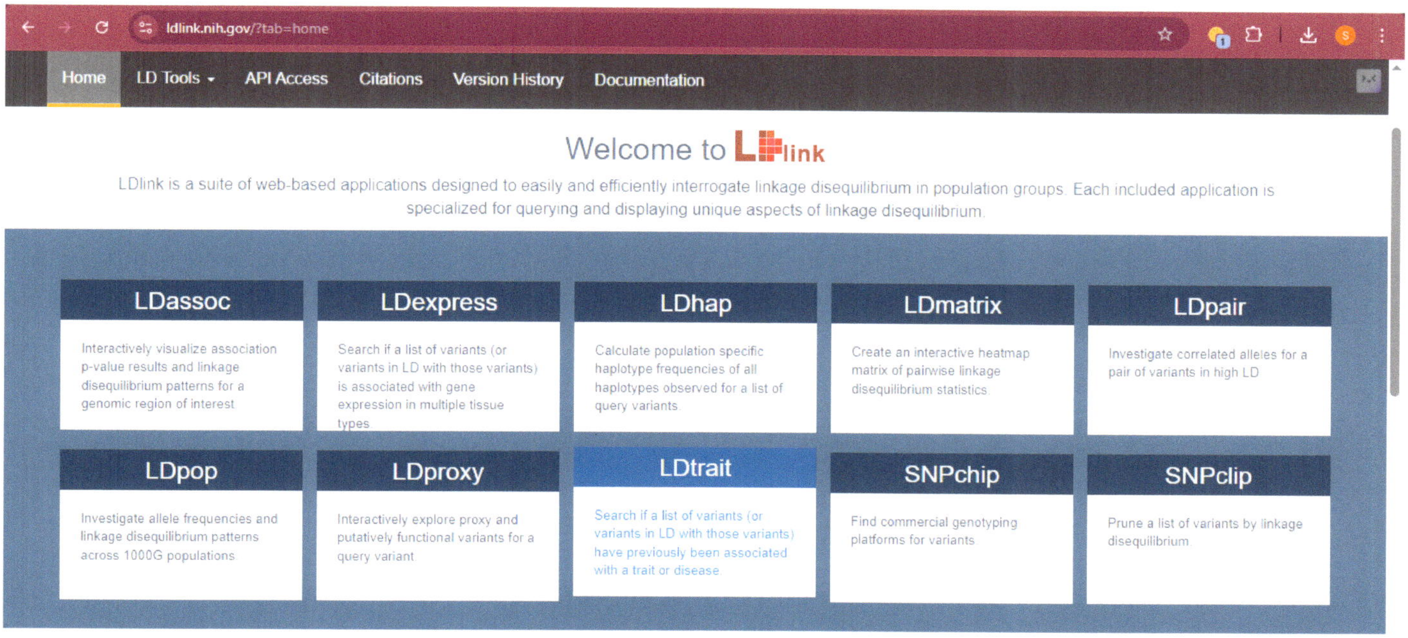

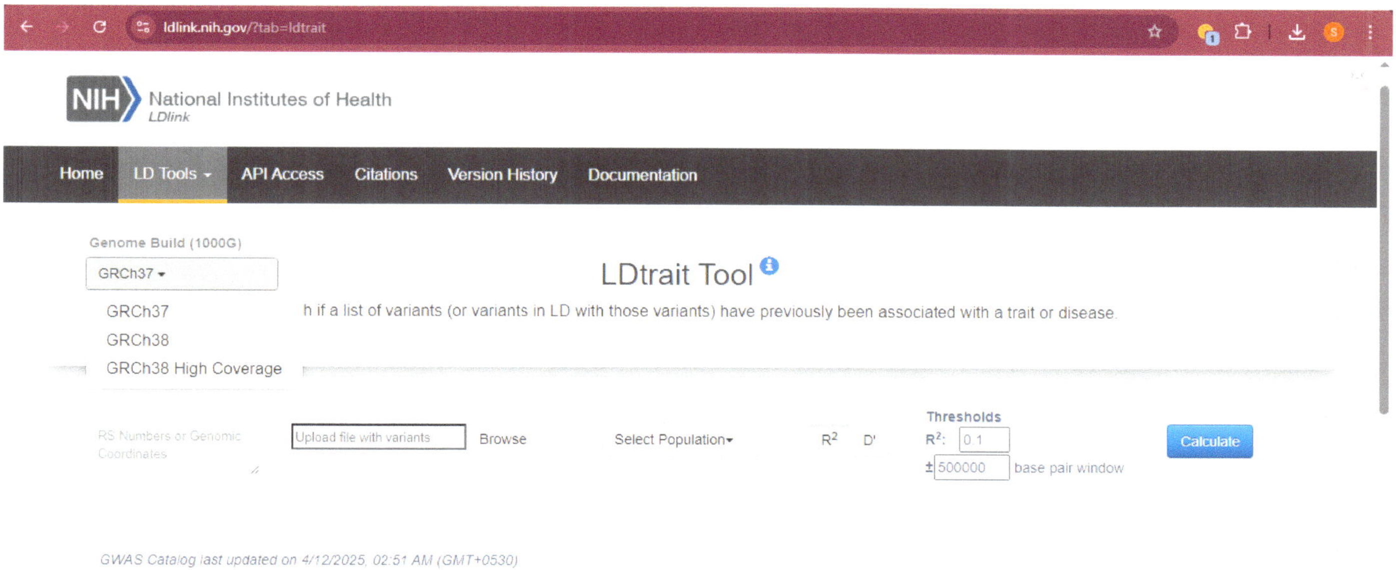

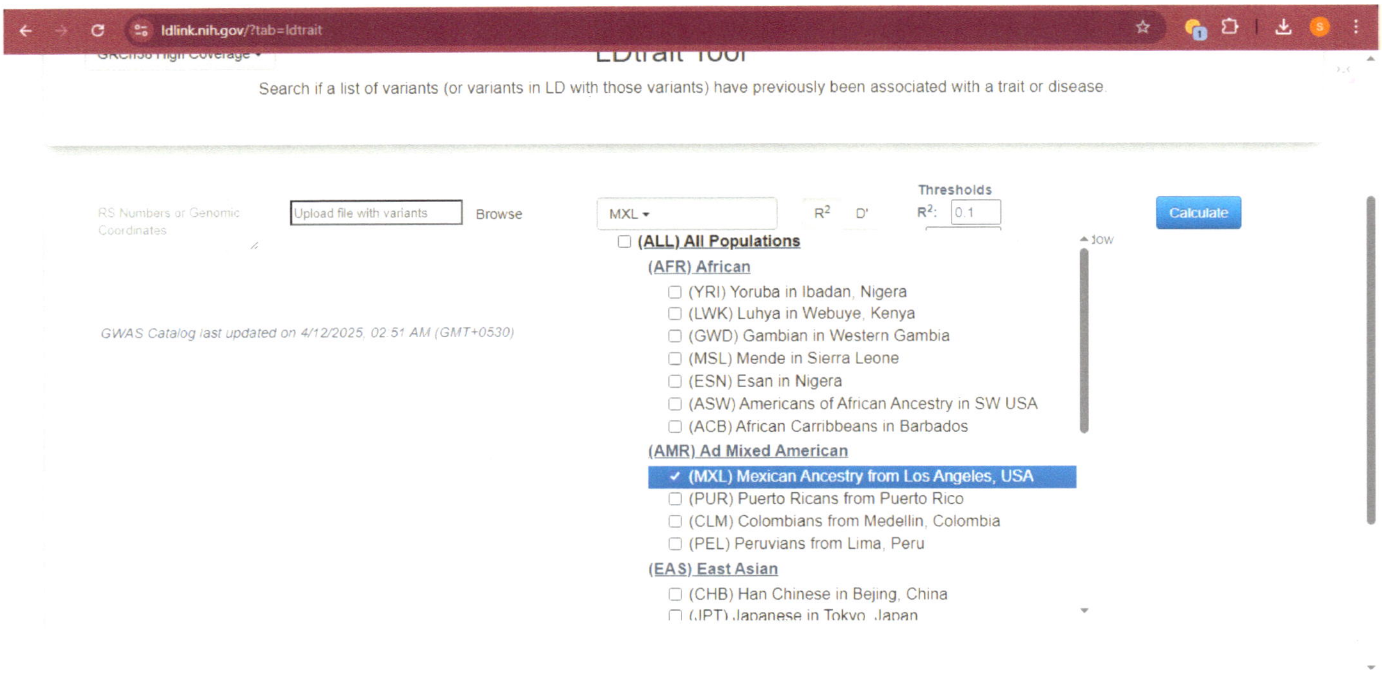
ldlink.nih.gov/?tab=ldtrait
Search if a list of variants (or variants in LD with those variants) have previously been associated with a trait or disease.
RS Numbers or Genomic Coordinates
Upload file with variants
Browse
MXL
R2
D'
Thresholds
R2: 0.1
Calculate
GWAS Catalog last updated on 4/12/2025, 02:51 AM (GMT+0530)
(ALL) All Populations
(AFR) African
(YRI) Yoruba in Ibadan, Nigera
(LWK) Luhya in Webuye, Kenya
(GWD) Gambian in Western Gambia
(MSL) Mende in Sierra Leone
(ESN) Esan in Nigera
(ASW) Americans of African Ancestry in SW USA
(ACB) African Carribbeans in Barbados
(AMR) Ad Mixed American
(MXL) Mexican Ancestry from Los Angeles, USA
(PUR) Puerto Ricans from Puerto Rico
(CLM) Colombians from Medellin, Colombia
(PEL) Peruvians from Lima, Peru
(EAS) East Asian
(CHB) Han Chinese in Bejing, China

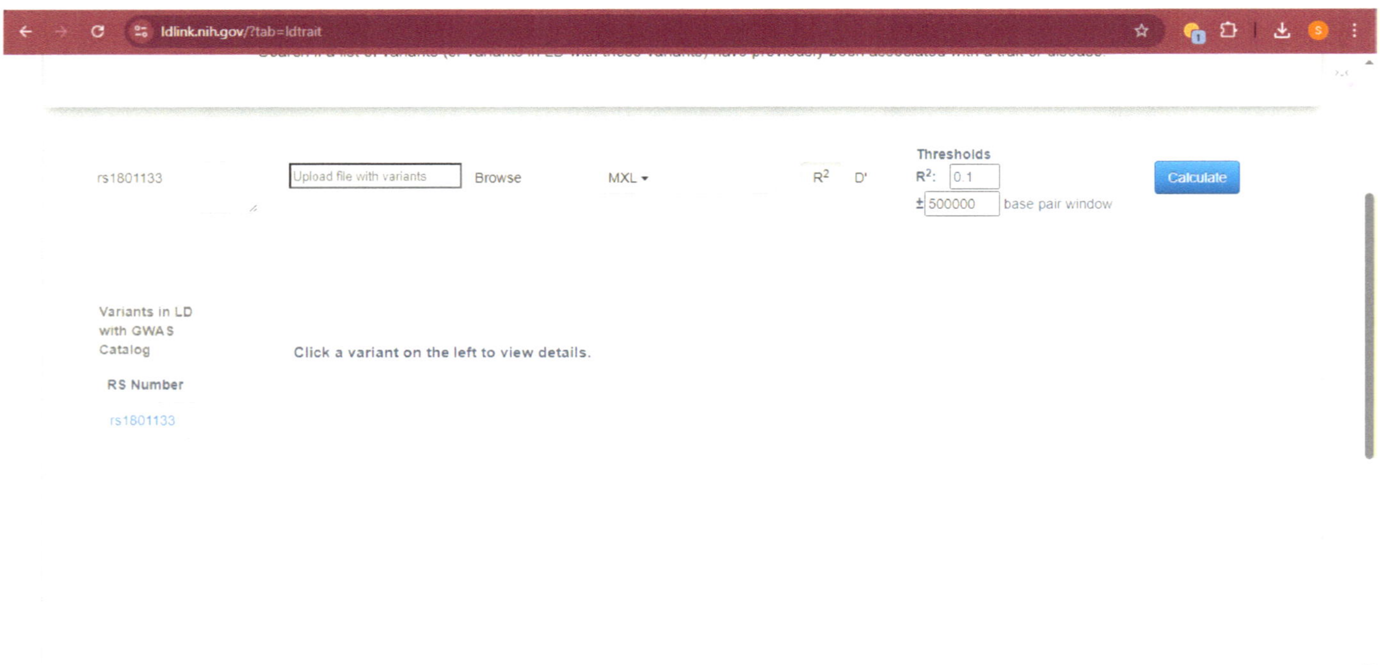
ldlink.nih.gov/?tab=ldtrait
rs1801133
Upload file with variants
Browse
MXL
R2
D'
Thresholds
R2: 0.1
± 500000 base pair window
Calculate
Variants in LD with GWAS Catalog
RS Number
rs1801133
Click a variant on the left to view details.

ldlink.nih.gov/?tab=ldtrait

rs1801133 | Upload file with variants | Browse | MXL ▾ | R^2 D'

Thresholds
R^2: 0.1
± 500000 base pair window

Calculate

Variants in LD with GWAS Catalog

Show 10 entries

Search:

Details for rs1801133

RS Number

rs1801133

GWAS Trait	PMID	RS Number	Position (GRCh38 High Coverage)	Alleles	R^2	D'	Risk Allele Frequency	Beta or OR	Effect Size (95% CI)	P-value	GWAS Catalog
Natriuretic peptide levels	21273288	rs1023252	chr1:11838976	G=0.859, T=0.141	0.144	1.0	0.260	0.200	0.16-0.24	$4x10^{-16}$	link
Platelet count	22139419	rs2336384	chr1:11986006	G=0.5, T=0.5	0.251	0.533	NR	2.172	1.42-2.9210^9/	$1x10^{-8}$	link
Eosinophil counts	30595370	rs12759042	chr1:12045275	G=0.438, T=0.562	0.188	0.462	NR	NA	NA	$5x10^{-33}$	link
Uncharacterized protein KIAA2013 levels	34648354	rs926270	chr1:11909729	G=0.375, T=0.625	0.163	0.556	0.510	0.130	0.1-0.16	$7x10^{-22}$	link
Pulse pressure x alcohol consumption	29912962	rs6668659	chr1:11862241	G=0.188, T=0.812	0.138	0.822	0.650	NA	NA	$1x10^{-17}$	link

ldlink.nih.gov/?tab=ldtrait

RS Number

rs1801133

GWAS Trait	PMID	RS Number	Position (GRCh38 High Coverage)	Alleles	R^2	D'	Risk Allele Frequency	Beta or OR	Effect Size (95% CI)	P-value	GWAS Catalog
Natriuretic peptide levels	21273288	rs1023252	chr1:11838976	G=0.859, T=0.141	0.144	1.0	0.260	0.200	0.16-0.24	$4x10^{-16}$	link
Platelet count	22139419	rs2336384	chr1:11986006	G=0.5, T=0.5	0.251	0.533	NR	2.172	1.42-2.9210^9/	$1x10^{-8}$	link
Eosinophil counts	30595370	rs12759042	chr1:12045275	G=0.438, T=0.562	0.188	0.462	NR	NA	NA	$5x10^{-33}$	link
Uncharacterized protein KIAA2013 levels	34648354	rs926270	chr1:11909729	G=0.375, T=0.625	0.163	0.556	0.510	0.130	0.1-0.16	$7x10^{-22}$	link
Pulse pressure x alcohol consumption interaction (2df test)	29912962	rs6668659	chr1:11862241	G=0.188, T=0.812	0.138	0.822	0.650	NA	NA	$1x10^{-17}$	link
Pulse pressure	38459180	rs6668659	chr1:11862241	G=0.188, T=0.812	0.138	0.822	NR	0.020	0.016-0.024	$1x10^{-11}$	link
Pulse pressure	38459180	rs6668659	chr1:11862241	G=0.188, T=0.812	0.138	0.822	NR	0.020	0.012-0.028	$9x10^{-10}$	link
Hip index	34021172	rs1801131	chr1:11794419	G=0.164, T=0.836	0.173	1.0	NR	0.019	0.012-0.025	$4x10^{-9}$	link
Hypertension	37947095	rs10864536	chr1:11764518	C=0.867, T=0.133	0.135	1.0	NR	NA	NA	$2x10^{-15}$	link
N-terminal pro B-type natriuretic peptide levels	29237677	rs12406089	chr1:11861124	C=0.812, G=0.188	0.138	0.822	0.709	0.201	0.17-0.23	$8x10^{-48}$	link

Showing 1 to 10 of 162 entries Previous 1 2 3 4 5 … 17 Next

RegulomeDB

Who Created It

- Developed by the **Snyder Lab at Stanford University**.

History and Purpose

- Designed to assess the **regulatory potential** of noncoding variants.
- Integrates data from ENCODE, Roadmap Epigenomics, and other epigenomic projects.

What You Can Discover

- SNPs located within regulatory elements such as promoters and enhancers.
- Transcription factor binding sites and chromatin accessibility data.
- Functional scores indicating regulatory potential.

Benefits

- Ideal for understanding how SNPs affect gene regulation.
- Supports the study of nutrigenomic traits influenced by gene regulation and expression in various tissues.

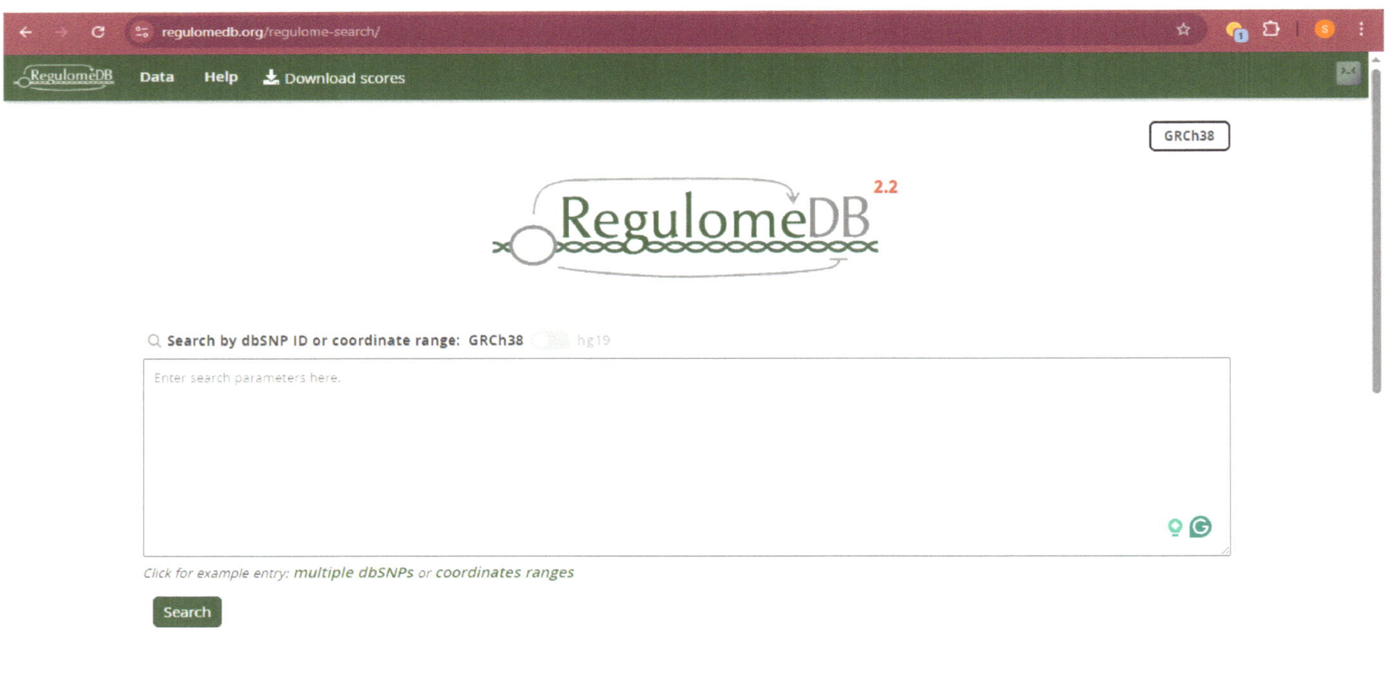

Key Databases for Searching SNPS and Trait Associations

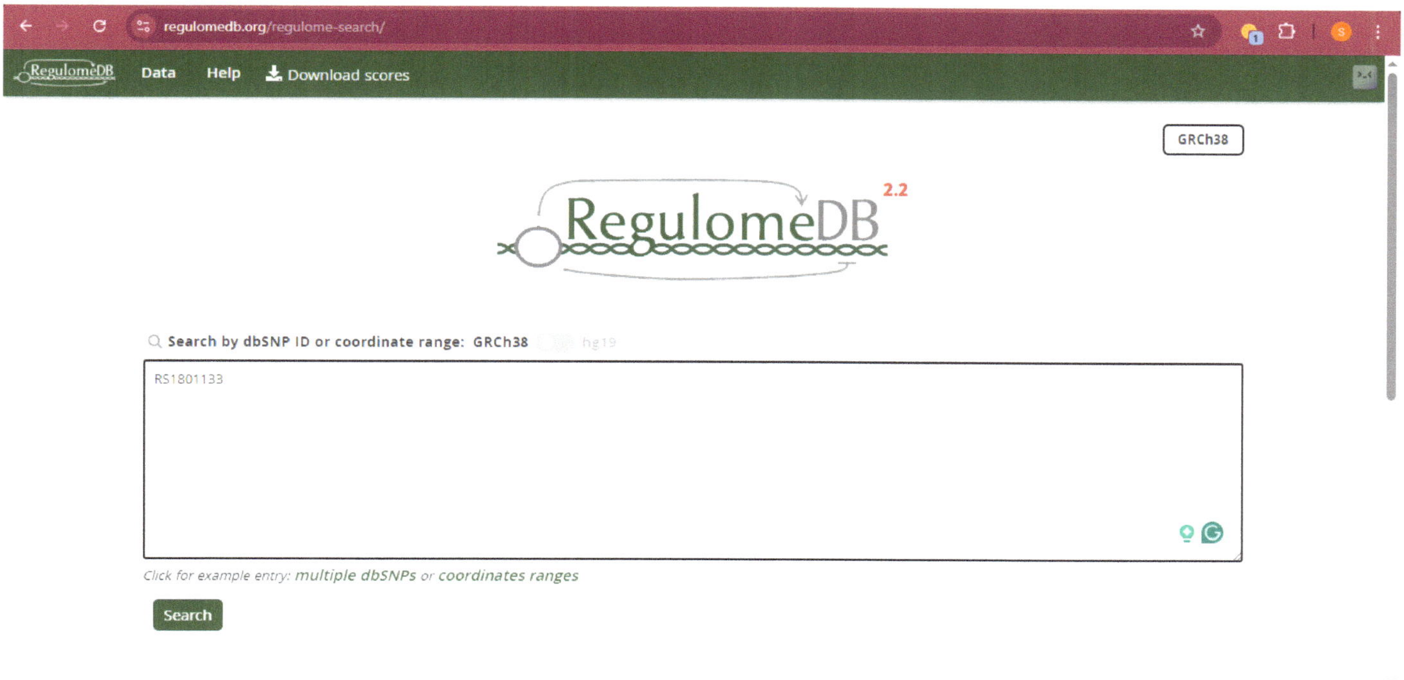

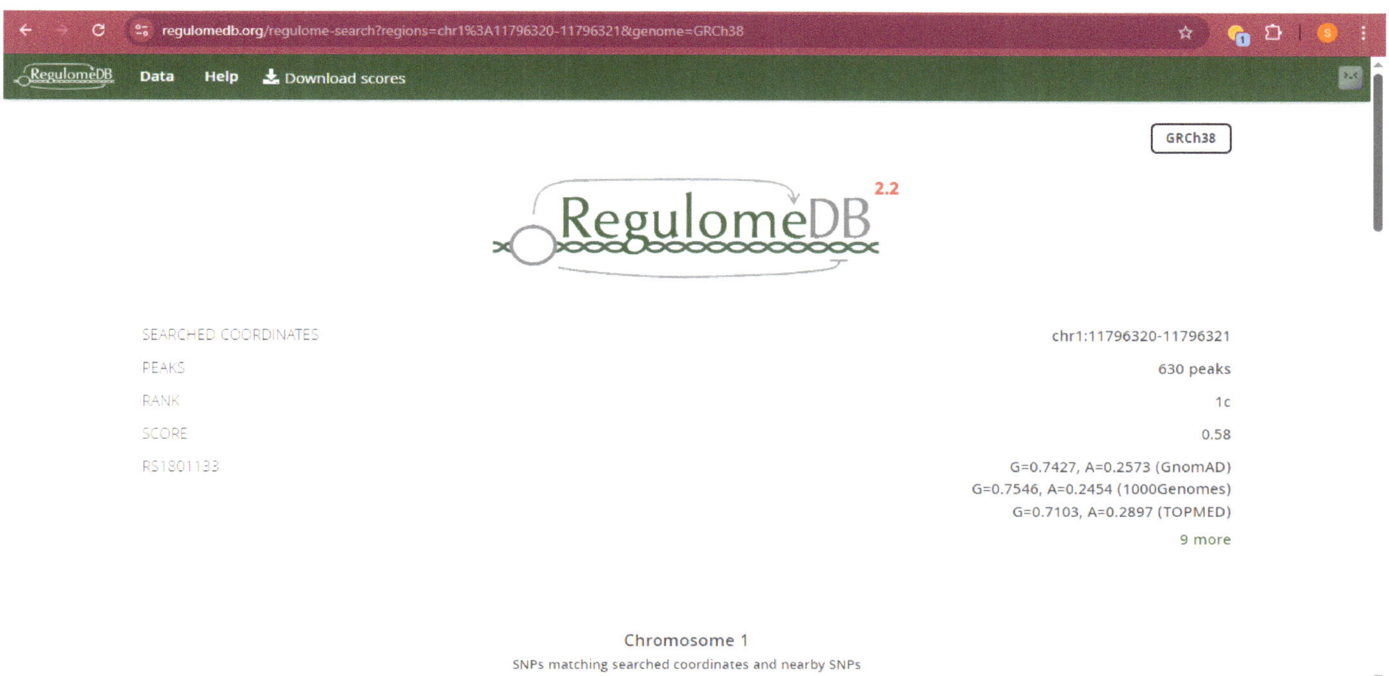

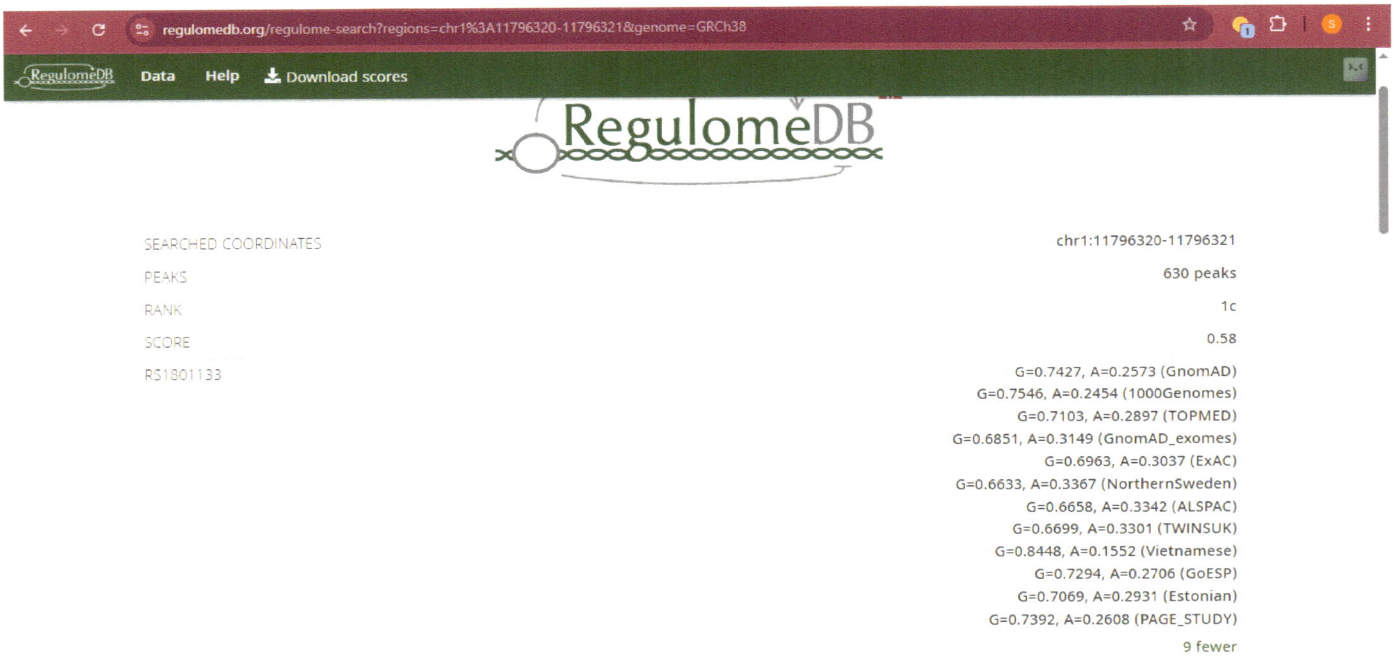
regulomedb.org/regulome-search?regions=chr1%3A11796320-11796321&genome=GRCh38
RegulomeDB
Data
Help
Download scores
RegulomeDB
SEARCHED COORDINATES
chr1:11796320-11796321
PEAKS
630 peaks
RANK
1c
SCORE
0.58
RS1801133
G=0.7427, A=0.2573 (GnomAD)
G=0.7546, A=0.2454 (1000Genomes)
G=0.7103, A=0.2897 (TOPMED)
G=0.6851, A=0.3149 (GnomAD_exomes)
G=0.6963, A=0.3037 (ExAC)
G=0.6633, A=0.3367 (NorthernSweden)
G=0.6658, A=0.3342 (ALSPAC)
G=0.6699, A=0.3301 (TWINSUK)
G=0.8448, A=0.1552 (Vietnamese)
G=0.7294, A=0.2706 (GoESP)
G=0.7069, A=0.2931 (Estonian)
G=0.7392, A=0.2608 (PAGE_STUDY)
9 fewer

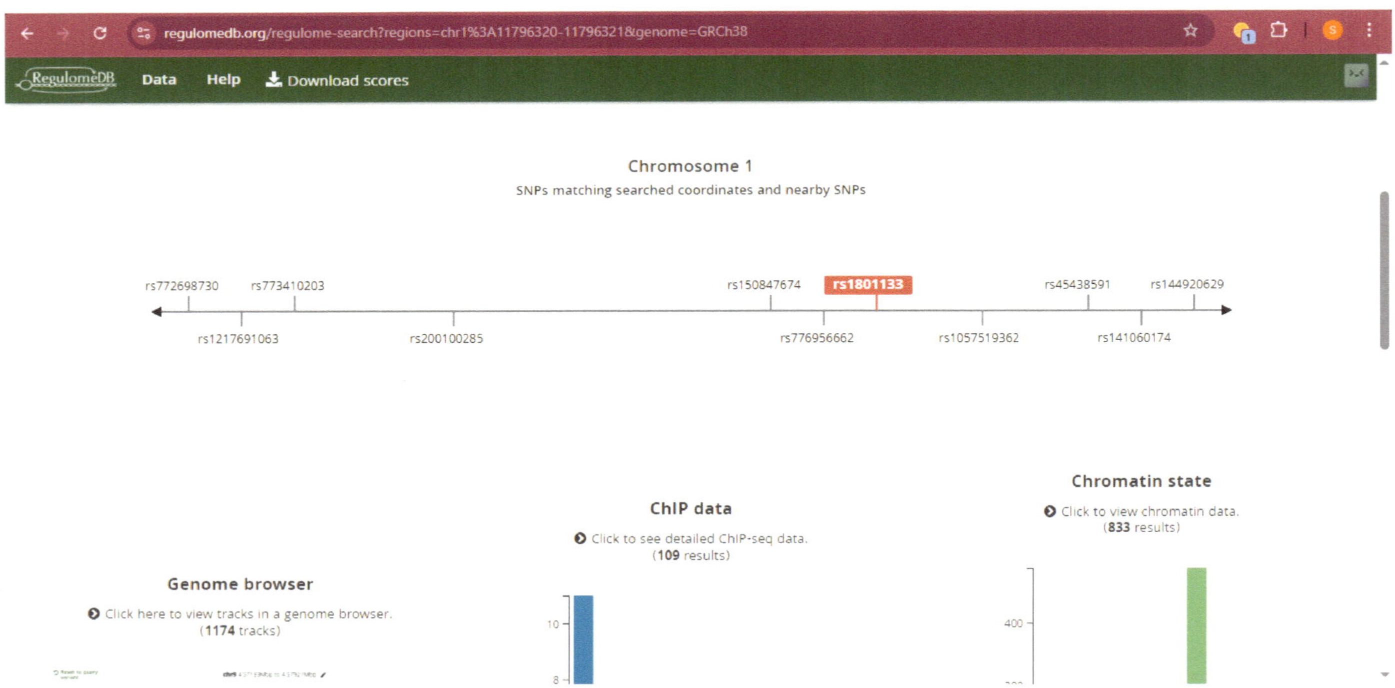
regulomedb.org/regulome-search?regions=chr1%3A11796320-11796321&genome=GRCh38
RegulomeDB
Data
Help
Download scores
Chromosome 1
SNPs matching searched coordinates and nearby SNPs
rs772698730
rs773410203
rs150847674
rs1801133
rs45438591
rs144920629
rs1217691063
rs200100285
rs776956662
rs1057519362
rs141060174
Genome browser
Click here to view tracks in a genome browser.
(1174 tracks)
ChIP data
Click to see detailed ChIP-seq data.
(109 results)
10
8
Chromatin state
Click to view chromatin data.
(833 results)
400

1000 Genomes Project

Who Created It

- An international collaboration including **The Broad Institute**, **Wellcome Trust Sanger Institute**, and **Baylor College of Medicine**, supported by NIH.

History and Purpose

- Started in **2008**, completed Phase 3 in **2015**.
- Aimed to provide a **comprehensive map of human genetic variation.**

What You Can Discover

- Over 80 million genetic variants including SNPs, small insertions/deletions (indels), and structural variants.
- Allele frequency data across 26 diverse human populations.
- Genotype data for thousands of individuals from various ethnic backgrounds.

Benefits

- A vital resource for population-based genetic studies.
- Provides reference data for both common and rare variants in human populations.
- Facilitates allele frequency comparison across ethnicities for nutrigenomic research.

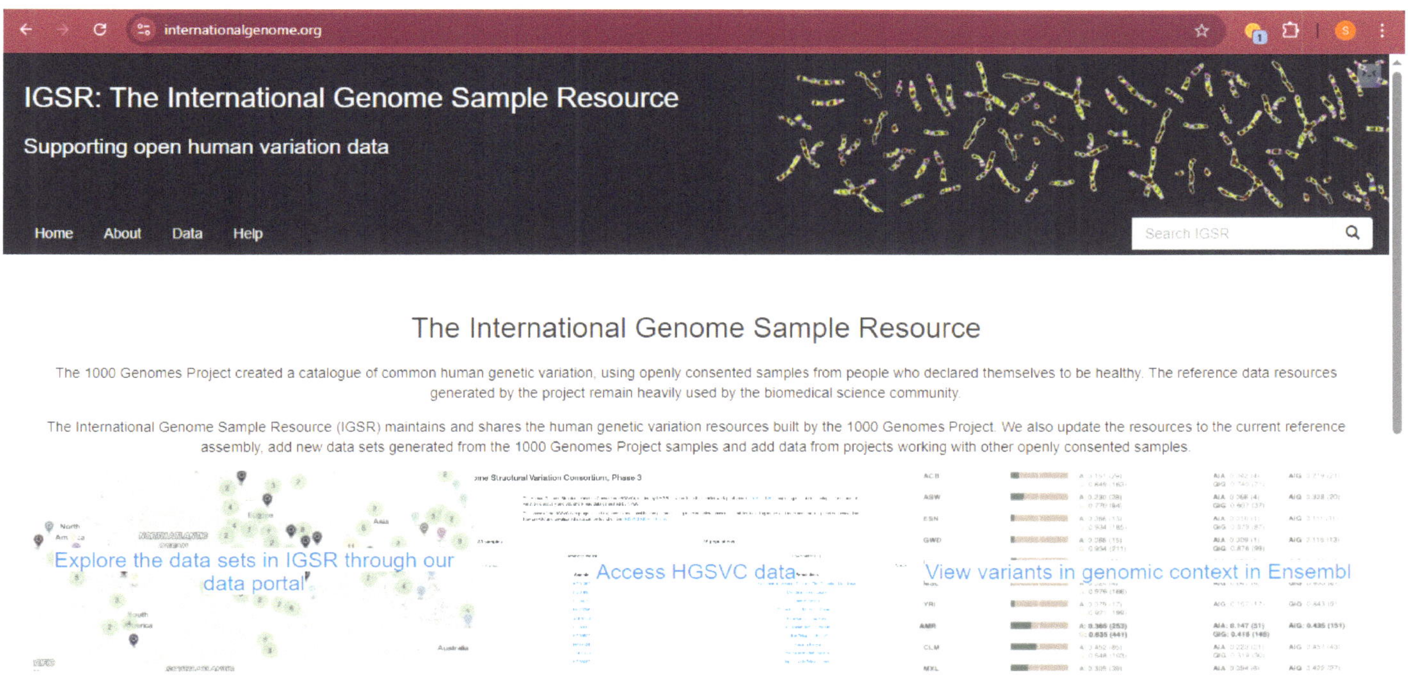

Summary of Key Databases for SNP Identification and Trait Associations

Database Name	Website Link	Description	How to Use It for SNP-Trait Associations
dbSNP	https://www.ncbi.nlm.nih.gov/snp/	A comprehensive database of single nucleotide polymorphisms (SNPs) maintained by NCBI.	Search by rsID, gene name, or chromosome location. Check allele frequencies, validation status, and genomic context.
GWAS Catalog	https://www.ebi.ac.uk/gwas/	A curated repository of genome-wide association studies (GWAS) linking SNPs with various traits and diseases.	Search for SNPs associated with traits like obesity, diabetes, or vitamin levels. Results include p-values, populations, and sample sizes.
Ensembl Genome Browser	https://www.ensembl.org/	A genome browser that provides detailed annotations of genes, variants, and regulatory elements.	Search genes or SNPs and view their locations, linkage disequilibrium, conservation, and trait annotations.
ClinVar	https://www.ncbi.nlm.nih.gov/clinvar/	Archive of clinically significant genetic variants and associated phenotypes.	Search SNPs with known clinical significance, especially in relation to disease risk. Useful for health-related nutrigenomic traits.
SNPedia	https://www.snpedia.com/	Wiki-style database of SNPs with health, trait, and ancestry annotations.	Search rsIDs to get a summary of known trait associations, often linked to scientific publications.
PhenoScanner	http://www.phenoscanner.medschl.cam.ac.uk/	A database of human genotype-phenotype associations including GWAS and expression quantitative trait loci (eQTL) data.	Explore SNP associations with multiple traits, gene expression, and methylation data.
LDlink	https://ldlink.nci.nih.gov/	A suite of web-based applications for exploring linkage disequilibrium and haplotype structures.	Identify SNPs in LD with a target SNP; useful for tagging SNPs or regional mapping.
RegulomeDB	https://www.regulomedb.org/	Annotates SNPs with known and predicted regulatory elements in the intergenic regions of the human genome.	Great for exploring regulatory SNPs affecting gene expression – useful in nutrigenomics.
1000 Genomes Project	https://www.internationalgenome.org/	Provides a comprehensive resource on human genetic variation across populations.	Check allele frequencies, variant distribution, and population-specific SNP prevalence.

Conclusion

The databases discussed in this chapter provide essential tools for researchers to explore, annotate, and interpret SNPs in the context of nutrigenomics. By integrating information from resources like dbSNP, GWAS Catalog, Ensembl, and others, scientists can better understand genetic diversity, identify functional variants, and develop targeted nutritional strategies. These bioinformatics platforms serve as the backbone of modern genetic research, empowering both basic and applied studies in human health and nutrition.

Questions

1. What is the primary focus of dbSNP?
2. How can you search for a specific SNP in dbSNP?
3. What type of information does dbSNP provide about SNPs?
4. What does the GWAS Catalog specialize in?
5. What types of traits can you find associated with SNPs in the GWAS Catalog?
6. What key statistical information does GWAS Catalog provide for each SNP-trait association?
7. Which database provides detailed gene, variant, and regulatory annotations through a genome browser?
8. What kind of trait annotations can you explore in the Ensembl Genome Browser?
9. How does Ensembl help researchers understand SNP conservation across species?
10. Which database archives clinically significant genetic variants?
11. Why is ClinVar valuable in nutrigenomics and health-related research?
12. Which platform allows a wiki-style browsing of SNP-trait associations?
13. How does SNPedia typically present its information about SNPs?
14. Which database can link SNPs to gene expression and methylation data?
15. What types of genotype-phenotype relationships can be explored using PhenoScanner?
16. What is the purpose of using LDlink when studying SNPs?
17. How does exploring linkage disequilibrium (LD) help in SNP-trait association studies?
18. Which database annotates SNPs with known and predicted regulatory elements?
19. How can RegulomeDB annotations help in understanding the functional effects of non-coding SNPs?
20. What kind of population-specific genetic information can the 1000 Genomes Project provide?

Answers

1. dbSNP is a comprehensive database of single nucleotide polymorphisms (SNPs) maintained by NCBI.
2. You can search by rsID, gene name, or chromosome location.
3. It provides allele frequencies, validation status, and genomic context.
4. The GWAS Catalog specializes in compiling genome-wide association study results linking SNPs with traits and diseases.
5. You can find traits like obesity, diabetes, vitamin levels, and other health-related traits.
6. It provides p-values, populations studied, and sample sizes for each association.
7. The Ensembl Genome Browser provides detailed annotations of genes, variants, and regulatory elements.
8. You can explore SNP locations, linkage disequilibrium, conservation, and trait-related information.
9. It helps by showing conservation scores and comparative genomics across different species.
10. ClinVar archives clinically significant genetic variants and associated phenotypes.
11. ClinVar helps identify SNPs linked to disease risks, which is crucial for nutrigenomic trait analysis.
12. SNPedia provides a wiki-style collection of SNP-trait summaries.
13. It presents summaries linked to health, trait, and ancestry information, often citing scientific publications.
14. PhenoScanner can link SNPs to multiple traits, gene expression levels, and methylation patterns.
15. You can explore how SNPs are associated with diseases, traits, and biological pathways.
16. LDlink helps researchers find SNPs that are in linkage disequilibrium with a target SNP.
17. Understanding LD can help identify causal variants and map regions associated with traits.
18. RegulomeDB annotates SNPs with information about regulatory elements, such as enhancers and promoters.
19. It helps researchers understand if a non-coding SNP might affect gene expression regulation.
20. The 1000 Genomes Project provides data on allele frequencies, variant distributions, and SNP prevalence across diverse global populations.

CHAPTER 5

OBESITY: THE INTERPLAY OF GENETICS, NUTRITION, AND EPIGENETICS

Introduction

Obesity is a complex, multifactorial condition that extends beyond excess body weight to encompass disruptions in energy balance, metabolism, and long-term health. This chapter begins by clearly defining obesity and distinguishing it from being overweight, followed by an overview of Body Mass Index (BMI) as a commonly used measure to assess population-level adiposity and obesity risk. Establishing these foundational concepts provides a clinical and epidemiological framework for understanding how obesity is identified, monitored, and interpreted in both research and practice.

Building on this foundation, the chapter then explores the **biological regulation of appetite and satiety**, focusing on the hormonal and neural mechanisms that govern hunger, fullness, and food intake. Hormones such as ghrelin and leptin, along with key genes involved in appetite signaling, are discussed to illustrate how genetic variation can influence eating behavior, satiety perception, and nutritional responses. These mechanisms operate early in the pathway toward weight gain, shaping daily food choices, portion control, and responsiveness to dietary interventions.

The chapter subsequently transitions to the genetic determinants of obesity and BMI**,** which represent downstream, cumulative outcomes of long-term energy imbalance. Unlike appetite- and satiety-related genetic variants that primarily affect eating behavior, obesity- and BMI-associated single-nucleotide polymorphisms (SNPs) reflect genetic influences on adiposity, fat distribution, energy expenditure, and metabolic efficiency over time. Separating these sections allows for conceptual clarity and emphasizes that obesity is not solely driven by appetite dysregulation but arises from the interaction of behavioral, metabolic, and genetic factors.

By structuring the chapter in this progressive manner—from definition and measurement, to hormonal and behavioral regulation, and finally to obesity and BMI genetics—readers are guided through a layered understanding of obesity biology. This approach supports precision nutrition by enabling nutritionists and healthcare professionals to distinguish between genetic factors influencing how individuals eat and those affecting how the body stores and utilizes energy, thereby informing more targeted and effective intervention strategies.

Definition of Obesity and How It Differs from Being Overweight

Obesity is a condition characterized by excessive body fat accumulation that may negatively impact health. It differs from being overweight, which generally refers to weighing more than what is considered normal for a person's height, but is not necessarily due to excess body fat. Overweight individuals may have extra muscle, bone, water, or fat, whereas obesity specifically indicates an excessive accumulation of body fat.

Obesity is typically assessed through a calculation called Body Mass Index (BMI), which takes into account a person's weight and height. The World Health Organization (WHO) classifies a BMI of 25 to 29.9 as overweight, and a BMI of 30 or above as obese. It's worth noting, however, that BMI is not a perfect measure since it does not distinguish between fat and muscle, nor does it account for fat distribution. Nevertheless, it remains a commonly used tool for assessing body weight status at a population level.

Real-life analogy: *Two people may weigh the same, yet have very different metabolic risks. A professional athlete with high muscle mass may fall into the "overweight" BMI range, whereas another individual with higher visceral fat may have obesity-related complications despite a similar BMI.*

Understanding Body Mass Index (BMI) as a Measurement Tool

Body Mass Index is calculated by dividing a person's weight (in kilograms) by the square of their height (in meters). The formula is:

$$\text{BMI} = \text{weight (kg)} / \text{height (m)}^2$$

Using this formula, people are categorized into different weight ranges:

- **Underweight**: BMI less than 18.5
- **Normal weight**: BMI 18.5 to 24.9
- **Overweight**: BMI 25 to 29.9
- **Obese**: BMI 30 and above

Despite its limitations, BMI is a simple and convenient screening tool that gives a quick indication of whether an individual falls into a healthy weight range.

Prevalence of Obesity: A Global Perspective

Obesity is a growing concern worldwide, with rates rising in nearly every country over the past few decades. It has become a significant public health issue due to its association with numerous health risks, such as heart disease, type 2 diabetes, and certain cancers. Here's a look at the obesity prevalence rates in India, the USA, and Europe:

Country	Prevalence of Obesity (%)	References
India	5.0 - 11.8	World Health Organization, 2021
USA	42.4	Centers for Disease Control and Prevention, 2020
Europe	16.5 - 35.0	European Health Information Gateway, 2019

The prevalence of obesity in India is relatively lower compared to Western countries. However, it is important to note that obesity rates in India are rapidly increasing, especially in urban areas. In contrast, the United States has one of the highest obesity rates globally, with nearly half of the adult population classified as obese. European countries show varied obesity rates, with some countries like the United Kingdom and Hungary having higher prevalence rates, while countries in Southern Europe, like Italy and France, report relatively lower obesity levels.

The causes of obesity are multifaceted, with genetics playing a crucial role. Specific genes have been identified that influence factors such as appetite, metabolism, and fat storage. However, genetic predisposition is not the sole cause of obesity. Environmental influences, including diet, physical activity, and lifestyle, are also critical contributors. For example, diets high in calorie-dense, nutrient-poor foods combined with sedentary lifestyles greatly increase obesity risk.

Impact of Obesity on Health and Well-being

Obesity is associated with a range of health complications, making it a major risk factor for chronic diseases such as cardiovascular disease, type 2 diabetes, certain cancers, and respiratory disorders. Additionally, obesity significantly impacts mental health, contributing to conditions like depression and anxiety, often exacerbated by social stigma and discrimination.

Economically, obesity places a significant burden on healthcare systems due to the increased need for medical treatment and management of associated health issues. Individuals with obesity often experience reduced quality of life, with limitations in mobility and daily activities. Given the rising rates of obesity, addressing this epidemic is essential for both individual health and societal well-being.

Understanding the interplay between genetics, nutrition, and epigenetics is key to developing targeted interventions for preventing and managing obesity. This chapter will explore the complex relationships among genetic predispositions, lifestyle factors, and the role of epigenetics, providing insight into how personalized nutrition can help mitigate obesity risks.

Genomics of Eating Behavior and Appetite Regulation

Eating behavior and appetite regulation are fundamental components of human health and survival, intricately linked to physiological, psychological, genetic, and environmental factors. These behaviors not only determine the choice, quantity, and timing of food consumption but also have profound implications for the management of weight, metabolic health, and chronic diseases. Recent advances in molecular genetics, behavioral sciences, and neuroimaging have shed light on the complex mechanisms governing why, how, and when we eat.

Appetite regulation is a multidimensional process that includes both homeostatic mechanisms, which maintain energy balance, and hedonic influences, which drive the consumption of pleasurable and palatable foods. This regulation involves intricate feedback loops between the brain, gut, and hormones, with genetic predispositions playing a pivotal role in modulating these interactions.

The following sections explore the multifaceted dimensions of eating behavior and appetite regulation, with a focus on:

- **Homeostatic and Hedonic Mechanisms**: Understanding how energy needs and food rewards influence eating behavior.
- **Genetic Contributions**: Examining how specific genetic variants shape appetite, taste preferences, and susceptibility to disordered eating.
- **Developmental and Environmental Influences**: Investigating how prenatal exposures, early taste experiences, and family dynamics shape long-term eating patterns.
- **Assessment and Methodologies**: Reviewing tools and approaches for studying eating behavior and its genetic underpinnings.
- **Implications for Health and Disease**: Linking eating behavior to obesity, metabolic syndrome, and chronic diseases.
- **Future Directions**: Highlighting emerging research and personalized interventions for managing appetite-related disorders.

Homeostatic and Hedonic Mechanisms

Homeostasis ensures that our body maintains a balance in energy intake and expenditure. The brain, gut, and hormones interact to regulate hunger (the physiological need for energy) and satiety (the sensation of fullness).

The human body maintains energy balance through a sophisticated interplay of hormones that regulate appetite, satiety, and metabolism. Among these, **ghrelin** and **leptin** are two pivotal players. Ghrelin, often referred to as the "hunger hormone," signals the brain to stimulate appetite and initiate food intake. In contrast, *leptin*, known as the "satiety hormone," signals when energy stores are sufficient, suppressing appetite to maintain energy balance. Understanding these hormones is critical for addressing conditions like obesity, eating disorders, and metabolic diseases. This chapter explores the roles of ghrelin and leptin in energy homeostasis, their molecular mechanisms, and their potential as therapeutic targets.

Hunger regulating hormones

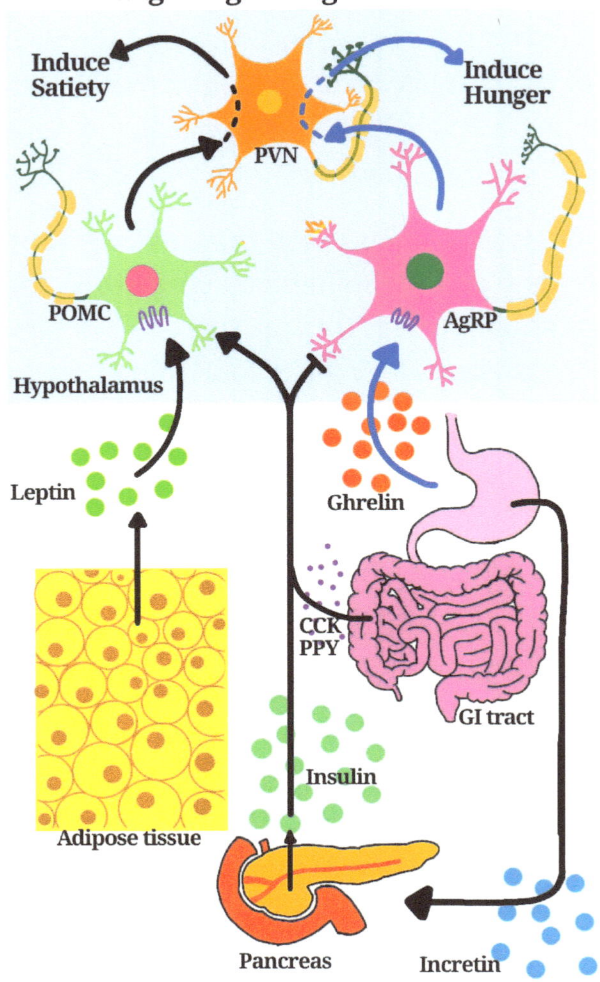

The Role of Ghrelin

What is Ghrelin?

Ghrelin is a hormone primarily secreted by the stomach but is also produced in smaller amounts in the pancreas and brain. Its levels increase before meals and decrease after eating, making it a key regulator of meal initiation. Beyond appetite regulation, ghrelin also influences glucose metabolism, sleep patterns, and taste perception.

Mechanism of Action

Ghrelin binds to the **growth hormone secretagogue receptor (GHS-R1a)** in the hypothalamus, particularly in the arcuate nucleus. This interaction stimulates the release of neuropeptides like neuropeptide Y (*NPY*) and agouti-related protein (AgRP), which promote hunger and food intake.

Example: *When you skip breakfast, your ghrelin levels rise, leading to increased hunger and a stronger urge to eat at lunchtime.*

Key Functions

- **Stimulates Appetite**: Prepares the body for food intake by enhancing hunger sensations.
- **Regulates Glucose Metabolism**: Influences blood sugar levels by reducing insulin release.
- **Influences Gastric Emptying**: Promotes efficient digestion, aiding nutrient absorption.

Clinical Relevance of Ghrelin

In individuals with conditions like **Prader-Willi syndrome**, elevated ghrelin levels contribute to hyperphagia (excessive eating) and obesity. Conversely, in **Anorexia Nervosa**, ghrelin levels may rise as a compensatory mechanism to stimulate appetite.

Prader-Willi Syndrome (PWS) is a rare genetic disorder caused by the loss of function of specific genes on chromosome 15. It is characterized by weak muscle tone (hypotonia), poor growth, insatiable appetite leading to obesity, developmental delays, and behavioral issues. PWS results from the absence of paternal genes in the affected region, often due to deletion, maternal uniparental disomy, or imprinting defects.

Anorexia Nervosa is a serious eating disorder characterized by an intense fear of gaining weight, a distorted body image, and excessive restriction of food intake. Individuals with anorexia often have dangerously low body weight and may engage in extreme dieting, over-exercising, or other behaviors to lose weight. It can lead to severe physical and mental health complications, including malnutrition, organ damage, and depression, and requires comprehensive medical and psychological treatment.

The Role of Leptin

What is *Leptin*?

Leptin is secreted by adipose tissue and serves as a long-term regulator of energy balance. It provides feedback to the brain about energy stores, signaling when fat reserves are sufficient. When *leptin* levels are high, it reduces food intake and increases energy expenditure to maintain homeostasis.

Mechanism of Action

Leptin binds to its receptor (*LEPRb*) in the hypothalamus, particularly in the arcuate nucleus. This interaction stimulates pro-opiomelanocortin (*POMC*) neurons and inhibits *NPY* and AgRP neurons, creating a sense of satiety.

Example: *After a calorie-dense meal, Leptin levels rise, signaling the brain to reduce appetite and prevent overeating.*

Key Functions

- **Regulates Energy Stores**: Acts as a feedback mechanism to maintain energy homeostasis.
- **Influences Metabolic Rate**: Enhances energy expenditure to prevent excessive fat accumulation.
- **Supports Reproductive Health**: Ensures sufficient energy reserves for reproductive functions.

Clinical Relevance

In many individuals with obesity, high circulating *Leptin* levels fail to suppress appetite due to a condition known as *Leptin* resistance. This impaired response disrupts energy regulation, leading to:

- Persistent hunger despite excess fat stores.
- Reduced energy expenditure, promoting further weight gain.

Hedonic Mechanisms: How Pleasure Drives Eating Behavior

Hedonic eating is driven by the pursuit of pleasure rather than physiological hunger. This type of eating is strongly linked to the brain's reward system, which involves the release of dopamine and other neurotransmitters. These signals create feelings of enjoyment and satisfaction when consuming certain foods, particularly those high in sugar, fat, and salt. While this mechanism evolved to help humans seek out calorie-dense foods for survival, in the modern world, it can lead to overeating and metabolic issues.

Leptin and Ghrelin in Appetite Regulation

Leptin, a hormone released by fat cells (adipocytes), plays a crucial role in signaling the brain about the body's fat stores. It is primarily involved in the long-term regulation of appetite and energy balance. Interestingly, low levels of *Leptin* act as a powerful trigger to stimulate appetite, as the body perceives this as a signal of insufficient energy reserves. In contrast, obesity is typically associated with high *Leptin* levels and a condition known as *Leptin* resistance, where the brain fails to respond effectively to *Leptin*'s satiety signals. This resistance is thought to be due to defects in the transport mechanism that moves *Leptin* from the bloodstream into the hypothalamus.

Ghrelin, on the other hand, is secreted by the stomach and serves as a short-term appetite regulator. It undergoes a unique post-translational modification, involving the addition of an octanoyl fatty acid group. This modification is essential for its biological activity and may also help ghrelin cross the blood-brain barrier to act on appetite-regulating centers in the hypothalamus.

Beyond *Leptin* and ghrelin, other hormones and peptides contribute to appetite regulation. Peptide tyrosine tyrosine (PYY), a gut hormone, reduces appetite and promotes satiety, while various gut peptides further modulate food intake. Additionally, adipocytokines, signaling molecules derived from fat tissue, play a crucial role in the intricate hormonal network governing appetite control and energy homeostasis. This complex interplay highlights the multifaceted regulation of energy balance and its implications for conditions such as obesity and metabolic disorders.

Key Genes Involved in Appetite Regulation and Satiety

Several genes play a critical role in regulating appetite, satiety, and energy balance, ultimately influencing body mass index (BMI) and obesity risk. These genes encode proteins that interact with hormonal and neural pathways to modulate food intake and metabolism. Understanding the genetic variants, particularly single-nucleotide polymorphisms (SNPs), provides insight into individual susceptibility to obesity and metabolic disorders.

The table below highlights key genes and their associated SNPs, detailing their functions and roles in appetite and weight regulation:

Gene	SNP (RSID)	Function	Role
LEP	***rs7799039***	**Regulates energy balance by inhibiting hunger.**	**Signals to the brain about fat stores.**
LEPR	***rs1137101***	**Mediates *Leptin*'s effects on appetite and energy balance.**	**Enhances hunger suppression and energy regulation.**
MC4R	***rs17782313***	**Plays a crucial role in appetite suppression and energy expenditure.**	**Critical for regulating body weight and energy balance.**
FTO	***rs9939609***	**Associated with increased appetite and higher risk of obesity.**	**Increases susceptibility to obesity by affecting food preferences.**
NPY	***rs16147***	**Stimulates hunger and reduces energy expenditure.**	**Key player in promoting appetite in response to fasting.**
POMC	***rs28932472***	**Precursor to melanocortins that regulate satiety.**	**Contributes to the production of peptides influencing satiety.**
GHRL	***rs696217***	**Stimulates hunger and promotes food intake.**	**Drives food intake during fasting states.**
SH2B1	***rs4788102***	**Regulates *Leptin* and insulin signaling pathways.**	**Impacts appetite and energy homeostasis via signaling pathways.**
UCP2	***rs660339***	**Regulates energy expenditure and may affect satiety.**	**Modulates metabolic efficiency and energy regulation.**
TBC1D1	***rs2279027***	**Influences glucose metabolism and food preferences.**	**Involved in nutrient sensing and energy expenditure.**

These genetic variations contribute to differences in appetite regulation, metabolic efficiency, and obesity susceptibility among individuals. Identifying such genetic markers can aid in the development of personalized nutrition and weight management strategies.

In the next section, we'll unravel the genetic blueprint behind appetite regulation, exploring how these genes impact food intake, metabolism, and obesity risk

LEP Gene: The Master Regulator of Hunger and Energy—A Journey Through Evolution

Imagine two mice, both small and furry but with one glaring difference: one is morbidly obese, and the other is not. Researchers at a lab in the 1950s were puzzled. What made these mice so different? As they investigated, they found something fascinating—a hormone that would later be named *Leptin*. Derived from the Greek word *"Leptos,"* meaning thin, *Leptin* was like a traffic signal for our body's energy use, hunger, and even fat storage.

This is the story of *Leptin*, a hormone produced in fat cells that communicates with the brain to help regulate hunger and energy balance. Over the years, researchers have investigated the evolutionary history of *Leptin* and its crucial role in human health.

The Discovery of *Leptin*: A Serendipitous Breakthrough

In the 1950s, scientists discovered two strains of genetically distinct mice. These mice had strikingly similar problems: they were obese, lethargic, and infertile. Surprisingly, their excessive weight gain was not solely due to overeating—it was linked to a genetic mutation. The genes responsible for this phenomenon were later named obese (ob/ob) and diabetic (db/db).

When scientists later isolated the *obese* gene, they discovered it encoded *Leptin*, a hormone that acts as the body's energy regulator. When fat stores are sufficient, *Leptin* signals the brain to reduce appetite and increase energy expenditure. Conversely, when energy reserves are low, *Leptin* levels drop, triggering hunger to restore balance. However, in mice with mutations in the *Leptin* gene or its receptor, this signaling system was disrupted, leading to uncontrolled eating and severe obesity.

What Makes *Leptin* Unique?

Leptin is not just a "hunger hormone"; it's much more. This protein hormone belongs to the cytokine family—a group of molecules involved in cell signaling. It's like a message courier delivering updates about your body's energy reserves.

For example:

- *After a large meal, Leptin levels rise, signaling satiety and reducing the drive to eat.*
- *During fasting or prolonged calorie restriction, Leptin levels drop, prompting the brain to seek food and conserve energy.*

Beyond hunger regulation, *Leptin* also plays a role in growth, reproduction, metabolism, and immune function, highlighting its broader impact on overall health.

A Shared Blueprint Across Species

One of the most intriguing aspects of *Leptin* is its **evolutionary conservation** across species. From humans to lizards to fish, *Leptin* has retained its core functions. While the amino acid sequence of *Leptin* differs across species, its 3D structure and function remain surprisingly similar.

- **In frogs**, *Leptin* regulates food intake and energy use, much like it does in humans. Experiments show that injecting *Leptin* in frogs suppresses hunger—a trait likely critical for survival during periods of scarcity.
- **In mammals**, *Leptin* helps regulate long-term energy balance by influencing hypothalamic neurons in the brain.

Think of *Leptin* as nature's way of ensuring species survive by balancing food consumption and energy use.

***Leptin* and Modern Health Challenges**

In humans, *Leptin* plays a critical role in maintaining a healthy weight. But what happens when the system malfunctions?

- ***Leptin* Deficiency**: A rare condition in which the body does not produce *Leptin*, leading to excessive hunger and severe obesity. Fortunately, it can be effectively treated with *Leptin* injections.
- ***Leptin* Resistance**: A much more common issue, particularly in obesity, where the brain becomes less responsive to *Leptin*'s satiety signals. As a result, individuals continue to feel hungry despite having adequate fat stores, making weight management difficult.

Researchers believe that understanding *Leptin*'s role in energy regulation could unlock new therapeutic strategies for obesity and metabolic diseases, offering hope for more effective interventions in the future.

Why Should Nutritionists Care About *Leptin*?

For nutritionists, *Leptin* provides a crucial lens into the biological foundations of hunger, satiety, and weight regulation. By acknowledging the genetic and hormonal influences on appetite, practitioners can create personalized interventions. For example:

- **Tailored Diet Plans**: Clients with ***Leptin* resistance** may benefit from a **low-carb, high-protein diet**, which helps stabilize hunger hormones and improve satiety.
- **Behavioral Coaching**: Understanding *Leptin*'s role can help explain **why some individuals struggle more with hunger than others**, leading to more **empathetic and effective counseling**.

The Impact of *rs7799039*: A Key *Leptin* Gene Variant

Genetic differences in the ***LEP* gene** can significantly affect appetite regulation. A study on overweight men explored how the ***rs7799039* polymorphism** influenced feelings of hunger and fullness after meals, yielding fascinating insights:

1. **Fullness Ratings:** Individuals with the "AA" genotype reported feeling fuller for longer compared to those carrying the "G" allele (either "GA" or "GG").

2. **Future Food Cravings:** Those with the "G" allele" were more likely to feel hungry again sooner, even after a large meal, compared to "AA" individuals.

These findings suggest that *rs7799039* influences appetite regulation, potentially contributing to overeating tendencies in certain individuals.

How This Relates to Everyday Life

To understand this better, let's consider two friends, Sarah and John. Sarah has the "AA" genotype, and John carries the "G" allele of rs7799039. After a hearty lunch, Sarah feels satisfied and doesn't think about food for hours. However, John finds himself peeking into the fridge just an hour later, wondering what he could snack on next. This subtle genetic difference may help explain their contrasting post-meal behaviors.

Why Does This Matter?

Understanding genetic variations like *rs7799039* is crucial for several reasons:

1. **Personalized Nutrition:** If an individual is genetically predisposed to feeling less full after meals, nutritionists can recommend strategies such as increasing fiber and protein intake to enhance satiety.
2. **Obesity Prevention:** Identifying individuals with higher genetic risks for overeating can allow for early interventions, reducing the likelihood of weight gain and associated health issues.
3. **Better Understanding of Obesity:** While lifestyle factors play a significant role, genetic influences like *rs7799039* remind us that some aspects of eating behavior are biologically hardwired.

Moving Forward

Though the research highlights the importance of the *LEP* gene in appetite regulation, it's important to remember that genetics is just one piece of the puzzle. Factors such as diet, physical activity, sleep patterns, and stress levels also shape hunger and satiety. The key is integrating genetic insights with practical lifestyle strategies to create sustainable, healthier eating habits.

Real-World Application

For individuals with the "G" allele of *rs7799039*, here are practical strategies to help manage hunger effectively:

1. **Choose Satiating Foods:** Opt for meals rich in protein and fiber, as they promote longer-lasting fullness.
2. **Practice Mindful Eating:** Pay attention to portion sizes and eat slowly to give your brain time to process fullness signals.
3. **Maintain Regular Meal Timing:** Stick to a consistent eating schedule to regulate hunger hormones effectively.

LEP Gene and Its Influence on Appetite and Satiety in Schizophrenia

Building on the broader understanding of the *LEP* gene and its impact on appetite regulation, this section delves into how the gene's polymorphism, *rs7799039*, manifests in a unique context: **schizophrenia**. Individuals with schizophrenia often face heightened risks of metabolic disturbances, including obesity and related complications. Given its pivotal role in hunger and satiety, the *LEP* gene offers valuable insights into the genetic underpinnings of appetite regulation in this population.

LEP Gene in Schizophrenic Patients: Key Findings

A study conducted on 577 schizophrenic patients in Taiwan revealed a significant association between the *rs7799039* polymorphism of the *LEP* gene and metabolic traits such as body mass index (BMI) and waist circumference (WC)—both critical indicators of obesity.

Key findings include:

1. **Association with BMI and WC:** Individuals carrying the "AA" genotype of *rs7799039* had a higher likelihood of increased BMI and WC compared to those carrying the "G" allele.
2. **Blood Pressure (BP):** The "AA" genotype was also linked to differences in blood pressure, further contributing to the metabolic complexities observed in schizophrenia.
3. **Risk Factor:** Approximately 58% of the study population carried the "AA" genotype, showing a 10% higher chance of being overweight and a 7% higher likelihood of central obesity than those carrying the "G" allele.

Genetic and Environmental Interplay

The metabolic adversities in schizophrenic patients are often exacerbated by antipsychotic medications, which are known to induce weight gain and glucose dysregulation. However, the study found that the associations between *rs7799039* and obesity-related traits persisted even after adjusting for medication patterns and BMI. This indicates that genetic predispositions play a substantial role in appetite and satiety regulation, independent of environmental factors.

Real-Life Example: Appetite Regulation in Schizophrenia

To better understand the implications of the *LEP* gene in appetite regulation for schizophrenia patients, consider two individuals:

- *Anna, who carries the "AA" genotype, struggles with persistent hunger cues despite eating regular meals. She often finds herself snacking late at night, which contributes to weight gain.*
- *Michael, with the "G" allele, experiences more manageable hunger signals and tends to feel satiated after meals, making it easier for him to maintain a stable weight.*

This contrast underscores how rs7799039 influences appetite regulation, shaping dietary behaviors and metabolic health outcomes in schizophrenia.

Clinical Implications for Appetite Regulation

1. **Personalized Nutrition Plans:** For individuals with the "AA" genotype, integrating high-fiber and protein-rich meals into their diets can help prolong satiety. Foods like lentils, beans, and leafy greens may help curb excessive hunger.
2. **Behavioral Interventions:** Mindful eating strategies—such as eating slowly, chewing thoroughly, and minimizing distractions during meals—can be particularly effective in managing hunger for those genetically predisposed to increased appetite.
3. **Medical Monitoring:** Schizophrenic patients carrying the "AA" genotype may benefit from regular metabolic screenings to monitor and manage risks early, particularly for high BMI, central obesity, and elevated blood pressure.

Why This Matters?

Individuals with schizophrenia often face a dual challenge: managing their mental health while also navigating an increased risk of metabolic disorders. The *LEP* gene provides a window into understanding how genetic factors influence appetite regulation in this vulnerable group. By tailoring interventions to genetic predispositions, clinicians and nutritionists can support these individuals in achieving better health outcomes.

Genetic Fiber Connection: How *rs7799039* Influences Appetite and Satiety

Expanding on the role of *rs7799039* in the *LEP* gene, researchers have explored how dietary fiber, specifically soluble fiber from **Plantago ovata husk (Po-husk)**, interacts with this polymorphism to influence metabolic outcomes. Since this SNP is located in the promoter region of the *LEP* gene, it plays a role in regulating *Leptin* expression, a key hormone in satiety signaling.

Fiber Meets Genetics: Key Findings

A study examined how participants with different *rs7799039* genotypes (GG, GA, and AA) responded to an eight-week dietary intervention involving Po-husk supplementation alongside a low-saturated-fat diet.

Key results included:

1. **Total Cholesterol Levels**:
    - Individuals with the GG genotype experienced a 4.4% reduction in total cholesterol (TC) levels after consuming Po-husk.
    - In contrast, the placebo group showed only a 1.1% reduction in TC.
    - The AA and GA carriers showed minimal changes, highlighting the genetic-specific response.

2. ***Leptin* Signaling and Cholesterol**:
   - The GG genotype may disrupt *Leptin*-mediated cholesterol regulation, aligning with earlier findings of *Leptin*'s involvement in lipid metabolism.
3. **Implications for Satiety**:
   - While the study primarily focused on cardiovascular markers, the role of *Leptin* in appetite control suggests that such dietary fibers could indirectly influence satiety, especially in GG carriers.

Real-Life Application: Sarah and David's Fiber Journey

Meet Sarah and David, both committed to improving their diet and managing their weight through healthier food choices. They each begin incorporating **psyllium husk (Po-husk)** into their meals—known for its cholesterol-lowering effects and ability to promote satiety through soluble fiber. However, their results differ dramatically due to their genetic profiles.

- *Sarah carries the GG genotype for a gene variant linked to enhanced fiber responsiveness. As she continues this dietary intervention, she experiences a noticeable reduction in LDL cholesterol and finds herself feeling full for longer after meals—helping her reduce overall caloric intake and maintain better dietary adherence.*
- *David, on the other hand, has the AA genotype, which is associated with a diminished physiological response to soluble fiber. Despite following the same regimen as Sarah, David sees minimal changes in his cholesterol levels and does not benefit from the same increase in satiety.*

This real-world example highlights how genetics can shape individual responses to dietary interventions, emphasizing the potential for personalized nutrition strategies based on genetic makeup.

Implications for Personalized Nutrition

These findings highlight the importance of tailoring dietary interventions based on genetic profiles. For individuals with the GG genotype of *rs7799039*, specific recommendations could include:

- **Increasing Soluble Fiber Intake**: Foods like psyllium husk or oat bran could be prioritized to enhance satiety and improve metabolic markers.
- **Focused Nutritional Counseling**: Personalized strategies could help optimize *Leptin* function and manage appetite more effectively.

For individuals with the AA genotype, other interventions, such as higher protein or fat-rich satiety-promoting foods, might be explored to compensate for a potentially lesser response to fiber.

While *Leptin* plays a critical role in appetite suppression by signaling energy reserves, it doesn't work alone. The brain relies on multiple pathways to regulate hunger, and one of the most important is the melanocortin system. At the center of this system is the *MC4R* gene, which helps balance energy intake and expenditure. Now, let's take a closer look at *MC4R* and its role in appetite regulation.

MC4R rs17782313: Appetite and Satiety Regulation

The melanocortin-4 receptor (*MC4R*) plays a pivotal role in regulating appetite and energy balance. This receptor is part of the melanocortin system in the brain, which integrates signals from hormones like *Leptin* and insulin to control hunger and energy expenditure. Variants in the *MC4R* gene, such as *rs17782313*, are associated with an increased risk of obesity, making this gene a key focus for understanding appetite regulation.

The Science Behind *MC4R*

MC4R is highly expressed in the hypothalamus, a region of the brain responsible for energy homeostasis. When activated, *MC4R* suppresses appetite and boosts energy expenditure. However, mutations or polymorphisms—such as *rs17782313*—can disrupt this system, leading to dysregulated hunger signals and overeating.

Key Findings on *rs17782313*

The SNP *rs17782313*, located near the *MC4R* gene, has been extensively studied for its association with obesity and eating behaviors:

1. **Impact on Appetite**: Individuals carrying the risk allele of *rs17782313* tend to consume more calories and show a preference for energy-dense foods due to disrupted melanocortin signaling.
2. **Satiety Challenges**: Those with the risk allele may experience delayed satiety, meaning they feel full only after consuming larger quantities of food.

Real-Life Example

Consider two siblings, Emma and Jake. Emma carries the risk allele for rs17782313, while Jake does not. During family meals:

- *Emma often eats beyond fullness and gravitates towards high-carb, high-fat foods like pasta and desserts.*
- *Jake, on the other hand, feels satisfied after moderate portions and doesn't experience the same strong cravings.*

This contrast illustrates how genetics can influence appetite regulation and food preferences.

Research Insights

1. **Brazilian Study**: In a study of severely obese Brazilian patients, *MC4R* variants, including *rs17782313*, were linked to early-onset obesity and increased hunger signals. The findings highlight how such genetic factors may predispose individuals to obesity when combined with high-calorie diets.
2. **European Cohort**: Another study involving European populations found that *rs17782313* carriers were more likely to consume high-fat and high-sugar foods, reinforcing the link between this SNP and altered dietary preferences.

Implications for Personalized Nutrition

Understanding the role of *MC4R rs17782313* in appetite and satiety opens doors for tailored interventions:

- **Dietary Strategies**: Individuals with the risk allele may benefit from structured meal plans emphasizing low-calorie, high-satiety foods like vegetables and lean proteins. Incorporating portion control techniques and slow eating can help manage hunger signals effectively.
- **Behavioral Interventions**: Mindfulness-based approaches to eating, such as focusing on hunger cues and avoiding emotional eating, can be especially useful for those with genetic predispositions affecting appetite.

Another key player is the *FTO* (Fat Mass and Obesity-Associated) gene, one of the most significant genetic contributors to obesity. While *MC4R* primarily affects hunger signaling within the melanocortin pathway, *FTO* modulates appetite, satiety responsiveness, and energy balance through a different mechanism. Now, let's delve into the *FTO* gene and its role in appetite regulation.

FTO Gene and Appetite Regulation

The *FTO* (Fat Mass and Obesity-Associated) gene is one of the most studied genetic factors in obesity. Its role in appetite and satiety has been well-documented, particularly through its impact on food intake behavior and energy homeostasis. The *rs9939609* single nucleotide polymorphism (SNP) within the *FTO* gene has been repeatedly associated with increased food intake, diminished satiety, and higher body mass index (BMI).

The Role of *FTO* in Appetite and Satiety

The *FTO* gene is expressed in key areas of the brain, such as the hypothalamus, which is central to hunger and satiety regulation. The hypothalamus processes hormonal signals like ghrelin (a hunger-stimulating hormone) and *Leptin* (a satiety hormone). Variants of the *FTO* gene, such as *rs9939609*, disrupt the brain's ability to process these signals efficiently, leading to overeating and weight gain.

Key Mechanisms of Action

1. **Expression in the Hypothalamus:**
   - The *FTO* gene is highly active in hypothalamic nuclei, including the arcuate, paraventricular, and ventromedial nuclei, which regulate hunger and satiety.
   - Food deprivation increases *FTO* expression, suggesting it is sensitive to energy demands.
2. **Influence on Satiety Responsiveness:**
   - Individuals with the A allele of *rs9939609* show reduced responsiveness to satiety cues, meaning they need larger meals to feel full.
   - Studies in children and adults demonstrate a direct link between this genetic variant and diminished satiety responses, leading to overeating.
3. **Hormonal Modulation:**
   - *FTO* impacts levels of appetite-regulating hormones such as ghrelin, enhancing hunger perception, especially in A allele carriers.
4. **Epigenetic Interactions:**
   - The *FTO* gene's effects may involve DNA demethylation, a process affecting the expression of other genes linked to metabolism and hunger regulation.
   - This suggests that *FTO*'s impact on obesity extends beyond just food intake—it may also alter metabolism and energy utilization.

Findings Related to *rs9939609*

1. **Increased Energy Intake:**
   - Carriers of the A allele consume higher amounts of energy, favor calorie-dense foods, and show stronger preferences for high-fat and high-sugar options.
   - In children, the AA genotype was linked to an average weight difference of 3 kg compared to TT homozygotes.
2. **Blunted Satiety Responses:**
   - Postprandial satiety responses are significantly lower in individuals with the A allele, both in children and adults (hunger and satiety *FTO*).
   - Reduced satiety leads to prolonged eating and increased portion sizes, contributing to weight gain.
3. **Interaction with Other Genes:**
   - Epistatic interactions between *FTO rs9939609* and genes such as *LEPR* (*Leptin* Receptor) and DNMT3B (DNA Methyltransferase 3B) suggest that genetic and epigenetic mechanisms collectively influence hunger and satiety regulation.

Research Highlights

Children's Study on the *FTO* Gene and Satiety

Researchers studied a cohort of 3,337 children from the UK, aged between 8 and 11 years, to understand why some kids are more prone to overeating and weight gain than others, even in similar environments. They focused on a specific gene called ***FTO*** and its variation known as ***rs9939609*** to explore its role in appetite and satiety.

What the Scientists Found

1. **The "A" Allele and Appetite**:
   - Some children carried a version of the *FTO* gene called the **A allele**, which made it harder for them to feel full after eating.
   - These children had weaker internal signals telling them to stop eating, leading to a tendency to eat larger portions.
2. **Satiety Responsiveness**:
   - Satiety refers to the feeling of fullness after eating. Scientists assessed this by using questionnaires about eating habits.
   - Children with the **A allele** were less responsive to these fullness cues, meaning they often continued eating even when their bodies had consumed enough.
3. **Connection to Weight**:
   - The researchers found that these children were more likely to weigh more, partly because their genes influenced how much food they ate.
   - This link between the *FTO* variant and reduced satiety occurred independently of their body size or fat levels (known as "adiposity"). It showed that the gene had a direct effect on their appetite regulation.

Why Is This Important?

This study highlights how genetics can influence a child's eating behaviors, making them more likely to overeat and gain weight. It's not just about eating habits or willpower; there's a biological basis for these tendencies.

For parents and caregivers:

- Children with this genetic predisposition may benefit from strategies to help them recognize when they're full.
- Offering meals rich in fiber and protein, which promote fullness, can help them manage their appetite.

- Teaching mindful eating habits, such as eating slowly and paying attention to hunger cues, can also be beneficial.

By uncovering how genes like *FTO* affect appetite, scientists can create targeted interventions to help children maintain a healthy weight.

Adult Experimental Study on the *FTO* Gene and Satiety

A group of 103 adults participated in a research study to understand how a specific variation in the ***FTO*** gene (***rs9939609***) affects feelings of fullness after eating— known as postprandial satiety. The aim was to understand whether genetic differences could explain why some individuals tend to eat more or feel less satisfied after meals.

What the Scientists Found

1. **The "A" Allele and Satiety**:
   - Adults carrying the **A allele** of the *FTO* gene had noticeably weaker sensations of fullness after eating compared to those without this allele.
   - This reduced satiety response suggests a higher likelihood of consuming larger portion sizes or eating for longer durations.
2. **The AA Genotype**:
   - Among the participants, those with two copies of the **A allele** (AA genotype) experienced the weakest satiety responses. This group reported feeling less full after meals compared to people with one or no copies of the allele.
   - The diminished satiety response was significant enough to stand out in the study, emphasizing the impact of the AA genotype on appetite regulation.
3. **Postprandial Satiety**:
   - Postprandial satiety plays a vital role in appetite control by signaling the body to stop eating after sufficient energy intake.
   - In **A allele** carriers, this signaling pathway appears less efficient, potentially due to impaired communication between the gut and brain, increasing the risk of overeating.

Why Is This Important?

This study provides direct experimental evidence that genetic variation in the *FTO* gene can influence satiety perception — a key factor in long-term energy balance and weight management.

For adults, this insight is particularly relevant because it highlights a biological factor that could contribute to weight management challenges.

The Bigger Picture

This research highlights how genes like ***FTO*** influence eating behaviors and weight regulation, even in adulthood. By understanding the biological factors behind hunger and satiety, personalized strategies can be developed to support healthier eating habits and weight management for those genetically predisposed to weaker satiety responses.

Personalized Nutrition Insights for *FTO rs9939609* and Appetite Regulation

The *FTO* gene variant *rs9939609* is one of the most extensively studied genetic markers associated with appetite regulation, satiety response, and obesity risk. Evidence suggests that individuals with this variant may exhibit distinct responses to dietary interventions, influencing their ability to manage weight effectively.

This section highlights key findings from two pivotal studies that explored how the *FTO rs9939609* variant interacts with diet composition — followed by practical, evidence-based dietary recommendations.

Study 1: Macronutrient Interaction in a Calorie-Restricted Diet

Study Overview

A 10-week randomized intervention study investigated how obese individuals with different *FTO rs9939609* genotypes responded to two distinct hypo-energetic diets:

- Low-fat, high-carbohydrate (LF) diet
- High-fat, low-carbohydrate (HF) diet

The primary aim was to determine whether macronutrient composition influenced weight loss outcomes and metabolic parameters across *FTO* genotypes.

Key Findings

1. **Diet Adherence:**
    - Carriers of the A allele had a higher dropout rate when on the HF diet, suggesting lower tolerability or satiety with higher-fat regimens.
    - Conversely, A allele carriers exhibited better adherence and completion rates on the LF diet, likely due to improved appetite control and greater satiety effects from higher carbohydrate content.
2. **Metabolic Changes:**
    - Among TT genotype individuals, the LF diet led to:
        1. Smaller reductions in resting energy expenditure (REE) — preserving metabolic rate during calorie restriction.
        2. Greater improvements in markers of insulin resistance (HOMA-beta and HOMA-IR).

- No significant genotype-dependent differences were observed in overall weight loss or fat mass reduction across both dietary interventions.

Conclusion

- The low-fat, high-carbohydrate (LF) diet appears to be more suitable for A allele carriers in terms of adherence and appetite regulation during weight loss interventions.
- TT genotype individuals may derive additional metabolic benefits from the LF diet, supporting its broader applicability in weight management strategies.

Study 2: Interaction of Dietary Fat, Carbohydrates, and Physical Activity with *FTO*

Study Overview

This cross-sectional study investigated how macronutrient intake, fiber consumption, and physical activity levels interact with the *FTO rs9939609* variant to influence BMI. The study analyzed data from 4,839 participants in the Malmö Diet and Cancer study.

The study aimed to evaluate whether lifestyle factors could modify the genetic risk of obesity associated with the A allele of *FTO*.

Key Findings

1. **High-Fat Diet Impact:**
    - A allele carriers consuming a high-fat diet had significantly higher BMIs compared to TT carriers.
    - On a low-fat diet, BMI differences across genotypes were negligible, suggesting that reducing dietary fat can mitigate the effects of the A allele.
2. **Carbohydrate and Fiber Intake:**
    - Low-carbohydrate diets were also associated with higher BMIs in A allele carriers.
    - These findings underscore the importance of maintaining adequate carbohydrate intake — ideally from whole-food, fiber-rich sources — for effective weight management in genetically susceptible individuals.
3. **Physical Activity:**
    - Sedentary individuals with the A allele showed the highest BMIs, indicating that low physical activity levels exacerbate genetic susceptibility to obesity.

Conclusion

High-fat diets and physical inactivity amplify obesity risk for A allele carriers. A low-fat, high-carbohydrate, fiber-rich diet combined with regular physical activity effectively counteracts this genetic predisposition. This research provides strong evidence that personalized nutrition and lifestyle interventions can effectively mitigate genetic risk factors for obesity.

Integrated Dietary Insights for *FTO rs9939609*

By synthesizing the findings from these studies, a tailored nutritional approach emerges:

1. **Prioritize a Low-Fat, High-Carbohydrate Diet:**
   - Ideal macronutrient breakdown: 20–25% of energy from fat, 60–65% from carbohydrates.
   - Opt for complex carbohydrates (whole grains, legumes, vegetables) over refined carbs to improve satiety and energy balance.
2. **Focus on Fiber-Rich Foods:**
   - Incorporate plenty of fiber from fruits, vegetables, and whole grains to enhance fullness and regulate appetite.
   - Fiber contributes to delayed gastric emptying, prolonged satiety, and better appetite regulation — particularly beneficial for individuals with diminished satiety signals linked to the A allele.
3. **Lean Protein Sources:**
   - Include lean proteins such as chicken, fish, tofu, or beans to support muscle preservation and satiety during weight management.
   - Protein can further modulate appetite regulation and reduce overeating tendencies.
4. **Moderate Physical Activity:**
   - Regular exercise is essential, particularly for A allele carriers, to offset the BMI increase associated with a sedentary lifestyle.
5. **Avoid High-Fat Diets:**
   - Minimize dietary fat intake, particularly from saturated fats and energy-dense processed foods, as A allele carriers show greater susceptibility to weight gain under high-fat dietary conditions.
6. **Behavioral Practices:**
   - Encourage mindful eating practices to enhance interoceptive awareness of hunger and fullness cues.
   - Portion control, slower eating pace, and structured meal timing may assist in managing the weaker satiety response characteristic of the *FTO* risk genotype.

Conclusion

These insights demonstrate the importance of aligning dietary strategies with genetic predispositions. For individuals with the *FTO rs9939609* variant, focusing on a low-fat, high-carbohydrate, and fiber-rich diet, along with maintaining an active lifestyle, can significantly improve appetite regulation, metabolic health, and long-term weight management outcomes.

Summary of Major *FTO* SNPs and Their Effects

SNP Variant	Population	High-Risk Allele	Normal Allele	Key Findings	Reference
rs9939609	European, Asian, and global populations	A	T	A allele is associated with reduced satiety responsiveness and higher energy intake, leading to increased risk of obesity and overeating in children and adults.	Wardle et al., 2008; Den Hoed et al., 2009
rs1421085	European and multi-ethnic populations	C	T	The C allele alters gene regulation related to appetite control, impairing satiety signals and increasing obesity susceptibility.	Claussnitzer et al., 2015
rs8050136	European and North American populations	A	C	A allele is associated with higher BMI and altered responses to hunger and satiety cues, impacting appetite regulation.	Frayling et al., 2007
rs17817449	European populations	G	T	G allele correlates with increased energy intake and reduced satiety responsiveness, contributing to weight gain and obesity risk.	Dina et al., 2007

NPY Gene and Appetite Regulation

The *NPY* (Neuropeptide Y) gene is a key regulator in appetite and energy homeostasis. Neuropeptide Y, the protein encoded by this gene, is one of the most potent stimulators of appetite in humans and animals. Variations in the *NPY* gene have been linked to differences in appetite, satiety, and body weight regulation, making it an essential focus in the study of eating behaviors and obesity.

The Role of *NPY* in Appetite and Satiety

NPY is expressed primarily in the hypothalamus, a brain region critical for hunger and energy balance. It interacts with other appetite-regulating hormones, such as *Leptin* and ghrelin, to modulate food intake. Genetic variants influencing *NPY* activity can alter these regulatory pathways, leading to increased hunger, reduced satiety, and a higher risk of weight gain.

Key Mechanisms of Action:

1. Hypothalamic Expression:
   - *NPY* is highly expressed in the arcuate nucleus of the hypothalamus, where it acts to increase food-seeking behavior and reduce energy expenditure.
   - Fasting and caloric restriction significantly upregulate *NPY* expression, amplifying hunger signals and encouraging energy conservation.
2. Interaction with *Leptin*:
   - *Leptin*, a hormone produced by fat cells, inhibits *NPY* activity to suppress appetite.
   - Variations in the *NPY* gene may impair this regulatory feedback, resulting in persistent hunger signals.
3. Regulation of Ghrelin:
   - *NPY* also enhances the appetite-stimulating effects of ghrelin, a hormone secreted by the stomach.
   - Individuals with genetic variants that increase *NPY* expression may exhibit a stronger hunger response to ghrelin, further promoting food intake.
4. Energy Storage and Metabolism:
   - Beyond appetite regulation, *NPY* promotes energy storage by enhancing fat deposition and reducing thermogenesis (heat production).
   - This contributes to a positive energy balance, favoring weight gain, particularly in individuals with genetic predispositions affecting *NPY* pathways.

Research Highlights

NPY Polymorphisms and Appetite Regulation

Researchers have identified key genetic variants in the *NPY* gene, such as *rs16147*, which are associated with variations in appetite control and body weight. The following study illustrates the influence of *NPY* polymorphisms on hunger and satiety mechanisms:

Children's Study on *NPY* Gene Variants and Appetite

Study Design

A cohort of 1,500 children aged 6–10 years was studied to evaluate how *NPY* polymorphisms influence hunger and eating behaviors. Researchers focused on the *rs16147* SNP within the *NPY* gene.

Findings

1. Increased Hunger Signals:
    - Children carrying the T allele of *rs16147* exhibited stronger hunger signals compared to those with the C allele. This effect was further amplified during periods of caloric restriction, indicating a role in survival-driven feeding behavior.
2. Diminished Satiety:
    - T allele carriers had weaker satiety responses, leading to increased food intake and larger meal portions.
3. Higher BMI:
    - A positive correlation was observed between the T allele and BMI, mediated by increased food intake.

Why It Matters

This study demonstrates the contribution of *NPY* gene variants to appetite dysregulation in children. It underscores the importance of early nutritional strategies and behavioral interventions in individuals genetically predisposed to heightened hunger and reduced satiety.

<u>**Adult Study on *NPY* and Stress-Induced Eating**</u>

Study Design

A study involving 200 adults examined the interaction between *NPY* gene variants and stress-induced eating behaviors, with a particular focus on emotional overeating. The *rs16147* SNP within the *NPY* gene was the primary genetic variant investigated.

Findings

1. Stress-Driven Hunger and Cravings:
    - Individuals carrying the T allele of *rs16147* reported increased hunger sensations and stronger food cravings in response to psychological stress.
2. Preference for Calorie-Dense Foods:
    - T allele carriers exhibited a notable preference for calorie-rich foods, particularly those high in fat and sugar, during stressful situations.
3. Impact on Weight:
    - Over time, stress-related overeating contributed to higher weight gain in T allele carriers compared to non-carriers.

Why It Matters

This study highlights the influence of *NPY* genetic variation on emotional and stress-related eating behaviors. It emphasizes the potential importance of stress management and behavioral interventions as part of personalized weight control strategies in genetically susceptible individuals.

Implications for Personalized Nutrition

Given the central role of the *NPY* gene in appetite regulation, dietary and behavioral interventions can be tailored to mitigate its effects. Here are practical strategies for individuals with *NPY*-related appetite dysregulation:

Dietary Strategies:

1. High-Satiety Foods:
    - Emphasize nutrient-dense, high-fiber foods such as vegetables, legumes, and whole grains to promote fullness. Include lean proteins, which are more effective in suppressing appetite than carbohydrates or fats.
2. Small, Frequent Meals:
    - To counteract hunger spikes associated with *NPY* activity, opt for smaller, more frequent meals throughout the day.
3. Avoid Energy-Dense Foods:
    - Reduce the intake of high-fat, high-sugar foods that may be especially appealing to individuals with heightened *NPY*-driven appetite.

Behavioral Strategies:

1. Stress Management:
    - Adopt stress-reducing practices such as yoga, mindfulness, meditation, or regular physical activity to prevent stress-induced overeating.
2. Mindful Eating:
    - Encourage slower eating, paying attention to internal hunger and satiety cues to avoid excessive intake.
3. Portion Control:
    - Plan and control portion sizes in advance to reduce the likelihood of overeating during meals.

Role of Physical Activity

Regular physical activity plays a dual role in appetite regulation — modulating appetite hormones and reducing stress. Aerobic exercises, in particular, may temporarily suppress appetite and contribute to better energy balance in individuals with *NPY*-related appetite dysregulation.

POMC Gene: Appetite Regulation Through a Molecular Lens

The ***POMC*** **(Proopiomelanocortin)** gene plays a pivotal role in appetite regulation and energy balance, acting as a molecular switchboard that connects hormonal signals to the brain's control center for hunger. This is the story of *POMC* and its intricate role in human metabolism.

The Discovery of *POMC*: A Gateway to Understanding Appetite

The ***Leptin*-Melanocortin Pathway** represents a finely tuned system maintaining energy homeostasis. Within this pathway, ***POMC*** acts as a central regulator:

- *Leptin*, a hormone secreted by adipose tissue, signals energy sufficiency by binding to *Leptin* receptors in the hypothalamus.
- This stimulates *POMC* neurons to produce *α-MSH* (alpha-Melanocyte Stimulating Hormone), which activates *MC4R* (Melanocortin-4 Receptor), leading to appetite suppression.
- Concurrently, *Leptin* inhibits *NPY/AgRP* neurons, which are known to promote hunger.

This dual mechanism ensures appropriate regulation of food intake and energy balance. However, disruptions in *POMC* expression or *Leptin* signaling — often due to genetic mutations — can impair this system, leading to hyperphagia (excessive eating) and obesity.

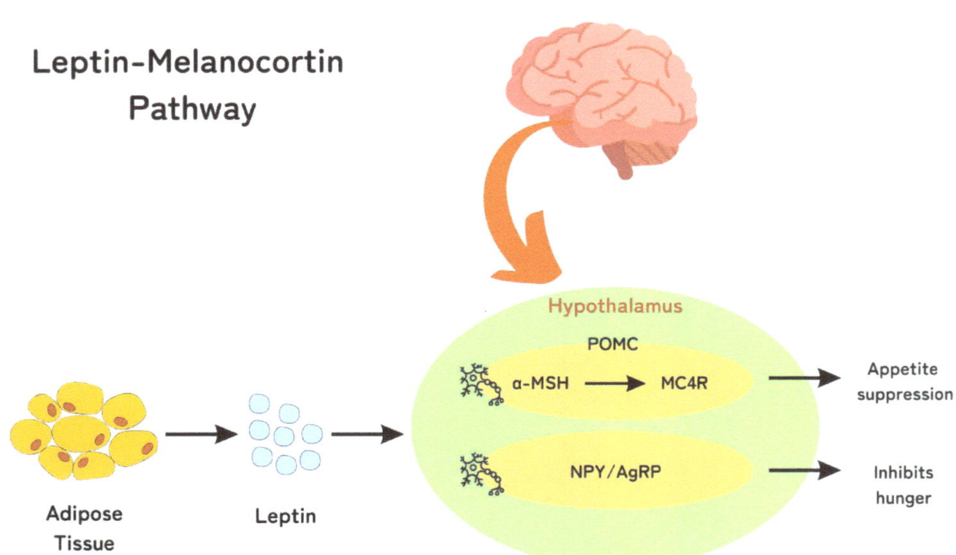

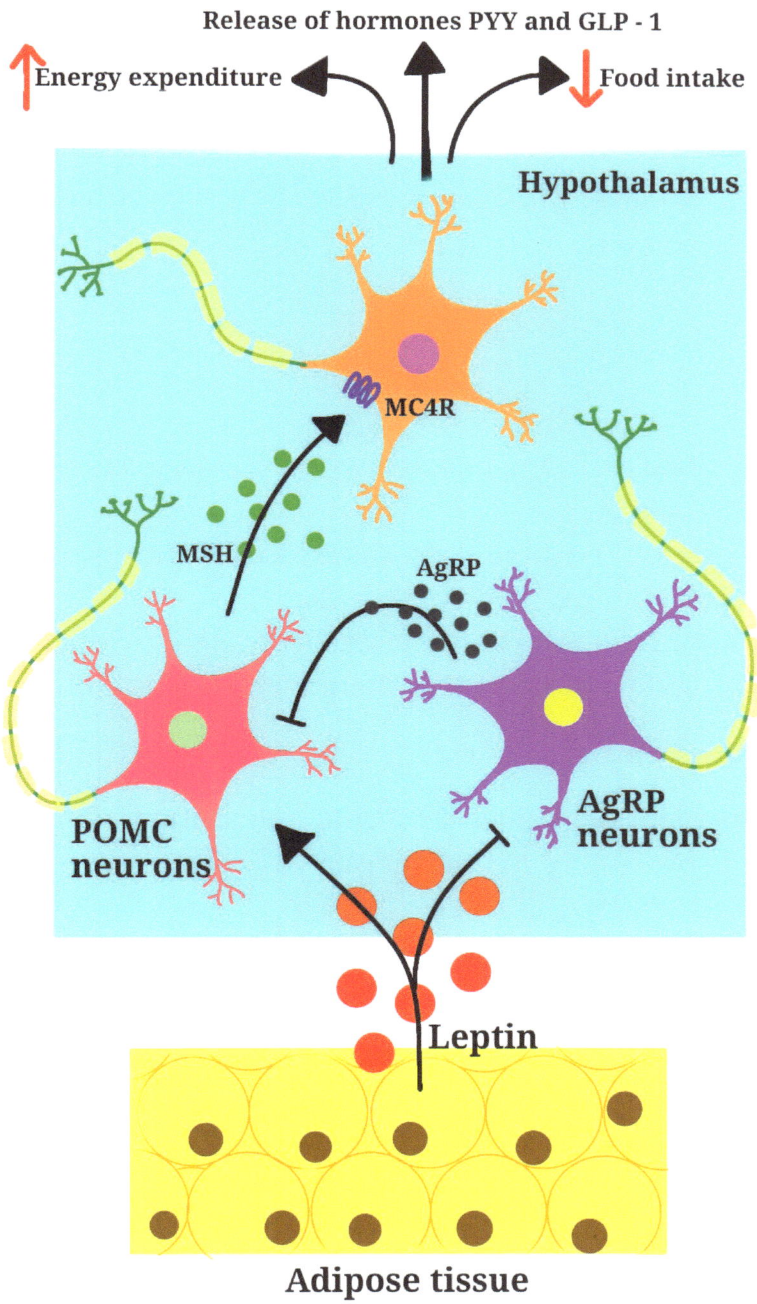

What Makes *POMC* Special?

POMC is not just a "hunger gene"; it plays multiple roles in the body. The peptides derived from *POMC* have diverse functions:

- **Hunger Regulation**: α-MSH suppresses appetite by activating *MC4R* in the brain.
- **Energy Balance**: *POMC*-derived peptides influence energy expenditure, ensuring that calorie intake matches energy needs.
- **Pigmentation**: Some *POMC* peptides, such as β-MSH, are involved in skin pigmentation.

This multi-functional gene is an evolutionary marvel, highlighting nature's efficiency in using a single gene for various essential processes.

POMC and Appetite Regulation: The Role of *rs28932472*

One of the notable SNPs in the *POMC* gene is ***rs28932472***, which has been linked to appetite regulation and obesity-related traits.

Research Findings

1. **Children's Study**:
    - **Lower Diastolic Blood Pressure**: Children with the C allele of *rs28932472* exhibited lower diastolic blood pressure.
    - **Higher LDL Cholesterol**: The same allele was associated with increased levels of low-density lipoprotein (LDL) cholesterol.
    - **Increased Risk of Altered Total Cholesterol**: Overweight children carrying this allele were found to have a 7.35-fold higher risk of altered total cholesterol levels.
2. **Implications for Adolescents**:
    - **Energy Dysregulation**: Mutations in *POMC* can disrupt normal appetite-suppressing signals, leading to overeating and weight gain.

POMC and Real-Life Scenarios

To put this into perspective, imagine two individuals, Amy and Liam, who are both children with similar lifestyles. Amy carries the C allele of *rs28932472*, while Liam does not. After a meal, Amy may struggle to feel full and might crave high-calorie foods, while Liam feels satisfied and avoids overeating. Over time, these subtle genetic differences could significantly affect their weight management and overall health.

POMC Variants and Their Broader Implications

Leptin-Melanocortin Pathway

POMC operates within the *Leptin*-melanocortin signaling axis, crucial for regulating appetite and energy expenditure:

- *Leptin*, secreted by adipose tissue, signals energy sufficiency to the hypothalamus.
- *POMC*-derived peptides (e.g., α-MSH) activate *MC4R*, leading to appetite suppression.
- Mutations in *POMC* disrupt this pathway, impairing the brain's ability to regulate hunger signals effectively.

Obesity and Cardiovascular Risk

Variants such as *rs28932472* have been associated with:

- Increased susceptibility to obesity.
- Elevated cholesterol levels (especially LDL).
- Greater risk for cardiovascular diseases.

Clinical Relevance

Understanding *POMC* polymorphisms can inform early interventions, particularly in at-risk children and adolescents. Personalized nutrition strategies, combined with lifestyle modifications, may help offset the genetic predisposition toward overeating and metabolic disorders.

Why Nutritionists Should Care About *POMC*

Understanding the role of *POMC* and its variants, such as *rs28932472*, provides nutritionists with valuable insight for developing personalized nutrition plans. Genetic factors influencing appetite regulation highlight the need for targeted dietary and behavioral strategies.

Real-Life Examples

Consider Arin, an adolescent who frequently reports feeling hungry soon after meals and struggles with portion control, despite consuming balanced home-cooked meals. Nutritional assessment reveals no major dietary deficiencies, yet weight gain and elevated LDL cholesterol are gradually emerging. Genetic screening identifies that Arin carries the C allele of the POMC rs28932472 variant, which is associated with altered appetite-suppressing signals.

Rather than attributing Arin's eating behavior to poor discipline, a nutritionist uses this genetic insight to design a plan focused on enhancing satiety, structuring meals, and building sustainable eating habits. This approach improves appetite control and metabolic markers, demonstrating how genetic awareness can directly inform effective nutritional counseling.

Key Implications for Nutritional Practice

- **Tailored Interventions**: Individuals with *POMC* mutations may respond better to diets rich in protein and fiber to enhance satiety and control hunger.
- **Behavioral Coaching**: Recognizing genetic predispositions allows nutritionists to offer customized coaching to prevent overeating and manage portion control.
- **Preventive Health**: Early identification of genetic risk factors enables proactive strategies to reduce the likelihood of obesity, dyslipidemia, and cardiovascular diseases.

Dietary Strategies

1. For individuals carrying risk variants in *POMC*, the following evidence-based strategies may be beneficial:

Strategy	Practical Recommendations
Choose Satiating Foods	Prioritize protein-rich and fiber-dense foods like lean meats, legumes, whole grains, and vegetables to promote fullness.
Mindful Eating Practices	Encourage slower eating, paying attention to hunger and satiety cues, to avoid overeating.
Regular Physical Activity	Incorporate aerobic and resistance exercises to regulate appetite hormones and maintain energy balance.

UCP2 Gene: The Appetite Regulator with a Metabolic Twist

Imagine a thermostat in your body that not only controls energy expenditure but also influences how much food you crave. The ***UCP2*** **(Uncoupling Protein 2)** gene plays a dual role in regulating energy balance and appetite, making it a fascinating target in nutrigenetics

What is *UCP2*?

UCP2 belongs to a family of mitochondrial proteins involved in energy metabolism. Unlike its close relative, UCP1, which is primarily involved in thermogenesis, *UCP2* has broader roles, including reducing oxidative stress and influencing appetite regulation through its effects on the hypothalamus.

- **Location**: Expressed in multiple tissues, including the brain, liver, and adipose tissue.
- **Function**: Acts as a mitochondrial proton carrier, dissipating the proton gradient to reduce ATP synthesis, which affects energy balance and metabolic efficiency.

UCP2 rs660339 and Appetite Regulation

One of the most studied polymorphisms in the *UCP2* gene is ***rs660339***, a missense mutation that results in a change from alanine to valine in the protein structure. This SNP has been linked to variations in appetite control, energy metabolism, and obesity risk.

Research Findings

1. **Children's Study**:
   - **Hunger Sensations**: Children carrying the T allele of *rs660339* reported higher hunger levels compared to those with the C allele.
   - **Increased Calorie Intake**: T allele carriers consumed more calories during meals, particularly in energy-dense foods.
   - **BMI Association:** A positive correlation was observed between the T allele and higher BMI, indicating a genetic tendency toward overeating.

2. **Adult Study**:
    - **Stress-Induced Eating**: Adults with the T allele were more likely to engage in emotional eating and preferred high-fat, high-sugar foods under stress.
    - **Weight Gain**: Long-term weight gain was more pronounced in T allele carriers, particularly in obesogenic environments with easy access to calorie-rich foods.

How *UCP2 rs660339* Impacts Appetite

The *UCP2* gene influences appetite regulation through its effects on hypothalamic neurons:

1. **Mitochondrial Activity in the Hypothalamus**: *UCP2* modulates the activity of neurons involved in energy sensing, particularly in the arcuate nucleus.
2. Regulation of Hunger Hormones: Altered mitochondrial efficiency affects the release of appetite-regulating hormones like ghrelin and *Leptin*.
3. **Oxidative Stress and Inflammation**: Increased oxidative stress due to inefficient *UCP2* function can disrupt appetite signaling pathways, contributing to overeating.

Real-Life Example

Imagine two friends, Arjun and Priya. Arjun carries the T allele of rs660339, while Priya does not. After a meal, Priya feels full and satiated, but Arjun continues to crave high-calorie snacks. Over time, this genetic predisposition could lead to significant differences in their body weight and metabolic health.

Practical Strategies for Individuals with *UCP2* Variants

Individuals with the T allele of *rs660339* may benefit from targeted nutrition and lifestyle strategies to control appetite and prevent overeating:

Dietary Approaches

- **High-Satiety Foods:** Prioritize protein-rich options (chicken, eggs, legumes) and fiber-dense foods (vegetables, fruits, whole grains) to enhance fullness.
- **Limit Energy-Dense Foods:** Reduce intake of high-fat, high-sugar snacks that may trigger overeating in T allele carriers.

Lifestyle and Behavioral Strategies

- **Regular Exercise:** Supports energy balance, regulates appetite hormones, and reduces stress-related food cravings.
- **Stress Management:** Incorporate stress-reducing practices such as mindfulness, yoga, or relaxation techniques to minimize emotional eating triggers.

TBC1D1 Gene: A Gatekeeper in Energy Use and Appetite Regulation

Imagine a gene that acts as a traffic controller, directing glucose and energy where they're most needed. The ***TBC1D1* (TBC1 Domain Family Member 1)** gene plays this role in energy metabolism and appetite regulation. It has gained attention for its influence on fat storage, glucose uptake, and food preferences, making it a crucial component in nutrigenetics.

What is *TBC1D1*?

TBC1D1 encodes a protein involved in glucose metabolism, specifically in skeletal muscle. It regulates GLUT4, a transporter responsible for glucose uptake into cells. Variations in this gene can alter metabolic efficiency and influence appetite regulation through energy balance mechanisms.

- **Location**: Highly expressed in skeletal muscle and adipose tissue.
- **Function**: Regulates glucose homeostasis, fat oxidation, and energy partitioning, which indirectly affects appetite.

TBC1D1 rs2279027 and Appetite Regulation

The ***rs2279027*** SNP in *TBC1D1* has been linked to variations in energy utilization and appetite, particularly in relation to dietary preferences and obesity risk.

Research Findings

1. **Impact on Food Preferences**:
    - **Increased Fat Preference**: Individuals with the T allele of *rs2279027* tend to prefer high-fat foods, likely due to altered energy signaling pathways.
    - **Reduced Carbohydrate Oxidation**: The T allele is associated with reduced reliance on carbohydrates as an energy source, encouraging the consumption of calorie-dense, fatty foods.
2. **Obesity Risk and Physical Activity**:
    - **Higher BMI**: Carriers of the T allele are at a greater risk of developing obesity due to the combined effects of increased fat intake and reduced energy expenditure.
    - **Lower Physical Activity Levels**: The SNP is associated with decreased motivation for physical activity, compounding its effect on weight gain.
3. **Energy Balance and Appetite**:
    - **Impaired Fat Oxidation**: Reduced ability to utilize stored fat as an energy source can lead to increased hunger and overeating.
    - **Altered *Leptin* Sensitivity**: T allele carriers may exhibit decreased sensitivity to *Leptin*, the hormone responsible for signaling satiety, further contributing to overeating.

How *TBC1D1 rs2279027* Impacts Appetite

TBC1D1 plays a key role in energy sensing, glucose metabolism, and appetite regulation. Variations like *rs2279027* can influence dietary behaviors and predispose individuals to specific eating patterns.

1. **Glucose Uptake in Muscles**: Impaired GLUT4 translocation reduces glucose utilization, shifting energy demands toward dietary fat.
2. ***Leptin* and Insulin Resistance**: Dysfunctional energy partitioning can disrupt hormonal signals, leading to increased hunger and fat storage.
3. **Dietary Feedback Loops**: Preference for high-fat foods can exacerbate energy imbalances, promoting further weight gain.

Real-Life Examples

Imagine two colleagues, Alex and Maya. Alex carries the T allele of rs2279027, while Maya does not. During lunch, Alex gravitates toward fatty dishes and feels hungrier sooner after eating, while Maya enjoys balanced meals and stays full for longer. Over time, this genetic difference may contribute to variations in body weight, metabolic health, and risk of obesity.

Practical Strategies for Individuals with *TBC1D1* Variants

For individuals with the T allele of *rs2279027*, personalized dietary and lifestyle strategies can help counteract genetic predispositions:

1. **Focus on Balanced Macronutrients**: Incorporate moderate amounts of healthy fats, complex carbohydrates, and lean protein to maintain energy balance.
2. **Encourage Regular Physical Activity**: Engage in activities that promote fat oxidation, such as aerobic exercises or strength training.
3. **Choose High-Satiety Foods**: Fiber-rich and protein-dense meals can help curb hunger and reduce cravings for high-fat foods.
4. **Monitor Caloric Intake**: Be mindful of portion sizes to avoid overeating, especially when consuming calorie-dense meals.

SH2B1 Gene: A Molecular Link Between Appetite and Metabolism

The ***SH2B1* (SH2B Adaptor Protein 1)** gene is a critical regulator of energy balance, linking appetite control with metabolic pathways. Variants in this gene, such as ***rs4788102***, have been associated with differences in appetite regulation, body weight, and metabolic efficiency. Let's delve into the role of *SH2B1* and how this SNP contributes to hunger and obesity.

What is *SH2B1*?

SH2B1 is an adaptor protein that enhances signaling of several key hormones, including:

- ***Leptin***: Signals satiety and energy sufficiency.
- **Insulin**: Regulates glucose uptake and metabolism.
- **Growth Hormone**: Influences growth and metabolic function.

It plays a pivotal role in hypothalamic signaling pathways, which control food intake and energy expenditure.

- **Location**: Highly expressed in the hypothalamus — the brain's appetite control center — as well as in peripheral metabolic tissues.
- **Function**: Amplifies *Leptin* and insulin signaling, critical for appetite suppression and energy regulation.

SH2B1 rs4788102 and Appetite Regulation

The *rs4788102* SNP, located in the *SH2B1* gene, has been extensively studied for its role in obesity and appetite-related traits.

Research Findings

Hunger and Satiety

1. **Increased Appetite**
    - **Genetic Insight**: The A allele of *rs4788102* is a "risk allele" associated with heightened hunger sensations.
    - **Mechanism**: *SH2B1* is known to enhance the signaling of *Leptin* and insulin in the brain, particularly in the hypothalamus, which is the primary center for hunger regulation. Alterations in *SH2B1* function due to the A allele may impair these signaling pathways, resulting in dysregulated hunger signals and an enhanced drive to eat.
    - **Clinical Implications**: Risk allele carriers report difficulty in managing hunger, leading to potential overeating behaviors.

2. **Weakened Satiety**
   - **Genetic Insight**: Risk allele carriers of *rs4788102* experience a reduced sense of fullness after eating.
   - **Mechanism**: *Leptin*, secreted by adipose tissue, communicates nutritional sufficiency to the brain. *SH2B1* normally amplifies *Leptin*'s action, enhancing satiety signaling. However, the presence of the A allele compromises *SH2B1* activity, weakening this feedback loop and predisposing individuals to chronic overeating.
   - **Clinical Relevance**: Individuals feel less satisfied after meals, leading to increased calorie intake over time.

Body Weight and Obesity

1. **Higher BMI**
   - **Genetic Insight**: Carriers of the A allele show a significant association with increased body mass index (BMI) and a predisposition to obesity, particularly during developmental stages such as childhood and adolescence.
   - **Mechanism**: The impaired *Leptin* and insulin signaling in risk allele carriers can lead to a positive energy balance—caloric intake exceeds expenditure—which translates into progressive weight gain.
   - **Population-Level Impact**: Early identification and preventive interventions focusing on diet and physical activity are crucial to mitigating long-term obesity risk.

2. **Fat Distribution**
   - **Genetic Insight**: Risk allele carriers often exhibit increased **central adiposity** (abdominal fat), a phenotype linked to a higher likelihood of developing metabolic disorders like type 2 diabetes and cardiovascular diseases.
   - **Mechanism**: Central adiposity may arise from altered energy storage preferences due to the interplay between *SH2B1* dysregulation and metabolic signaling pathways.
   - **Clinical Significance**: Greater central adiposity represents a double burden: it not only contributes to increased BMI but also exacerbates metabolic risks. Interventions focusing on lifestyle changes can reduce these adverse outcomes.

***Leptin* Resistance**

1. **Mechanism of Resistance**
   - **Genetic Insight**: *Leptin* resistance, frequently observed in A allele carriers, is a state where the brain's response to circulating *Leptin* levels is diminished. This results in a paradox: despite high levels of *Leptin* in the bloodstream (often seen in obesity), the brain fails to recognize satiety signals effectively.

- **Role of *SH2B1***: As a critical enhancer of *Leptin* receptor signaling, *SH2B1* variants such as the A allele impair the efficiency of *Leptin*'s appetite-suppressing action. This effect is compounded by the inability of *Leptin* to stimulate the hypothalamic pathways regulating energy balance.
- **Clinical Implications**: This resistance leads to a feedback failure — the body keeps signaling hunger despite sufficient fat stores. The result is chronic overeating, reduced energy expenditure, and a vicious cycle of weight gain.

How *SH2B1 rs4788102* Impacts Appetite

SH2B1 enhances the brain's ability to respond to *Leptin* and insulin signals. Variations in *rs4788102* can disrupt this signaling, leading to:

1. **Diminished *Leptin* Sensitivity**: The brain receives weaker signals to stop eating, resulting in persistent hunger.
2. **Altered Energy Balance**: Reduced insulin and *Leptin* efficiency may impair energy expenditure, promoting fat storage.
3. **Overeating in Stressful Conditions**: Risk allele carriers often show heightened susceptibility to emotional eating and cravings for high-calorie foods.

Real-Life Example

Imagine a family dinner where siblings Sarah and Rahul respond differently to the same meal. Sarah, a carrier of the A allele, feels hungry soon after eating and reaches for dessert. Rahul, who does not carry the risk allele, feels satisfied and skips the extra calories. These subtle but impactful genetic differences in SH2B1 signaling shape their respective appetite responses and long-term eating patterns.

Practical Strategies for Individuals with *SH2B1* Variants

For individuals with the A allele of *rs4788102*, targeted lifestyle modifications can help manage appetite and reduce obesity risk:

1. **Incorporate High-Satiety Foods**:
   - Protein-rich meals (e.g., lean meats, tofu, eggs).
   - Fiber-dense options (e.g., legumes, vegetables, and whole grains).
2. **Focus on Regular Meal Timing**:
   - Consistent eating schedules can help regulate hunger hormones and prevent overeating.
3. **Avoid Energy-Dense Foods**:
   - Limit intake of sugary and fatty snacks that exacerbate cravings.

4. **Engage in Stress Management**:
   - Activities like yoga or mindfulness can mitigate stress-induced eating.
5. **Encourage Physical Activity**:
   - Regular exercise improves *Leptin* sensitivity and overall energy balance.

GHRL rs696217: Appetite and Reward System Regulation

The **ghrelin gene (*GHRL*)** is crucial in appetite and energy balance regulation, producing the orexigenic peptide ghrelin, which stimulates hunger through the hypothalamus and modulates the brain's reward pathways. The *rs696217* single-nucleotide polymorphism (SNP), also referred to as Leu72Met, has been associated with various eating behaviors and metabolic traits, providing insight into the genetic underpinnings of appetite and reward-driven eating.

The Science Behind *GHRL* and *rs696217*

GHRL, located on chromosome 3p25-26, encodes the precursor for ghrelin, which influences hunger signaling and reward-related behaviors. The *rs696217* polymorphism results in an amino acid substitution (Leu72Met) within the gene's non-coding region. This SNP has been studied for its impact on the peptide's activity in energy homeostasis, food intake, and metabolic syndrome risk.

Key molecular pathways influenced by ghrelin include:

- **Hypothalamic signaling:** Ghrelin acts on the growth hormone secretagogue receptor (GHS-R1A) in the hypothalamus, enhancing hunger signals.
- **Reward pathways:** Ghrelin modulates the mesolimbic dopamine system, influencing reward-driven consumption of palatable foods like sweets and alcohol.

Findings Related to *rs696217*

The *rs696217* variant has been extensively studied in both human and rodent models, revealing its association with appetite and metabolic traits:

- **Impact on Appetite and Eating Behavior:**
  - Studies highlight increased appetite and a preference for energy-dense, high-sugar foods in carriers of the Met allele. This effect is linked to heightened ghrelin activity in reward circuits such as the ventral tegmental area (VTA) and nucleus accumbens.
  - In populations such as the Old Order Amish, the Met allele has been associated with higher fasting glucose levels and increased risk of metabolic syndrome, suggesting its influence extends beyond hunger to metabolic regulation.

- **Reward System and Sweet Preference:**
  - Research demonstrates that ghrelin, via the GHS-R1A receptor, increases sucrose consumption in rodents. GHS-R1A antagonism reduces both sucrose and alcohol intake, reinforcing the SNP's role in reward-seeking behavior.
  - Human cohort studies reveal a correlation between the *rs696217* variant and sweet consumption preferences, highlighting its potential impact on dietary choices and obesity risk.

Real-Life Example

Consider Jane and Alex, siblings with contrasting eating habits. Jane, who carries the Met allele of rs696217, gravitates towards sugary snacks and struggles with portion control. In contrast, Alex, who does not carry this variant, maintains a balanced appetite and rarely overeats. This genetic predisposition likely contributes to Jane's heightened sensitivity to food rewards, influencing her preference for high-calorie, energy-dense foods.

Research Insights

Japanese Study on Eating Disorders

Association Between Met Allele and Bulimia Nervosa (BN):

- **Genetic Insight**: The study highlights a significant association between the **Met allele of the preproghrelin (*GHRL*) gene** and increased susceptibility to **binge eating behaviors** in individuals with bulimia nervosa (BN).
- **Mechanism**: Ghrelin, commonly referred to as the "hunger hormone," is secreted by the stomach and acts on the hypothalamus to regulate appetite and energy homeostasis. In carriers of the Met allele, dysregulation of ghrelin secretion may impair hunger and satiety signaling, contributing to the compulsive eating patterns characteristic of BN.
- **Clinical Implications**: The findings suggest that individuals carrying the Met allele may benefit from targeted therapies aimed at restoring ghrelin balance, potentially alleviating binge-eating behaviors. Moreover, ghrelin regulation may serve as a potential biomarker for diagnosing or predicting susceptibility to BN.

Ghrelin and Sucrose Intake in Rodents (Landgren et al., 2011)

Role of Ghrelin in Reward-Driven Eating:

- **Preclinical Evidence**: Experimental studies in rodent models demonstrate that **peripheral ghrelin administration** significantly increases the consumption of sucrose and other sweetened solutions. These findings suggest that ghrelin plays a critical role not only in regulating hunger but also in driving reward-based eating behaviors.

- **Mechanism**: Ghrelin enhances the activity of the brain's reward centers, particularly the **dopaminergic pathways** in the ventral tegmental area (VTA) and nucleus accumbens. This neurobiological effect reinforces the motivation to consume calorie-dense, palatable foods, such as sweets.
- **Implications for Humans**: These findings underscore the potential of ghrelin as a target for interventions aimed at controlling sugar cravings and compulsive eating. Strategies aimed at modulating ghrelin signaling could reduce the consumption of highly palatable foods and aid in the management of diet-related disorders, including obesity and binge-eating syndromes.

Metabolic Syndrome in Old Order Amish Population

1. **Impact of *GHRL* Variants on Metabolic Syndrome:**

    - **Genetic Insight**: In the Old Order Amish population, carriers of the **Met allele** of the *GHRL* gene have demonstrated a higher prevalence of **metabolic syndrome** — a cluster of conditions that includes obesity, dyslipidemia, hypertension, and insulin resistance.
    - **Mechanism**: Variants in the ***GHRL* gene** affect the regulation of ghrelin, which in turn disrupts energy balance, lipid metabolism, and glucose homeostasis. This dysregulation increases the risk of metabolic syndrome.
    - **Lipid Profile Alterations**: Met allele carriers showed **elevated triglycerides and low HDL cholesterol**, further emphasizing the allele's role in predisposing individuals to metabolic complications.
    - **Clinical Implications**: Understanding the relationship between *GHRL* variants and metabolic syndrome could inform personalized treatment approaches, including dietary modifications and pharmacological strategies targeting ghrelin pathways.

Implications for Personalized Nutrition

Understanding the role of *GHRL rs696217* in appetite regulation offers opportunities for tailored interventions:

1. **Dietary Strategies:**

    - Individuals carrying the Met allele may benefit from nutrition plans that emphasize high-satiety, low-glycemic foods. Diets rich in fiber-containing vegetables, whole grains, and lean protein sources can help promote satiety and reduce susceptibility to reward-driven eating.
    - Structured meal timing and portion control are particularly important in mitigating tendencies towards overeating, especially in environments rich in palatable, high-sugar foods.

2. **Behavioral Interventions:**
   - Techniques like mindful eating and limiting exposure to food-related cues can be particularly effective for managing reward-driven hunger.
   - Cognitive-behavioral approaches focusing on impulse control may help reduce binge eating episodes.

Scientific Evidence for SNPs Associated with Obesity and BMI

In the previous chapter, we examined single nucleotide polymorphisms (SNPs) associated with appetite regulation and satiety, emphasizing how genetic variations influence eating behaviors and nutritional responses. This understanding highlighted the potential for tailoring dietary interventions based on individual genetic profiles, particularly regarding hunger cues, portion control, and satiety signaling.

Building upon that foundation, this section shifts focus to the genetic determinants of obesity and body mass index (BMI) — two complex and multifactorial phenotypes with substantial implications for public health and disease prevention. Identifying and understanding the SNPs associated with obesity and BMI is pivotal not only for unraveling the genetic predisposition to excess weight but also for developing targeted interventions. These SNPs provide valuable insights into the molecular pathways that regulate body weight, fat storage, and energy balance.

In the sections that follow, we will highlight key genes and their associated SNPs that play a significant role in influencing obesity risk and BMI variations. This exploration will underscore the importance of genetic insights in shaping precision nutrition approaches, enabling the design of personalized interventions to manage weight and promote metabolic health.

Table: Genetic Variants Associated with Obesity and BMI: An Overview

Gene	SNP	Population	Association	Reference
FTO	*rs9939609*	European, Asian, African, Hispanic	Increased BMI and obesity risk	Frayling et al., 2007; Dina et al., 2007
MC4R	*rs17782313*	European, Asian, African, Hispanic	Obesity susceptibility	Loos et al., 2008; Qi et al., 2008
LEP	*rs2167270*	European, Asian	Higher *Leptin* levels, BMI increase	Li et al., 2010; Mammès et al., 1998
LEPR	*rs1137101*	European, Asian, Hispanic	Obesity and BMI variation	Chagnon et al., 2000; Wu et al., 2010
TMEM18	*rs6548238*	European, Asian	Increased BMI	Thorleifsson et al., 2009
ADCY3	*rs713586*	European, Asian	Obesity susceptibility	Bonnefond et al., 2013
SH2B1	*rs7498665*	European, Asian	BMI and obesity risk	Boes et al., 2011

BDNF	*rs6265*	European, Asian	Obesity and eating behavior	Zhang et al., 2014; Speliotes et al., 2010
PCSK1	*rs6232, rs6235*	European	Obesity susceptibility	Benzinou et al., 2008
GNPDA2	*rs10938397*	European, Asian	Increased BMI and obesity risk	Willer et al., 2009
NEGR1	*rs2815752*	European, Asian	BMI and fat distribution	Thorleifsson et al., 2009
TMEM18	*rs7561317*	European, Asian	Obesity susceptibility	Thorleifsson et al., 2009
TNNI3K	*rs1514175*	European	BMI and obesity risk	Choquet et al., 2013
PPARG	*rs1801282*	European, Asian	Fat accumulation and BMI variation	Memisoglu et al., 2003
KCTD15	*rs29941*	European, Asian	Obesity risk	Willer et al., 2009
MAP2K5	*rs2241423*	European, Asian	Increased BMI	Speliotes et al., 2010

Now, let us delve into each gene and SNP in detail to understand their association with BMI and obesity.

The *FTO* Gene: Its Significance in Obesity Genetics

The discovery of the *FTO* (Fat Mass and Obesity-associated) gene as a major genetic contributor to obesity and Body Mass Index (BMI) regulation represents a landmark achievement in human genetic research. This finding emerged from the pioneering work of the Wellcome Trust Case Control Consortium (WTCCC), which initially conducted a genome-wide association study (GWAS) aimed at identifying susceptibility genes for type 2 diabetes. Interestingly, the strongest association observed during this study was not directly related to diabetes, but instead to BMI, shifting the scientific focus from glucose metabolism to the genetic basis of obesity.

Key Insights:

1. **Initial Association with Type 2 Diabetes:**
    - The *FTO* gene variants were first identified in connection with type 2 diabetes risk. However, subsequent analyses clarified that this association was largely mediated through BMI, indicating that increased adiposity, rather than intrinsic glucose dysregulation, was the primary link.
2. **Identification of SNP *rs9939609*:**
    - SNP *rs9939609* — located within the first intron of the *FTO* gene emerged as a particularly strong marker associated with higher BMI and an increased risk of obesity. This SNP became the most widely studied obesity-related genetic variant.

3. **Validation Across Diverse Cohorts:**
    - The association between *FTO* variants and BMI was robustly validated across multiple large-scale cohorts, involving over 38,000 individuals from diverse ethnic backgrounds and age groups. These findings established the universal relevance of *FTO* in obesity risk across populations.
4. **Impact on Fat Mass from Early Childhood:**
    - Importantly, the impact of *FTO* genetic variants on fat mass and body weight regulation was evident from early childhood. Studies reported measurable differences in adiposity among carriers of the risk allele as early as seven years of age, underscoring its early-life effects.
5. **High Expression in the Brain:**
    - Biological evidence further supported the role of *FTO* in energy balance, as the gene exhibited high expression levels in specific brain regions, particularly the hypothalamus — a key center for appetite regulation and energy homeostasis.

This discovery of the *FTO* gene not only transformed our understanding of the genetic underpinnings of obesity but also catalyzed a new wave of research focused on elucidating the molecular mechanisms through which *FTO* variants influence energy intake, adiposity, and long-term weight regulation.

Research Study 1: *FTO* rs9939973: A Key Genetic Determinant of BMI and Obesity

Impact on BMI and Obesity

- **Initial Discovery**: The rs9939973 variant within the *FTO* gene was identified as strongly associated with increased Body Mass Index (BMI) in the landmark study by Frayling et al., published in *Science*. This association was discovered during a genome-wide association study (GWAS) aimed at identifying genetic factors linked to type 2 diabetes. Subsequent analysis showed the association was mediated through BMI rather than directly influencing diabetes risk.
- **Effect Size**: Carriers of the risk allele (A) of rs9939973 exhibited a significant increase in BMI. Notably:
    - Homozygous individuals (A/A) were, on average, 3 kilograms heavier than non-carriers (T/T).
    - The risk allele conferred a 1.67-fold increased risk of obesity, underscoring its substantial effect size.
- **Validation Across Cohorts**: This variant was validated in 13 independent cohorts encompassing over 38,000 participants of European descent, demonstrating its robust association with BMI and obesity risk across populations and age groups.

Biological Mechanism

- **Fat Accumulation**: The effect of rs9939973 on BMI is primarily attributed to increased fat mass rather than changes in lean body mass. This was supported by anthropometric and dual-energy X-ray absorptiometry (DEXA) studies showing that the risk allele was associated with higher subcutaneous and visceral fat deposits.
- **Expression in Brain Regions**: The *FTO* gene is highly expressed in the brain, particularly in areas involved in energy homeostasis, such as the hypothalamus. This suggests its role in appetite regulation and energy expenditure.

Early-Onset Impact

- The influence of rs9939973 on BMI is evident from childhood. Longitudinal studies demonstrated that children harboring the risk allele displayed increased BMI as early as 7 years of age. This genetic effect persisted into adulthood, highlighting the long-term impact of *FTO* variants on weight regulation.

Population-Level Implications

- **Global Prevalence**: The risk allele of rs9939973 is prevalent across multiple populations, though its frequency varies. It was observed in 39% of Europeans, 52% of Yorubans, and 14% of East Asians.
- **Population Attributable Risk**: Although the variant accounts for approximately 1% of the variance in BMI at the population level, it contributes to 20.4% of the attributable risk for obesity, reflecting its considerable public health relevance.

Research Highlights

1. **Anthropometric Evidence**: Studies indicated that the rs9939973 variant was associated with increased weight, higher waist circumference, and elevated fat mass across all age groups.
2. **Mechanistic Insights**: The variant is implicated in pathways regulating appetite control and energy homeostasis, offering potential targets for personalized interventions aimed at obesity prevention and management.

Research Study 2: Validation Across Diverse Populations — Strengthening the Role of *FTO* rs9939973 in Obesity

- **Strengthened Evidence**: A study published in *BMC Medical Genetics* further substantiates the association of the rs9939973 variant in the ***FTO* gene** with increased Body Mass Index (BMI) and obesity. This study highlights its role as one of the strongest genetic determinants of obesity across various populations.

- **Effect Magnitude**: The risk allele (A) was associated with an average increase in BMI of 0.4–0.6 kg/m^2 per allele. Homozygous carriers of the A allele exhibited a 1.66-fold higher risk of obesity compared to non-carriers.

Validation in Diverse Populations

- Expanding beyond initial studies focused primarily on European populations, this research incorporated data from African and Asian cohorts, confirming the universality of the rs9939973 variant's impact on adiposity.
- **Ethnic Variations**: While the effect size of the variant on BMI remained relatively consistent across populations, notable differences in allele frequency were observed:
    - Higher prevalence in Europeans and African populations
    - Lower frequency in East Asian populations

These variations have important implications for population-level risk assessments and public health strategies.

Mechanisms Underlying the Association

- **Appetite Regulation**: The *FTO* rs9939973 variant influences brain regions responsible for hunger and satiety signals, particularly the hypothalamus. This leads to an increased propensity for overconsumption of calorie-dense foods.
- **Energy Expenditure**: Carriers of the risk allele demonstrate alterations in basal metabolic rate, contributing to weight gain.

Early and Longitudinal Effects

- The association between rs9939973 and obesity is evident from early childhood, reinforcing the gene's role in the developmental trajectory of obesity. Its effects are sustained across different life stages, contributing to long-term weight gain and obesity risk.

Population-Level Implications

- **Global Perspective**: The rs9939973 risk allele contributes significantly to the heritability of obesity. It explains approximately 1.5% of BMI variance in European populations, with a slightly lower impact in non-European groups due to allele frequency differences.
- **Public Health Relevance**: This variant has a significant attributable risk for obesity in populations with a high prevalence of the risk allele, making it a target for population-based interventions.

Research Highlights

1. **Meta-Analysis Evidence**: This study consolidates findings from multiple cohorts, emphasizing rs9939973's strong association with BMI and obesity risk.
2. **Interaction with Lifestyle Factors**: The genetic predisposition conferred by rs9939973 is exacerbated by environmental factors such as high-calorie diets, reduced physical activity, and sedentary behaviors, emphasizing the importance of lifestyle modifications in genetically susceptible individuals.

Research Study 3: Findings Related to *FTO* Gene rs9939973 in the Japanese Population

- **Significant Association in a Non-European Population**: Expanding the global understanding of the *FTO* gene's role in obesity, a study conducted in a Japanese cohort identified the rs9939973 variant as significantly associated with severe obesity (BMI ≥ 30 kg/m^2). This finding highlights its relevance in non-European populations where obesity prevalence and genetic architecture differ.
- **Effect Size**: Individuals carrying the risk allele (A) of rs9939973 showed an increased likelihood of obesity, with an odds ratio (OR) of 1.32 in additive models. The association remained robust even after adjusting for age and gender.
- **Validation Across Multiple SNPs**: Rs9939973 was among 15 SNPs located in a linkage disequilibrium (LD) block (~50 kb) that demonstrated a strong association with obesity phenotypes. This LD block also included *rs9939609*, a well-established obesity-related SNP.

Biological Mechanism

- **Gene Expression**: The *FTO* gene, including the rs9939973 variant, is predominantly expressed in the hypothalamus — a key brain region involved in energy homeostasis, appetite control, and satiety regulation.
- **Phenotypic Effects**: The study revealed that the risk allele of rs9939973 correlates with higher BMI due to increased fat accumulation, aligning with findings in European populations.

Population-Level Implications

- **Unique Impact in Asians**: While rs9939973 is associated with obesity in Japanese individuals, its effect size is smaller compared to European populations. This discrepancy may be attributed to differences in BMI distributions and lifestyle factors across populations.
- **Prevalence of the Risk Allele**: The frequency of the rs9939973 risk allele was lower in Japanese compared to Caucasian populations, which could influence its overall contribution to obesity risk in this group.

Research Highlights

1. Case-Control Evidence: The study compared 927 severely obese individuals (BMI ≥ 30 kg/m^2) to 1,527 normal-weight controls (BMI < 25 kg/m^2), identifying rs9939973 as a significant contributor to obesity in the Japanese.
2. Consistent LD Block: The SNP resides in a genomic region with high linkage disequilibrium, reinforcing its biological relevance in obesity-related pathways. https://pubmed.ncbi.nlm.nih.gov/18379722/?dopt=Abstract

Research Study 4: Findings Related to *FTO* Gene rs9939973 in the Mexican Population

Impact on BMI and Obesity

- **Association with Obesity**: In a study of the Mexican Mestizo population, the *rs9939609* variant, in strong linkage disequilibrium with rs9939973, was identified as a significant risk factor for obesity, particularly class III obesity (BMI ≥ 40 kg/m^2). The association was robust across additive and dominant genetic models, with odds ratios (OR) of 2.42 and 2.80, respectively, indicating a strong genetic predisposition.
- **Risk Allele Frequencies**: The frequency of the A allele in the Mexican population (20.5%) was lower than in European populations but higher than in Amerindian groups, reflecting the mixed ancestry of the Mexican Mestizo population.

Mechanisms Underlying the Association

- **Gene Expression in Adipose Tissue**: *FTO* mRNA levels were significantly higher in the subcutaneous adipose tissue of class III obese individuals compared to lean individuals. This upregulation was more pronounced in carriers of the risk allele (A), suggesting a role for *FTO* expression in fat accumulation and obesity development.
- **Metabolic Effects**: In non-obese individuals, the risk allele was nominally associated with lower fasting insulin levels and altered homeostasis model assessment (HOMA) indices, indicating potential effects on glucose metabolism independent of obesity.

Population-Level Implications

- **Admixture Adjustment**: The study accounted for the genetic admixture of the Mexican population, confirming that the association between *FTO* variants and obesity was not confounded by population stratification.
- **Disparities in Obesity Prevalence**: The prevalence of class III obesity in Mexico was found to be lower than in European populations, which may influence the observed genetic effects.

Research Highlights

1. **Case-Control Evidence**: The study included 788 unrelated Mexican Mestizo individuals, with a significant association observed between the A allele and obesity phenotypes, especially in the class III obesity group.
2. **Functional Insights**: Elevated *FTO* expression in adipose tissue among risk allele carriers provides mechanistic support for its role in energy storage, fat metabolism, and obesity development.

Research Study 5: Findings Related to *FTO* Gene *rs9939609* in the Roma/Gypsy Population

Impact on BMI and Obesity

- **Association with Obesity**: The *FTO rs9939609* variant showed a significant association with Body Mass Index (BMI) and other obesity indices, including waist circumference (WC) and waist-to-hip ratio (WHR), in the Roma/Gypsy population. The odds ratio (OR) for obesity among carriers of the risk allele (A) was 1.55 (95% CI: 1.129–2.128; p = 0.007), even after adjusting for age, sex, and smoking status.
- **Effect Size**: Homozygous carriers of the risk allele (AA) had a mean BMI of 28.45 kg/m^2, 3.5 units higher than non-carriers (TT homozygotes), and their waist circumference was 7.1 cm larger on average.
- **Prevalence of Obesity**: Among the Roma population, 55.9% of females and 46.6% of males were classified as overweight or obese, highlighting a high burden of obesity.

Biological Mechanism

- **Fat Accumulation**: The association of *rs9939609* with obesity is believed to stem from its effect on fat mass rather than lean body mass. Adjusting for BMI weakened the association of the SNP with central obesity metrics like WC and WHR, further supporting this hypothesis.
- **Energy Homeostasis**: The *FTO* variant may affect overall energy balance, contributing to increased fat accumulation over time.

Population-Level Implications

- **Genetic Predisposition in Isolated Populations**: The Roma population exhibited a minor allele frequency (MAF) of 0.47 for *rs9939609*, comparable to European populations (0.40–0.45) and higher than Asian populations. This highlights the genetic predisposition to obesity within this population due to its genetic background and socioeconomic factors.
- **Admixture and Evolutionary Considerations**: The allele frequency in Roma likely reflects their mixed ancestry and historical genetic drift, emphasizing the need for population-specific genetic studies.

Research Highlights

1. **Case-Control Evidence**: The study stratified the Roma population into obesity cases (BMI ≥ 25 kg/m^2) and controls, observing significant differences in allele frequency between the groups.
2. Anthropometric Insights: Carriers of the A allele consistently showed higher BMI, WC, and WHR values, emphasizing the genetic impact of *rs9939609* on obesity-related traits.

Research Study 6: Findings Related to *FTO* Gene *rs9939609* in the Multiethnic Children

Key Findings:

This study investigated the role of genetic variants, including *FTO rs9939609*, in influencing obesity traits among children from diverse ethnic backgrounds.

- **Genetic Variants Analyzed:** The research focused on 17 single nucleotide polymorphisms (SNPs) located in 16 genes previously associated with body mass index (BMI) through genome-wide association studies (GWAS).
- **Study Population:** The sample comprised 298 children from various racial and ethnic backgrounds, including European American, African American, Hispanic, and Asian American groups.
- **Cumulative Genetic Risk Score (GRS):** A composite score, aggregating risk alleles from the analyzed SNPs, was calculated for each individual. The GRS showed a positive correlation with BMI, waist circumference, and fat mass, indicating that children with a higher number of risk alleles tended to have greater obesity-related measurements.
- **Ethnic Differences:** The strength and significance of associations between specific SNPs and obesity traits varied across different ethnic groups, suggesting potential interactions between genetic predispositions and environmental or lifestyle factors unique to each group

Research Highlights:

- This study highlights the relevance of considering genetic predisposition when addressing childhood obesity, particularly in multiethnic populations.
- The findings support the potential for personalized interventions that account for an individual's genetic risk profile, thereby improving the effectiveness of obesity prevention and treatment strategies.

Research Study 7: Findings Related to *FTO* Gene *rs9939609* in Childhood and Adult Obesity

Impact on BMI and Obesity

- **Association with BMI**: SNP *rs9939609* in the ***FTO* gene** was strongly associated with BMI in both childhood and adulthood. Each copy of the risk allele (A) was linked to an increase of approximately 0.36 kg/m^2 in BMI, with homozygous individuals carrying two copies of the A allele showing an average increase of 3 kg in weight compared to those without the risk allele.

- **Odds Ratios**: Homozygous carriers had a 1.67-fold higher risk of obesity compared to non-carriers. For overweight individuals, the risk was increased by 1.38-fold per risk allele.

Validation Across Cohorts

- **Meta-Analysis Evidence**: This association was validated across 13 cohorts involving 38,759 participants. The statistical confidence of this association was robust, with a p-value of 3×10^{-35} across all studies, and showed no evidence of heterogeneity among cohorts.
- **Global Frequency of the Risk Allele**: The A allele was present in 39% of Europeans, 52% of Yorubans, and 14% of East Asians, indicating its varying contribution to obesity risk across populations.

Age-Dependent Effects

- **Early Childhood Impact**: In longitudinal studies, the association of *rs9939609* with BMI was evident from the age of 7 years and persisted through adolescence and adulthood. At age 11, the A allele was associated with a BMI increase of 0.4 kg/m^2 and a 1.35-fold increased risk of obesity.
- **Absence at Birth**: No association was observed between *rs9939609* and birth weight, indicating that its effects emerge after birth.

Mechanisms of Action

- **Fat Accumulation**: The association of the A allele with BMI was largely due to increased fat mass rather than changes in lean body mass. This was confirmed through dual-energy X-ray absorptiometry (DEXA) scans in children, where fat mass was significantly elevated in carriers of the risk allele.
- **Brain Expression**: The *FTO* gene showed high expression in the hypothalamus — a key brain region involved in appetite control and energy homeostasis — suggesting its role in promoting increased food intake and energy storage.

Population-Level Implications

- The *rs9939609* SNP accounted for approximately 1% of the variance in BMI across populations.
- In European populations, it contributed to 20.4% of the population-attributable risk for obesity, highlighting its considerable role in obesity prevalence.

Research Study 8: Findings Related to *FTO* Gene *rs9939609* in the Chinese population

Key Findings:

- **Association with BMI and Obesity:** The study found that the A allele of *rs9939609* is significantly associated with increased BMI and a higher risk of obesity in Chinese children. Specifically, each additional A allele corresponded to an increase in BMI and an elevated likelihood of being overweight or obese.
- **Metabolic Traits:** Beyond BMI, the A allele was also linked to higher levels of serum triglycerides and insulin, indicating a broader impact on metabolic health.
- **Prevalence of the A Allele:** The frequency of the A allele in this Chinese cohort was lower compared to European populations, which may contribute to differences in obesity prevalence and genetic risk factors between ethnic groups.

Implications:

- The study indicates that the *FTO rs9939609* variant plays a similar role in childhood obesity in the Chinese population as observed in European populations.
- However, the lower frequency of the risk allele in Chinese children may influence the overall genetic risk for obesity in this group.

Diet-Gene Interaction Studies

Thus far, multiple studies have consistently demonstrated a strong association between the *FTO* gene variant *rs9939609* and increased body mass index (BMI) and obesity risk across diverse populations, including both children and adults.

Building on this evidence, the following section will explore research investigating how dietary factors may influence weight management and metabolic outcomes in individuals carrying this specific *FTO* SNP.

Findings Related to *FTO* Gene *rs9939609* and Macronutrient-Specific Diets in Obese Europeans

Study Overview

- **Objective**: This study investigated the impact of the *FTO rs9939609* variant on weight loss and metabolic changes during a 10-week randomized hypo-energetic diet intervention, comparing high-fat (HF) and low-fat (LF) diets.
- **Participants**: A total of 771 obese European adults were randomized to either an HF diet (40–45% energy from fat) or an LF diet (20–25% energy from fat). Anthropometric and metabolic parameters were measured before and after the intervention.

Key Findings

1. **Dietary Impact and Genetic Interaction**:
   - **Dropout Rates**: Carriers of the A allele had higher dropout rates when assigned to the HF diet compared to the LF diet (AA: 28.3% vs. 16.9%, respectively). TT genotype individuals showed lower dropout rates on the HF diet.
   - **Weight Loss**: No significant effect of *rs9939609* on weight loss, fat mass reduction, or waist circumference changes was observed between the HF and LF diet groups.
2. **Resting Energy Expenditure (REE)**:
   - TT genotype individuals exhibited a smaller reduction in REE on the LF diet compared to the HF diet (75 kcal/day difference; p=0.006), indicating a potential advantage of LF diets for this group.
3. **Insulin Sensitivity and Secretion**:
   - TT carriers showed greater improvements in insulin secretion (HOMA-b, p=0.008) and insulin resistance (HOMA-IR, p=0.047) on the LF diet compared to the HF diet. A allele carriers did not exhibit significant differences between diets.
4. **Overall Compliance**:
   - Participants on the LF diet had a higher compliance rate, particularly among A allele carriers, suggesting that macronutrient composition may influence adherence to dietary interventions.

Population-Level Implications

- These findings emphasize the relevance of personalized nutrition, where diet plans may be optimized based on genetic profiles.
- For TT genotype individuals, LF diets may offer additional metabolic benefits and better preservation of energy expenditure during weight loss.
- A allele carriers, despite not showing superior metabolic responses, demonstrated better compliance with LF diets, suggesting its practical utility for weight management.

Research Highlights

1. **Macronutrient Composition Matters**: The interaction between *rs9939609* and dietary fat and carbohydrate content underscores the importance of personalized nutrition.
2. **Behavioral Factors and Compliance**: The higher dropout rates among A allele carriers on HF diets suggest that genetic predisposition may also influence dietary preferences, tolerances, and adherence — factors crucial for long-term weight management.

Findings Related to *FTO* Gene *rs9939609* and Diet in Obesity

Impact of Macronutrient Composition on BMI

Research exploring the interaction between dietary patterns and the *FTO* gene variant *rs9939609* has provided valuable insights into the role of macronutrient composition in modulating obesity risk.

- **High-Fat Diet**: In individuals following an energy-adjusted high-fat diet, carriers of the risk allele (A) showed significantly higher BMI compared to non-carriers. AA carriers had an average BMI of 26.3 kg/m² compared to 25.3 kg/m² for TT carriers ($p = 0.0001$).
- **Low-Carbohydrate Diet**: Among individuals with a low-carbohydrate diet, AA carriers exhibited a mean BMI of 26.8 kg/m² compared to 25.4 kg/m² for TT carriers ($p < 0.0001$). The risk allele significantly increased obesity risk in this group.

Gene-Diet Interactions

- **Fat Intake**: The study identified a significant interaction between fat intake and *FTO* genotype on BMI ($p = 0.04$). AA carriers consuming high-fat diets were 2.47 times more likely to be obese compared to TT carriers.
- **Carbohydrate Intake**: A similar interaction was observed for carbohydrate intake ($p = 0.001$). High carbohydrate intake mitigated the BMI differences across *FTO* genotypes, while low carbohydrate intake exacerbated the risk of obesity for AA carriers.

Behavioral and Lifestyle Factors

- **Physical Activity**: Low levels of leisure-time physical activity amplified the BMI differences associated with *FTO* genotypes. Inactive AA carriers had a significantly higher BMI compared to active individuals with the same genotype.
- **Underreporting of Energy Intake**: A higher proportion of AA carriers were classified as underreporters of energy intake, particularly among obese individuals. This suggests potential biases in dietary self-reporting influenced by genotype.

Clinical Implications

- **Personalized Dietary Advice**: These findings emphasize the need for tailored dietary recommendations based on *FTO* genotype. Reducing fat intake and increasing carbohydrate intake may mitigate the genetic predisposition to obesity among AA carriers.
- **Lifestyle Modifications**: Encouraging physical activity could reduce the obesogenic effects of the *FTO* variant, offering an additional intervention strategy.

Research Highlights

- This study underscores the complex interplay between genetic predisposition, dietary macronutrient composition, and lifestyle factors in determining obesity risk.
- The findings provide strong support for the integration of precision nutrition approaches — incorporating genetic screening and personalized dietary advice — in the prevention and management of obesity.

Dietary Recommendations for Individuals with *FTO rs9939609* Variant

Based on the findings from the research studies, tailored dietary interventions for individuals with the ***FTO rs9939609* variant** can significantly influence weight management and metabolic health. The following evidence-based recommendations outline optimal dietary and lifestyle approaches for individuals carrying the *FTO rs9939609* variant.

1. Low-Fat Diet (LF) Benefits

- **Ideal for A Allele Carriers**: Individuals with the A allele (including AA and AT genotypes) exhibit better adherence and compliance with low-fat diets compared to high-fat diets. The LF diet minimizes dropout rates and may help sustain dietary changes.
- **Metabolic Advantages for TT Genotype**:
    - TT carriers on LF diets experience smaller reductions in resting energy expenditure (REE) compared to high-fat diets, helping preserve metabolic rate during weight loss.
    - Improvements in insulin sensitivity and secretion (HOMA-b and HOMA-IR) were more pronounced in TT carriers on LF diets, reducing the risk of metabolic disorders.

Dietary Strategy:

- Focus on **20–25% of total energy from fat**, with a preference for unsaturated fats found in nuts, seeds, and fatty fish.
- Emphasize lean proteins and high-fiber foods such as whole grains, vegetables, and legumes to enhance satiety.

2. High-Carbohydrate Diet Considerations

For A Allele Carriers

- Higher carbohydrate intake appears to mitigate the impact of the risk allele on BMI, helping to balance weight outcomes across genotypes.
- Carbohydrates provide an efficient energy source, especially when combined with regular physical activity, reducing fat accumulation in A allele carriers.

Dietary Strategy:

- Target **45–55% of total energy from carbohydrates**, prioritizing complex carbohydrates like whole grains, vegetables, and fruits.
- Limit refined sugars and processed carbohydrates to prevent spikes in blood glucose and insulin.

3. Avoidance of High-Fat Diets

For A Allele Carriers

- Consumption of high-fat diets significantly increases obesity risk in A allele carriers, with studies indicating a 2.47-fold higher likelihood of obesity compared to TT carriers.
- This risk is particularly pronounced in individuals with low levels of physical activity.

Dietary Strategy:

- Limit fat intake to no more than **30% of total energy**, focusing on reducing saturated fats found in red meats, full-fat dairy, and fried foods.

4. Encourage Physical Activity

- **Amplifying Benefits of Dietary Interventions**:
  - Physical activity reduces BMI differences associated with *FTO* genotypes and offsets the negative effects of low activity levels, particularly in A allele carriers.
- **Behavioral Influence**: Active lifestyles complement high-carbohydrate diets, enhancing energy utilization and reducing fat storage.

Lifestyle Strategy:

- Recommend at least **150 minutes of moderate-intensity aerobic activity** per week, combined with strength training exercises twice a week.

5. Structured Meal Planning to Improve Adherence

Addressing Underreporting of Energy Intake

- A allele carriers, particularly those with obesity, are prone to underreporting caloric intake, potentially hindering weight-loss progress.

Behavioral Strategies

- Implement structured meal plans and portion control techniques to support accurate energy intake monitoring.
- Utilize smaller plates, pre-portioned meals, and food diaries or nutrition tracking apps to facilitate dietary adherence.

Summary of Dietary Recommendations

Genotype	Recommended Diet	Macronutrient Focus	Lifestyle Add-ons
AA/AT	Low-fat, high-carbohydrate	20–25% fat, 45–55% carbohydrates	Encourage physical activity and meal tracking for adherence.
TT	Low-fat diet	20–25% fat, lean proteins, high fiber	Focus on improving metabolic health and maintaining exercise routines.

These recommendations highlight the importance of tailoring dietary and lifestyle interventions to the genetic predispositions of individuals with the *FTO rs9939609* variant, optimizing weight management and metabolic outcomes.

Having explored the role of the *FTO* gene in obesity, we now turn our attention to another important genetic determinant — the Melanocortin 4 Receptor (*MC4R*) gene — which has also been widely studied for its role in appetite regulation and energy balance.

Real-Life Example: Understanding the *FTO rs9939609* Polymorphism

Consider Alex, a 32-year-old working professional with a predominantly sedentary lifestyle. Alex and a colleague of similar age follow comparable daily routines, consume similar amounts of food, and engage in limited physical activity. Despite these similarities, Alex consistently experiences early hunger after meals and gradual weight gain, while the colleague maintains a relatively stable body weight.

Genetic analysis shows that Alex carries two copies of the A risk allele (AA genotype) of the *FTO rs9939609* polymorphism, whereas the colleague carries the TT genotype. The A allele is associated with reduced satiety signaling and increased appetite, particularly for energy-dense foods. As a result, Alex's brain receives weaker fullness signals after eating, increasing the likelihood of higher energy intake under identical environmental conditions.

When Alex adopts a low-fat, high-fiber diet, follows structured meal timing, and incorporates regular physical activity, appetite control improves, and weight gain stabilizes. This example illustrates that *FTO*-related genetic susceptibility influences obesity risk, but does not determine outcome, emphasizing the importance of lifestyle modification in genetically predisposed individuals.

The *MC4R* Gene: Its Significance in Obesity Genetics

The melanocortin-4 receptor (*MC4R*) gene has been a focal point in obesity genetics, given its critical role in energy homeostasis and appetite regulation. Initially, rare mutations in *MC4R* were identified as one of the most common monogenic causes of severe early-onset obesity. However, with advancements in genome-wide association studies (GWAS), common variants within or near the *MC4R* gene have also been recognized as important contributors to polygenic obesity.

Among these variants, single nucleotide polymorphisms (SNPs) such as *rs17782313* and rs12970134 have been extensively studied and consistently associated with increased Body Mass Index (BMI) and obesity risk across diverse ethnic populations.

Key Insights from the Discovery of *MC4R* SNPs

MC4R rs17782313: A Significant Genetic Factor in Obesity

Impact on BMI and Obesity

- **Initial Discovery:** The ***rs17782313*** variant, located 188 kb downstream of the *MC4R* gene, was first identified through GWAS as a significant determinant of BMI. Loos et al. (2008) and others reported a strong association between this SNP and increased obesity risk.
- **Effect Size:** Individuals carrying the risk allele (C) exhibit higher BMI values and an increased risk of obesity. Individuals homozygous for the C allele may weigh up to 1.5 kg more than non-carriers and have a 1.25-fold increased risk of developing obesity.
- **Validation Across Populations:** This variant has been extensively replicated in multiple cohorts, including European, Asian, and Hispanic populations, with consistent effects on BMI and adiposity.

Biological Mechanism

- **Involvement in Appetite Regulation:** *MC4R* is a key player in the central melanocortin system, which regulates energy intake and expenditure. The *rs17782313* risk allele has been linked to increased appetite and a preference for high-energy foods.
- **Brain Expression Patterns:** The *MC4R* gene is highly expressed in the hypothalamus, where it modulates satiety signals via interactions with *Leptin* and pro-opiomelanocortin (*POMC*) pathways.

Early-Onset Impact

- The effects of ***rs17782313*** on BMI are observable from **early childhood**, with significant weight gain evident as early as **5 years of age**.
- In longitudinal studies, children carrying the risk allele demonstrated increased food intake and reduced satiety responses, predisposing them to long-term obesity.

Population-Level Implications

- **Global Prevalence:** The risk allele (C) has varying frequencies across populations:
    - **European:** ~22%
    - **East Asian:** ~42%
    - **African:** ~9%
- **Population Attributable Risk:** The *rs17782313* allele accounts for approximately **0.4-0.6% of BMI variance** at the population level, making it one of the strongest common genetic predictors of obesity.

Real-Life Example

Consider an individual carrying two copies of the **C allele** of *rs17782313*. Compared to a non-carrier, they may have an increased appetite, a preference for calorie-dense foods, and a higher likelihood of weight gain, particularly when exposed to an energy-rich diet.

Research Highlights

- **Anthropometric Evidence:** *rs17782313* is consistently associated with increased weight, waist circumference, and obesity risk across multiple studies.
- **Mechanistic Insights:** This SNP may disrupt normal *MC4R* signaling, reducing satiety and increasing caloric intake, thereby promoting weight gain.

MC4R rs12970134: A Strong Determinant of Fat Mass and Obesity

Impact on BMI and Obesity

- **Initial Discovery:** The **rs12970134** SNP, located near the *MC4R* gene, was identified through GWAS as a significant determinant of BMI and adiposity.
- **Effect Size:** Individuals carrying the risk allele (A) exhibit a higher BMI by approximately 0.2–0.3 kg/m^2 and have an estimated 1.21-fold increased risk of developing obesity compared to non-carriers.
- **Validation Across Populations:** These findings have been consistently replicated across diverse ethnic groups, including European, Asian, and Hispanic populations, confirming the robust association of rs12970134 with increased adiposity.

Biological Mechanism

- **Regulation of Energy Balance:** *MC4R* is a critical receptor in the hypothalamic control of hunger and satiety. Variants like **rs12970134** may influence food intake by **altering neuronal signaling** in response to metabolic cues.
- **Neural and Hormonal Interactions:** This SNP has been associated with elevated circulating levels of ghrelin, a key appetite-stimulating hormone, suggesting that carriers of the risk allele may experience increased hunger and altered appetite regulation.

Early-Onset Impact

- The influence of the rs12970134 risk allele is evident from early life. Children carrying this allele tend to exhibit higher hunger scores and increased caloric intake compared to non-carriers, predisposing them to early weight gain and obesity development.

Population-Level Implications

- **Global Prevalence:** The risk allele (A) has been observed in varying frequencies:
    - **European:** ~30%
    - **East Asian:** ~50%
    - **African:** ~20%
- **Population Attributable Risk:** This SNP accounts for approximately 0.3% of the variance in BMI at the population level, making it a notable contributor to the genetic risk of obesity.

Real-Life Example

An individual carrying the A allele of rs12970134 may experience heightened hunger sensations and a greater tendency to overconsume food, particularly in environments with easy access to calorie-dense, highly palatable foods.

Research Highlights

- **Appetite Regulation:** rs12970134 is linked to increased hunger perception and greater food intake, making it a target for behavioral and pharmacological interventions.
- **Energy Expenditure:** In addition to its role in appetite regulation, this SNP may also influence basal metabolic rate (BMR), contributing to individual differences in energy expenditure and overall energy balance.

Findings Related to *MC4R* Gene Polymorphisms among Different Population

Research Study 1 — Chinese Population

Key Findings

Association with BMI and Obesity:

- ***rs17782313*:** The C allele of *rs17782313* has been significantly associated with increased BMI and a higher risk of obesity among Chinese individuals. A meta-analysis reported an odds ratio (OR) of 1.18 (95% CI: 1.15–1.21, $p < 0.001$) for obesity risk associated with this allele.
- **rs12970134:** The A allele of rs12970134 is linked to higher BMI and an elevated risk of overweight/obesity in Chinese children and adolescents. Specifically, each additional A allele

corresponded to an increase in BMI ($\beta = 0.33$ kg/m^2, 95% CI: 0.02–0.63, $p = 0.025$) and a higher likelihood of being overweight or obese (OR = 1.21, 95% CI: 1.03–1.44, $p = 0.025$).

Impact on Appetite and Food Intake

- **rs12970134:** This variant has been associated with increased food responsiveness and beverage intake among overweight and obese Chinese children. Carriers of the A allele exhibited higher scores for food responsiveness and greater beverage consumption. Mediation analysis suggested that food responsiveness partially mediates the effect of rs12970134 on beverage intake.

Gene-Environment Interactions

- **Physical Activity and Sedentary Behaviors:** The association between rs12970134 and BMI appears to be influenced by lifestyle factors. The effect of the A allele on increased BMI was more pronounced in children engaging in less than 1 hour of physical activity per day and those with 2 or more hours of sedentary behavior daily. This highlights the interplay between genetic predisposition and environmental factors in obesity risk.

Combined Genetic Effects

- ***FTO* and *MC4R* Interaction:** Research exploring the combined effects of risk variants in both *FTO* and *MC4R* genes reported that individuals carrying risk alleles at both loci had a higher susceptibility to obesity, suggesting a potential synergistic interaction between these genes.

Prevalence of Risk Alleles

- The frequency of the risk alleles for *rs17782313* and rs12970134 in the Chinese population is lower compared to European populations. This difference in allele prevalence may contribute to variations in obesity rates and genetic susceptibility between ethnic groups.

Implications

These findings indicate that *MC4R* gene polymorphisms, particularly *rs17782313* and rs12970134, play a significant role in influencing BMI, obesity risk, and related behaviors in the Chinese population. The interaction between these genetic factors and environmental influences, such as physical activity and dietary habits, underscores the importance of a comprehensive approach to obesity prevention and intervention that considers both genetic and lifestyle components.

Research Study 2 — Indian Population

Association with Obesity

- ***rs17782313*:** Studies investigating the *rs17782313* polymorphism in the Indian population have yielded mixed results. Some research indicates a potential association with increased body weight among children, while other studies have not found a significant link to obesity. For instance, one study reported that the *MC4R* variant (*rs17782313*) predicted increased body weight among children, but was not associated with other adiposity measures.

Prevalence of Risk Alleles

- The frequency of the risk alleles for *MC4R* polymorphisms in the Indian population varies across different studies, and further research is needed to establish definitive prevalence rates.

Implications

- The inconsistent findings suggest that while *MC4R* polymorphisms may influence body weight in certain subsets of the Indian population, their overall impact on obesity risk requires further investigation.

Research Study 3 — Findings from Different Populations on *MC4R* Gene Polymorphisms

European Population

Association with Obesity

- ***rs17782313* and rs12970134:** These polymorphisms have been consistently associated with increased BMI and obesity risk in European populations. A meta-analysis reported that the *rs17782313* variant is significantly associated with obesity risk, with an odds ratio (OR) of 1.18.

Prevalence of Risk Alleles

- The risk alleles of these *MC4R* polymorphisms are relatively common in European populations, contributing substantially to the genetic predisposition to obesity within this population.

Implications

- The strong and consistent association between *MC4R* variants and obesity risk underscores the importance of considering genetic factors in obesity prevention, management, and personalized intervention strategies in European populations.

African Population

Association with Obesity

- ***rs17782313*: Research on the association between *MC4R* polymorphisms and obesity in African populations is limited and has produced inconclusive results. Some studies conducted in African American cohorts have reported no significant association between *rs17782313* and obesity risk.

Prevalence of Risk Alleles

- The frequency of *MC4R* risk alleles in African populations appears to be lower compared to European populations, which may influence the genetic susceptibility to obesity in this group.

Implications

- The lack of a consistent association suggests that *MC4R* polymorphisms may have a limited impact on obesity risk in African populations, and that other genetic or environmental factors could play a more significant role.

Other Populations (East Asians and Hispanics)

Association with Obesity

- ***rs17782313* and rs12970134:** Studies in various populations, including East Asians and Hispanics, have demonstrated associations between these *MC4R* polymorphisms and increased BMI or obesity risk. However, the strength of these associations varies across different ethnic groups, reflecting genetic diversity and population-specific factors.

Prevalence of Risk Alleles

- The prevalence of *MC4R* risk alleles differs among populations, influencing the degree of genetic predisposition to obesity.

Implications

- Understanding the population-specific effects of *MC4R* polymorphisms is crucial for developing tailored public health strategies and interventions to combat obesity globally.

Conclusion

MC4R gene polymorphisms, particularly *rs17782313* and rs12970134, demonstrate variable associations with obesity across different populations. These population-specific differences highlight the significance of considering ethnic diversity and genetic backgrounds in evaluating obesity risk. Integrating genetic information into personalized prevention and intervention strategies may enhance the effectiveness of obesity management across diverse demographic groups.

Dietary Recommendations for Individuals with *MC4R rs17782313* Variant

Research Study 1: *MC4R* Gene *rs17782313* and Dietary Intake in Women

Key Findings

- **Genetic Variant Analyzed:** The study focused on the ***MC4R rs17782313*** polymorphism and its association with dietary intake, weight change, and diabetes risk.
- **Study Population:** The research involved **two large U.S. cohorts of women**, including **37,059 participants from the Nurses' Health Study** and **44,181 participants from the Health Professionals Follow-up Study**.
- **Associations with Obesity and Diet:**
    - **Higher Energy and Fat Intake: Individuals carrying the C allele** exhibited significantly **higher total energy intake** and **increased fat consumption** compared to non-carriers.
    - **Long-Term Weight Gain: *MC4R rs17782313* carriers** experienced **greater weight gain over a 20-year period**, which was associated with an **increased risk of developing type 2 diabetes.**
    - **Food Preferences:** Carriers of the **C allele** demonstrated a **preference for fatty foods**, potentially contributing to obesity risk.

Implications

This study provides **strong evidence** that ***MC4R rs17782313*** **plays a significant role in obesity by influencing dietary habits and energy intake**. The findings highlight the importance of **genetic screening and personalized nutrition strategies** for individuals carrying this variant. Tailored interventions that **limit dietary fat intake and promote healthier food choices** could help **mitigate obesity risk and prevent type 2 diabetes** in genetically predisposed individuals.

Nutritional Recommendations

- **Limit dietary fat intake**: Since ***MC4R*** **carriers tend to consume more fat**, limiting fat intake to **<25% of total energy** can help manage weight gain.
- **Increase protein and fiber intake**: Emphasizing high-protein and fiber-rich foods may enhance satiety and reduce overall caloric intake.
- **Monitor total energy intake**: Structured meal planning and portion control can help prevent overeating tendencies associated with this variant.

Research Study 2: *MC4R* Genotype, Dietary Protein, and Appetite Regulation

Key Findings

- **Genetic Variant Analyzed:** The study focused on the *MC4R* rs7227255 polymorphism and its interaction with dietary protein intake on appetite regulation.
- **Study Population:** The research followed 700 overweight or obese adults enrolled in the POUNDS Lost clinical trial, a two-year randomized controlled weight-loss study.
- **Associations with Appetite and Protein Intake:**
    - **Increased Hunger with High Protein Diets:** Individuals carrying the A allele of rs7227255 experienced greater increases in appetite and food cravings when consuming a high-protein diet.
    - **Lower Appetite with Low-Protein Diets:** *MC4R* variant carriers on a low-protein diet reported lower appetite levels, suggesting that high protein intake might trigger increased hunger in individuals with this genetic variation.

Nutritional Recommendations

- **Moderate Protein Intake:** Individuals carrying the A allele should avoid extremely high-protein diets (>30% of total energy) to prevent increased appetite.
- **Balance Macronutrients Distribution:** A diet composed of lean protein, complex carbohydrates, and healthy fats may help regulate hunger and promote sustainable weight loss.
- **Strategic Meal Timing:** Distributing protein intake evenly throughout the day can help regulate hunger hormones and support sustainable weight management in *MC4R* variant carriers.

Research Study 3: *MC4R* Gene and Dietary Fat Quality in Metabolic Syndrome

Key Findings

- **Genetic Variant Analyzed:** The study examined *MC4R* polymorphisms and their interaction with dietary fat quality on metabolic syndrome risk.
- **Study Population:** Research was conducted on an Iranian cohort assessing dietary fat intake and *MC4R*-related metabolic disturbances.
- **Associations Between Fat Intake and Metabolic Health:**
    - **Increased Metabolic Syndrome Risk with Saturated Fats:** *MC4R* variant carriers consuming higher saturated fats had a greater risk of developing metabolic syndrome.
    - **Protective Effect of Unsaturated Fats:** Replacing saturated fats with unsaturated fats (such as those found in nuts, seeds, and olive oil) significantly reduced metabolic risks.
    - **Stronger Gene-Diet Interaction:** *MC4R* risk allele carriers showed better metabolic outcomes on diets low in saturated fats, highlighting a strong interaction between genetic predisposition and dietary fat quality.

Nutritional Recommendations

- **Limit Saturated Fat Intake:** Restrict saturated fat consumption to less than 7% of total energy intake to mitigate the risk of metabolic syndrome.
- **Emphasize Unsaturated Fats:** Prioritize olive oil, avocado, nuts, and fatty fish as primary fat sources to support metabolic health.
- **Limit Processed and Fried Foods:** Avoid trans fats commonly found in processed and fried foods, which can exacerbate metabolic disturbances in *MC4R* variant carriers.

Research Study 4: *MC4R rs17782313* and Dietary Carbohydrates in Obese Women

Key Findings

- **Genetic Variant Analyzed:** The study focused on the *MC4R rs17782313* polymorphism and its interaction with carbohydrate intake on BMI and metabolic outcomes.
- **Study Population:** Overweight and obese women were assessed to determine how carbohydrate intake modifies genetic predisposition to obesity.
- **Associations Between Carbohydrate Intake and BMI:**
    - **Higher Carbohydrate Intake Increases BMI:** Individuals carrying the *rs17782313* risk allele exhibited higher BMI and waist circumference when consuming higher carbohydrate diets.
    - **Enhanced Weight Loss with Carbohydrate Restriction:** *MC4R* variant carriers benefited more from reducing carbohydrate intake, leading to greater weight loss.
    - **Improved Insulin Sensitivity with Lower Carbohydrate Intake:** Reducing carbohydrates improved insulin sensitivity, particularly in individuals carrying the *MC4R* risk allele.

Nutritional Recommendations

- **Reduce Simple Carbohydrate Intake:** Minimize refined carbohydrates, such as white bread, pastries, and sugary drinks, to stabilize blood sugar levels and prevent excessive fat accumulation.
- **Emphasize Complex Carbohydrates:** Increase fiber intake from whole grains, legumes, and vegetables to promote satiety and support metabolic health.
- **Consider Moderate Carbohydrate Restriction:** A diet with 40–45% carbohydrates may be optimal for weight management in *MC4R* carriers, as lower carbohydrate intake enhances insulin sensitivity and supports fat loss.

Summary of Dietary Recommendations

Genotype	Recommended Diet	Macronutrient Focus	Lifestyle Add-ons
MC4R Variant Carriers	Low-fat, balanced diet	20–25% fat, 45–55% carbohydrates	Encourage physical activity and portion control.
Non-Variant Carriers	Balanced diet	25–35% fat, 45–55% carbohydrates	Maintain regular physical activity.

Conclusion

Research findings emphasize the significance of personalized nutrition strategies for individuals carrying *MC4R* gene variants. The presence of *MC4R* polymorphisms influences appetite regulation, food preferences, energy intake, and metabolic health. Tailoring macronutrient composition — particularly reducing saturated fat intake and moderating carbohydrate consumption — can optimize weight management and reduce the risk of metabolic disorders in genetically predisposed individuals.

These insights reinforce the emerging role of nutrigenetics in obesity prevention and treatment. Understanding gene-diet interactions provides a valuable framework for developing individualized dietary recommendations, enhancing the effectiveness of nutritional interventions in combating obesity and its related metabolic complications.

The *LPL* Gene: Its Significance in Obesity Genetics

Lipoprotein lipase (LPL) is a critical enzyme in lipid metabolism, primarily responsible for hydrolyzing triglycerides in lipoproteins into free fatty acids and glycerol. This process plays a fundamental role in energy balance, fat storage, and lipid utilization. Given its involvement in lipid processing, variations in the LPL gene have been extensively studied for their potential association with obesity and Body Mass Index (BMI).

Genome-wide association studies (GWAS) have identified several single-nucleotide polymorphisms (SNPs) within the LPL gene that influence fat distribution, obesity risk, and metabolic health.

LPL rs328: A Protective Variant Against Obesity

Impact on BMI and Obesity

Initial Discovery: The rs328 polymorphism in the LPL gene results in a missense mutation (S447X), leading to a truncated enzyme with enhanced lipolytic activity. GWAS have identified this variant as protective against obesity and metabolic disorders.

Effect Size: Individuals carrying the minor allele (X allele) exhibit lower triglyceride levels, increased HDL cholesterol, and a reduced risk of obesity. Studies suggest that the S447X mutation is associated with a BMI reduction of approximately 0.3–0.5 kg/m^2.

Validation Across Populations: The protective effects of rs328 have been replicated in multiple populations, including European, Asian, and Hispanic cohorts.

Biological Mechanism

- **Enhanced Lipolysis:** The S447X mutation increases LPL enzyme efficiency, promoting better clearance of triglycerides from the bloodstream.
- **Improved Fat Utilization:** This variant is linked to enhanced fatty acid oxidation and reduced adiposity, contributing to lower BMI and a healthier metabolic profile.

Population-Level Implications

Global Prevalence: The frequency of the protective X allele varies across populations:

- European: ~15%
- East Asian: ~10%
- African: ~5%

Population Attributable Risk: The rs328 variant contributes to approximately 0.4% of the variation in BMI, making it a relevant genetic factor in lipid metabolism and obesity prevention.

Real-Life Example

An individual carrying the X allele of rs328 may have a lower likelihood of developing obesity due to enhanced lipid clearance and metabolic efficiency. This genetic advantage is particularly beneficial in high-fat dietary environments, where efficient fat metabolism can mitigate weight gain.

LPL rs13702: A Key Regulator of Fat Distribution

Impact on BMI and Obesity

Initial Discovery: The rs13702 variant, located in the 3′ untranslated region of the LPL gene, has been associated with variations in lipid levels, fat distribution, and obesity risk.

Effect Size: Individuals carrying the minor allele (T) exhibit reduced triglyceride levels, increased HDL cholesterol, and a lower risk of obesity. The estimated effect on BMI is a reduction of ~0.2–0.4 kg/m^2.

Validation Across Populations: Multiple studies confirm the association between rs13702 and improved lipid profiles, with consistent effects observed across European and Asian populations.

Biological Mechanism

- **MicroRNA Regulation:** The T allele disrupts a microRNA binding site, leading to increased LPL expression and enhanced triglyceride metabolism.

- **Improved Lipid Clearance:** This variant promotes more efficient fat utilization, reducing adiposity and obesity risk.

Population-Level Implications

Global Prevalence:

- European: ~25%
- East Asian: ~20%
- African: ~10%

Population Attributable Risk: The rs13702 variant explains approximately 0.3% of BMI variation, underscoring its role in lipid metabolism and obesity susceptibility.

Real-Life Example

A person with the T allele of rs13702 may have a lower predisposition to obesity due to enhanced fat metabolism and lower triglyceride accumulation, making dietary fat intake less impactful on weight gain.

Research Highlights

- **Anthropometric Evidence:** Both rs328 and rs13702 are consistently associated with lower BMI, reduced waist circumference, and improved lipid profiles.
- **Mechanistic Insights:** These variants enhance LPL activity, leading to better lipid clearance and reduced fat accumulation, offering potential therapeutic targets for obesity management.

Findings Related to LPL Gene Polymorphisms Among Different Populations

European Population

- **Association with Obesity:** The LPL rs328 and rs13702 variants have been linked to lower BMI and a reduced risk of metabolic disorders in European cohorts.
- **Implications:** Genetic screening can guide obesity prevention strategies focusing on lipid metabolism.

Asian Population

- **Association with Obesity:** Similar protective effects of rs328 and rs13702 have been observed, although allele frequencies differ from European populations.
- **Implications:** Personalized dietary recommendations could leverage these genetic variations to optimize lipid metabolism and weight management.

African Population

- **Association with Obesity:** The prevalence of protective LPL variants is lower in African populations, potentially influencing obesity risk differently.
- **Implications:** Further research is needed to explore additional genetic and environmental factors affecting obesity in African populations.

Conclusion

The LPL gene plays a significant role in lipid metabolism and obesity risk. Variants such as rs328 and rs13702 demonstrate protective effects against obesity by enhancing triglyceride metabolism and promoting better fat utilization. Understanding these genetic factors provides valuable insights for developing personalized nutrition strategies and metabolic health interventions aimed at reducing obesity risk across diverse populations.

The *LEPR* Gene: Its Significance in Obesity Genetics

The identification of the ***LEPR*** **(*Leptin* Receptor) gene** as a key regulator of obesity and **Body Mass Index (BMI)** is a significant advancement in the field of molecular genetics. The *LEPR* gene encodes the *Leptin* receptor, a crucial component in **energy homeostasis, appetite regulation, and fat metabolism**. Mutations and genetic variations in *LEPR* have been linked to ***Leptin*** **resistance, increased adiposity, and higher BMI**.

Genome-wide association studies (GWAS) have consistently identified *LEPR* polymorphisms as significant contributors to obesity risk and related metabolic disturbances, making the gene a focal point in obesity research and precision medicine.

Key Insights

Initial Association with Obesity and BMI

LEPR variants were first identified in **monogenic obesity**, where severe obesity resulted from mutations causing impaired *Leptin* signaling. Subsequent large-scale studies revealed that common ***LEPR*** **polymorphisms influence BMI and obesity risk** in the general population.

Discovery of SNP *rs1137101* (Q223R)

- The ***rs1137101*** **(Q223R) polymorphism** in the *LEPR* gene is one of the most extensively studied variants associated with obesity.
- The **A allele** of *rs1137101* has been linked to **higher BMI, increased fat mass, and *Leptin* resistance**.
- Studies have shown that individuals carrying the **AA genotype** have a **higher prevalence of obesity** compared to those with the GG genotype.

Validation Across Diverse Cohorts

- The association between ***LEPR rs1137101* and BMI** has been validated in multiple studies across different ethnicities, including **European, Asian, and African populations**.
- Meta-analyses confirm that **this SNP significantly contributes to obesity susceptibility**, emphasizing its role in global obesity trends.

Biological Mechanism

Leptin Resistance and Energy Regulation

- The *LEPR* gene encodes a receptor for ***Leptin*, a hormone secreted by adipose tissue that signals satiety**.
- Variants like ***rs1137101*** affect the receptor's ability to bind *Leptin*, leading to **impaired appetite control and persistent hunger**.
- Dysfunctional ***Leptin* signaling contributes to increased food intake**, reduced energy expenditure, and difficulty in weight management.

Expression in Hypothalamic Brain Regions

- The ***LEPR* gene is highly expressed in the hypothalamus**, the brain region responsible for **appetite control and energy balance**.
- Disruptions in *LEPR* function result in **altered hypothalamic signaling**, leading to excessive calorie intake and obesity.

Inflammatory Pathways and Obesity

- *LEPR* mutations have been linked to **chronic low-grade inflammation**, a key factor in obesity-related metabolic disorders.
- High *Leptin* levels in individuals with ***Leptin* resistance** contribute to **systemic inflammation**, increasing the risk of insulin resistance and metabolic syndrome.

Early-Onset Impact

LEPR Variants and Childhood Obesity

- Studies have demonstrated that **the impact of *LEPR* polymorphisms on BMI begins early in life.**
- Longitudinal studies show that children carrying the **risk allele of *rs1137101*** tend to have **higher BMI from an early age**.
- This genetic predisposition often persists into adulthood, influencing long-term obesity risk.

Population-Level Implications

Global Prevalence of *LEPR* Variants

- The **risk allele of *rs1137101* varies in frequency across populations**:
    - **Europeans (~39%)**
    - **Africans (~52%)**
    - **East Asians (~18%)**
- The **genetic contribution to obesity risk** is more pronounced in populations with a **higher prevalence of the risk allele**.

Public Health Significance

- The **population attributable risk (PAR) of obesity** due to *LEPR rs1137101* is estimated to be around **15-20%,** highlighting its relevance in obesity prevention strategies.
- Understanding ***LEPR*-associated obesity risk** can guide **personalized interventions and lifestyle modifications.**

Real-Life Example

Consider an individual who carries **two copies of the A allele of *rs1137101***. Compared to someone without the risk allele, they may have:

- **Higher circulating *Leptin* levels** but reduced receptor sensitivity, leading to **persistent hunger and overeating**.
- **Greater difficulty in losing weight** due to impaired energy balance and metabolic efficiency.
- **An increased risk of developing metabolic syndrome**, insulin resistance, and type 2 diabetes.

Research Highlights

Anthropometric and Metabolic Evidence

- Studies confirm that ***rs1137101* carriers** have increased **BMI, waist circumference, and fat percentage**.
- Individuals with ***Leptin* resistance exhibit altered energy metabolism**, leading to weight gain.

Mechanistic Insights

- ***Leptin* signaling disruption** is a critical factor in obesity, making ***LEPR* a potential therapeutic target**.
- **Gene-environment interactions** — such as dietary patterns and levels of physical activity — can influence the magnitude of obesity risk conferred by *LEPR* variants. Lifestyle modifications may either mitigate or exacerbate the genetic susceptibility.

Validation Across Diverse Populations

Strengthened Evidence

A study published in **BMC Medical Genetics** further substantiates the association between ***LEPR* *rs1137101* and BMI**. Key findings include:

- Each copy of the A allele was associated with an increase in BMI by approximately 0.4 to 0.6 kg/m^2.
- Homozygous carriers (AA genotype) had a 1.65-fold higher risk of developing obesity compared to non-carriers.

Ethnic Variations in Genetic Impact

- The effect size remained consistent across populations, but the **allele frequency varied**.
- The **highest prevalence was observed in African and European populations**, with a lower frequency in East Asians.

Mechanisms Underlying the Association

- **Appetite Dysregulation**: *LEPR* variants influence hunger signals, increasing susceptibility to **overeating**.
- **Basal Metabolic Rate Alterations**: Individuals carrying the **risk allele show lower metabolic efficiency**, leading to weight gain.

Global Perspective

- The ***rs1137101* risk allele contributes significantly to BMI heritability**, explaining **~1.5% of BMI variance in Europeans**.
- **Public health relevance**: Given the allele's strong link to obesity, it serves as a **potential target for early intervention strategies**.

Gene-Lifestyle Interaction

- The genetic risk associated with ***LEPR rs1137101*** is **exacerbated by modern lifestyles**, including **high-calorie diets and sedentary behavior**.
- **Targeted interventions**, such as **caloric restriction and exercise**, can mitigate genetic predisposition.

Conclusion

The *LEPR rs1137101* variant plays a critical role in the genetic architecture of obesity. While it contributes significantly to BMI variability and metabolic dysfunction, its impact is modifiable through personalized lifestyle interventions. Understanding gene-lifestyle interactions is essential for developing precision-based strategies to combat the growing global obesity epidemic.

TMEM18 rs6548238: A Key Genetic Determinant of Obesity and BMI

Introduction to *TMEM18* Gene Discovery

The *TMEM18* gene has emerged as a significant genetic factor influencing obesity and Body Mass Index (BMI), primarily identified through large-scale Genome-Wide Association Studies (GWAS).

TMEM18 encodes a transmembrane protein that is predominantly expressed in the hypothalamus and brainstem — regions critical for energy homeostasis, appetite control, and feeding behavior.

Uniquely, *TMEM18* is highly conserved across species, tracing back over 1500 million years, underscoring its evolutionary importance in body weight regulation.

Association with Obesity and BMI

The *TMEM18* gene was first identified in **the GIANT consortium GWAS study**, which found that ***rs6548238*** was strongly associated with increased **BMI and body weight**. This association was later replicated in **Icelandic and Swedish population studies**, confirming its role in **both childhood and adult obesity**.

Discovery of SNP rs6548238

- **SNP *rs6548238*** is located upstream of *TMEM18* and has been identified as a **risk variant for obesity**.
- The **C allele** of *rs6548238* is associated with an **increased risk of obesity**, while the **T allele** is linked to **lower BMI and reduced obesity risk**.
- The SNP was found to have a significant impact on BMI, particularly in **children and adolescents**, with the effect being **more pronounced in early life**.

Validation Across Diverse Cohorts

- The association between ***rs6548238* and obesity** has been validated in multiple cohorts, including studies in **Sweden, Iceland, and other European populations**.
- A study on **severely obese children in Sweden** showed that carriers of the **C allele** had **higher BMI** compared to non-carriers.
- These findings were further reinforced by studies that linked *rs6548238* to **increased fat accumulation and metabolic risk factors**.

Biological Mechanism of *TMEM18* rs6548238

Expression in Brain Regions

TMEM18 is highly expressed in neuronal cells throughout the brain, with its highest expression in the hypothalamus, a key regulator of energy balance, appetite, and metabolism.

Unlike some obesity-related genes, *TMEM18* does not show significant expression changes in response to fasting or increased caloric intake, suggesting a role in baseline energy homeostasis rather than short-term metabolic responses.

Impact on Energy Balance and Fat Mass

The C allele of *rs6548238* has been linked to higher body fat percentage, particularly in individuals with a genetic predisposition to obesity.

The SNP may influence neuronal function in appetite control regions, altering feeding behavior and energy expenditure.

Studies suggest that *TMEM18* affects cell migration in the brain, which could impact neural circuits involved in metabolism regulation.

Early-Onset Impact

The influence of *rs6548238* on BMI has been observed early in life, with significant effects detected in children as young as 6 years old.

In a study of 502 severely obese children and 527 healthy controls, the C allele was significantly associated with childhood obesity, suggesting a potential role in early weight gain.

Unlike some obesity genes that show stronger effects in adults, *TMEM18 rs6548238* has a more pronounced effect in childhood and adolescence, making it an important marker for early obesity risk prediction.

Population-Level Implications

Global Prevalence of *rs6548238* Risk Allele

The frequency of the **C allele** varies across populations:

- Swedish & European populations: ~18%
- Asian populations: Lower prevalence
- African populations: Minimal representation

This variation in allele frequency may contribute to ethnic differences in obesity prevalence and susceptibility.

Public Health and Clinical Relevance

Understanding the genetic impact of *TMEM18 rs6548238* offers critical insights for:

- Early identification of individuals at high risk for obesity
- Personalized interventions focusing on lifestyle modification and metabolic health
- Development of precision medicine approaches in obesity prevention and management

Further research is needed to explore how environmental factors — such as diet and physical activity — interact with *TMEM18* variants to influence obesity risk across different populations.

Conclusion

The consistent association of the *rs6548238* C allele with increased BMI and body fat across multiple populations, particularly in childhood, highlights its potential role in early-onset obesity. Furthermore, the gene's conserved evolutionary role and predominant expression in brain regions regulating appetite and energy balance suggest that *TMEM18* is a critical player in the neurobiological regulation of body weight. Recognizing the gene-environment interaction involving *TMEM18* offers opportunities for personalized interventions, especially in genetically susceptible individuals, to mitigate the rising global burden of obesity.

Questions

1. Which gene is *rs9939609* located in, and what trait is it associated with?
2. What is the main role of the *FTO* gene in obesity risk?
3. Which gene harbors the *rs17782313* SNP linked to appetite regulation?
4. What hormone does the *LEP* gene encode?
5. The rs2167270 variant is found in which obesity-related gene?
6. Which receptor gene carries *rs1137101*, associated with *Leptin* signaling?
7. What is the biological role of *TMEM18* in obesity?
8. Which SNP in *TMEM18* has been associated with BMI?
9. Which obesity-related gene contains rs713586, affecting energy metabolism?
10. What is the function of the *SH2B1* gene in energy balance?
11. Which neurotrophic factor gene contains rs6265, linked to obesity and eating behavior?
12. PCSK1 encodes which type of enzyme important for obesity risk?
13. GNPDA2 (rs10938397) is associated with which anthropometric trait?
14. Which gene harbors the rs1801282 polymorphism linked to obesity and insulin sensitivity?
15. Which gene's polymorphism rs29941 is implicated in obesity through neuronal development?
16. How does the *FTO rs9939609* risk allele contribute to increased food intake and obesity?
17. What is the functional mechanism of *MC4R rs17782313* in regulating satiety signals?
18. How does the *LEP* rs2167270 variant influence circulating *Leptin* levels and obesity predisposition?
19. Explain how *LEPR rs1137101* polymorphism affects *Leptin* receptor signaling and weight regulation.
20. Describe the role of *TMEM18* variants (rs6548238, rs7561317) in central nervous system regulation of body weight.
21. How does ADCY3 rs713586 polymorphism affect adiposity through cAMP signaling pathways?
22. What is the relationship between *SH2B1* rs7498665 variants and insulin signaling in obesity?
23. Discuss how BDNF rs6265 (Val66Met) influences eating behavior and BMI through brain-derived neurotrophic factor function.
24. How do PCSK1 polymorphisms (rs6232, rs6235) affect prohormone processing and obesity risk?
25. Explain how GNPDA2 rs10938397 contributes to obesity via carbohydrate metabolism.
26. What is the effect of NEGR1 rs2815752 on neuronal growth and its link to BMI regulation?
27. How does TNNI3K rs1514175 variant modulate energy metabolism and predisposition to obesity?
28. Explain the impact of PPARG rs1801282 (Pro12Ala) polymorphism on adipocyte differentiation and obesity susceptibility.
29. Describe how KCTD15 rs29941 interacts with hypothalamic pathways to influence BMI.
30. How does MAP2K5 rs2241423 variant affect MAPK signaling and obesity-related phenotypes?

Answers

1. *rs9939609* is in the *FTO* gene; it is associated with obesity and BMI.
2. *FTO* influences appetite regulation and preference for calorie-dense foods.
3. *rs17782313* is in the *MC4R* gene.
4. The *LEP* gene encodes *Leptin*.
5. rs2167270 is in the *LEP* gene.
6. *rs1137101* is in the *LEPR* gene (*Leptin* receptor).
7. *TMEM18* regulates neuronal development and hypothalamic appetite control.
8. *rs6548238* (and rs7561317) in *TMEM18* are linked to BMI.
9. rs713586 is in the ADCY3 gene.
10. *SH2B1* enhances *Leptin* and insulin signaling.
11. rs6265 is in the BDNF gene.
12. PCSK1 encodes a prohormone convertase ezyme.
13. rs10938397 in GNPDA2 is associated with BMI.
14. rs1801282 is in the PPARG gene.
15. rs29941 is in the KCTD15 gene.
16. *FTO rs9939609* increases food intake by altering hypothalamic satiety signaling.
17. *MC4R rs17782313* reduces melanocortin receptor activity, impairing satiety response.
18. *LEP* rs2167270 raises *Leptin* levels but contributes to *Leptin* resistance.
19. *LEPR rs1137101* alters receptor efficiency, reducing *Leptin* signaling and satiety.
20. *TMEM18* variants (rs6548238, rs7561317) affect hypothalamic gene expression controlling energy balance.
21. ADCY3 rs713586 reduces cAMP signaling, impairing *Leptin*/insulin pathways and increasing obesity risk.
22. *SH2B1* rs7498665 weakens insulin and *Leptin* receptor signaling, promoting insulin resistance and obesity.
23. BDNF rs6265 (Val66Met) disrupts activity-dependent BDNF secretion, altering appetite and reward pathways.
24. PCSK1 rs6232 and rs6235 impair prohormone processing (e.g., insulin, proglucagon), disrupting appetite and metabolism.
25. GNPDA2 rs10938397 affects the hexosamine pathway, promoting energy storage and adiposity.
26. NEGR1 rs2815752 influences hypothalamic neuronal growth, impacting feeding behavior and BMI.
27. TNNI3K rs1514175 alters mitochondrial energy metabolism, reducing efficiency and predisposing to obesity.
28. PPARG rs1801282 (Pro12Ala) modifies adipocyte differentiation and insulin sensitivity; some alleles lower obesity risk.
29. KCTD15 rs29941 affects hypothalamic transcriptional pathways regulating eating behavior and BMI.
30. MAP2K5 rs2241423 alters ERK5/MAPK signaling, impacting neuronal and adipocyte regulation of obesity traits.

References

1. Dalgaard, L. T., & Pedersen, O. (2001). Uncoupling proteins: Functional characteristics and role in the pathogenesis of obesity and type II diabetes. *Diabetologia, 44*(8), 946–965. https://doi.org/10.1007/s001250100579
2. Esterbauer, H., Oberkofler, H., Linnemayr, V., Iglseder, B., Hedegger, M., Aigner, L., ... Patsch, J. R. (2001). Uncoupling protein-2 gene variant is associated with obesity in middle-aged humans. *Nature Genetics, 28*(2), 178–183. https://doi.org/10.1038/88915
3. Rosskopf, D., Bornhorst, A., Rimmbach, C., Schwahn, C., Kayser, A., Kruger, A., ... Rettig, R. (2007). The Ala55Val polymorphism in the *UCP2* gene is associated with increased risk of obesity and hyperlipidemia. *Obesity, 15*(10), 1408–1416. https://doi.org/10.1038/oby.2007.165
4. Schäfer, A., Buettner, C., & Bollheimer, L. C. (2005). Role of *UCP2* in inflammatory and stress responses in obesity. *PLOS Biology, 3*(6), e132. https://doi.org/10.1371/journal.pbio.0030132
5. Chadt, A., & Al-Hasani, H. (2020). *TBC1D1* and TBC1D4—Two RabGTPase-activating proteins involved in insulin- and AMPK-mediated glucose transport regulation in skeletal muscle. *Frontiers in Endocrinology, 11,* 469. https://doi.org/10.3389/fendo.2020.00469
6. Stephens, J. M., & Sparks, L. M. (2015). *TBC1D1*: A new player in obesity and diabetes? *Adipocyte, 4*(4), 229–232. https://doi.org/10.4161/21623945.2014.974487
7. Macotela, Y., & Boucher, J. (2010). *TBC1D1*, a novel gene regulating muscle glucose metabolism, fat oxidation, and energy balance. *Journal of Endocrinology, 204*(1), 1–10. https://doi.org/10.1677/JOE-10-0238
8. Kowalski, G. M., & Bruce, C. R. (2014). The regulation of glucose metabolism: Implications and considerations for the impact of *TBC1D1* and TBC1D4 in metabolic diseases. *The Journal of Physiology, 593*(5), 1021–1027. https://doi.org/10.1113/jphysiol.2014.273656
9. Morris, D. L., Cho, K. W., & Rui, L. (2010). *SH2B1* and the regulation of energy balance and metabolism. *Trends in Endocrinology & Metabolism, 21*(11), 660–666. https://doi.org/10.1016/j.tem.2010.08.005
10. Boender, A. J., & van Rozen, A. J. (2016). *SH2B1* mutations and obesity. *Molecular and Cellular Endocrinology, 430,* 83–92. https://doi.org/10.1016/j.mce.2016.03.025
11. Yang, S., & Xu, L. (2017). Role of *SH2B1* in the central regulation of energy balance and body weight. *International Journal of Molecular Sciences, 18*(2), 391. https://doi.org/10.3390/ijms18020391
12. Clément, K., Meyre, D., Dina, C., Pelloux, V., & Froguel, P. (2011). Genetic variation in the *SH2B1* gene and its effect on obesity. *Nature Genetics, 43*(8), 715–719. https://doi.org/10.1038/ng.866
13. Ando, T., Komaki, G., Naruo, T., Okazawa, N., Takii, M., Kawai, K., ... Kurokawa, N. (2006). Possible role of preproghrelin gene polymorphisms in susceptibility to bulimia nervosa. *American Journal of Medical Genetics Part B: Neuropsychiatric Genetics, 141B*(9), 929–934. https://doi.org/10.1002/ajmg.b.30387

14. Landgren, S., Simms, J. A., Thelle, D. S., Strandhagen, E., Bergström, L., Helander, A., ... Engel, J. A. (2011). The ghrelin signalling system is involved in the consumption of sweets. *PLoS ONE, 6*(3), e18170. https://doi.org/10.1371/journal.pone.0018170
15. Steinle, N. I., Pollin, T. I., O'Connell, J. R., Mitchell, B. D., Shuldiner, A. R., & Snitker, S. (2005). Variants in the ghrelin gene are associated with metabolic syndrome in the Old Order Amish. *The Journal of Clinical Endocrinology & Metabolism, 90*(12), 6672–6677. https://doi.org/10.1210/jc.2005-0549
16. Hinney, A., Nguyen, T. T., Scherag, A., Friedel, S., Bronner, G., Müller, T. D., ... Hebebrand, J. (2007). Genome-wide association (GWA) study for early onset extreme obesity supports the role of fat mass and obesity associated gene (*FTO*) variants. *PLoS ONE, 2*(12), e1361. https://doi.org/10.1371/journal.pone.0001361
17. Villalobos-Comparán, M., Flores-Dorantes, M. T., Villarreal-Molina, M. T., Rodríguez-Cruz, M., García-Ulloa, A. C., Robles, L., ... Canizales-Quinteros, S. (2008). The *FTO* gene is associated with adulthood obesity in the Mexican population. *Obesity (Silver Spring), 16*(10), 2296-2301. https://doi.org/10.1038/oby.2008.367
18. Mačeková, S., Bernasovský, I., Gabriková, D., Bôžiková, A., Bernasovská, J., Boroňová, I., ... Carnogurská, J. (2012). Association of the *FTO rs9939609* polymorphism with obesity in Roma/Gypsy population. *American Journal of Physical Anthropology, 147*(1), 30-34. https://doi.org/10.1002/ajpa.21604
19. Smemo, S., Tena, J. J., Kim, K. H., Gamazon, E. R., Sakabe, N. J., Gomez-Marín, C., ... Nobrega, M. A. (2014). Obesity-associated variants within *FTO* form long-range functional connections with IRX3. *Nature, 507*(7492), 371–375. https://doi.org/10.1038/nature13138
20. Frayling, T. M., Timpson, N. J., Weedon, M. N., Zeggini, E., Freathy, R. M., Lindgren, C. M., ... McCarthy, M. I. (2007). A common variant in the *FTO* gene is associated with body mass index and predisposes to childhood and adult obesity. *Science, 316*(5826), 889-894. https://doi.org/10.1126/science.1141634
21. Grau, K., Hansen, T., Holst, C., Astrup, A., Saris, W. H. M., Arner, P., ... Sørensen, T. I. A. (2009). Macronutrient-specific effect of *FTO rs9939609* in response to a 10-week randomized hypo-energetic diet among obese Europeans. *International Journal of Obesity, 33*(11), 1227-1234. https://doi.org/10.1038/ijo.2009.159
22. Graff, M., Scott, R. A., Justice, A. E., Young, K. L., Feitosa, M. F., Barata, L., ... (CHARGE, EPIC-InterAct, PAGE Consortia). (2017). Genome-wide physical activity interactions in adiposity: A meta-analysis of 200,452 adults. *PLOS Genetics, 13*(4), e1006528. https://doi.org/10.1371/journal.pgen.1006528
23. Pan, H., Lino, C. H., Song, Y., Liu, J., Qi, L., & Chung, W. K. (2019). Common variants in *FTO* and near-*MC4R* are associated with obesity, type 2 diabetes, and lipid traits across racial/ethnic populations in the PAGE consortium. *Diabetes, 68*(6), 1121-1132. https://doi.org/10.2337/db18-1095
24. Vimaleswaran, K. S., Berry, D. J., Lu, C., Tikkanen, E., Pilz, S., Hiraki, L. T., ... Power, C. (2012). Causal relationship between obesity and vitamin D status: Bi-directional Mendelian

randomization analysis of multiple cohorts. *PLoS Medicine, 9*(2), e1001383. https://doi.org/10.1371/journal.pmed.1001383

25. Thompson-Smith, T., Luan, J., Zhao, X., Chen, W., ... & Wareham, N. J. (2023). Genome-wide interaction study of physical activity and sleep with obesity traits. *Nature Communications, 14,* 5980. https://doi.org/10.1038/s41467-023-41756-3
26. Wang, T. J., Pencina, M. J., Booth, S. L., Jacques, P. F., Ingelsson, E., Lanier, K., ... Vasan, R. S. (2012). Vitamin D deficiency and risk of cardiovascular disease. *Circulation, 126*(14), 1740-1748. https://doi.org/10.1161/CIRCULATIONAHA.112.111148
27. Huang, T., Zheng, Y., Hruby, A., Williamson, D. A., Bray, G. A., Shen, Y., ... Qi, L. (2017). Dietary protein modifies the effect of the *MC4R* genotype on 2-year change in appetite: The POUNDS Lost Trial. *Obesity (Silver Spring), 25*(4), 695-703. https://doi.org/10.1002/oby.21782
28. Alizadeh, S., Pooyan, S., Mirzababaei, A., Arghavani, H., Hasani, H., & Mirzaei, K. (2022). Interaction of *MC4R rs17782313* variants and dietary carbohydrate quantity and quality on basal metabolic rate and general and central obesity in overweight/obese women: A cross-sectional study. *BMC Endocrine Disorders, 22*(121). https://doi.org/10.1186/s12902-022-01023-5
29. Xi, B., Chandak, G. R., Shen, Y., Wang, Q., & Zhou, D. (2012). Association between common polymorphism near the *MC4R* gene and obesity risk: A systematic review and meta-analysis. *PLoS ONE, 7*(9), e45731. https://doi.org/10.1371/journal.pone.0045731
30. Walia, G. K., Saini, S., Vimal, P., Bhatia, K., Kumar, A., Singh, R., ... Gupta, V. (2021). Association of *MC4R* (*rs17782313*) gene polymorphism with obesity measures in Western India. *Diabetes & Metabolic Syndrome: Clinical Research & Reviews, 15*(3), 661-665. https://doi.org/10.1016/j.dsx.2021.03.013
31. Yang, Y., Gao, X. H., Tao, X. J., Gao, Q. H., Zhang, Y. H., & Yang, J. J. (2019). Combined effect of *FTO* and *MC4R* gene polymorphisms on obesity in children and adolescents in Northwest China: A case-control study. *Asia Pacific Journal of Clinical Nutrition, 28*(1), 177-182.
32. Song, J. Y., Song, Q. Y., Wang, S., Ma, J., & Wang, H. J. (2017). Physical activity and sedentary behaviors modify the association between melanocortin 4 receptor gene variant and obesity in Chinese children and adolescents. *PLoS ONE, 12*(1), e0170062. https://doi.org/10.1371/journal.pone.0170062
33. Wang, S., Song, J., Yang, Y., Chawla, N. V., Ma, J., & Wang, H. J. (2017). Rs12970134 near *MC4R* is associated with appetite and beverage intake in overweight and obese children: A family-based association study in Chinese population. *PLoS ONE, 12*(5), e0177983. https://doi.org/10.1371/journal.pone.0177983
34. Qi, L., Kraft, P., Hunter, D. J., & Hu, F. B. (2008). The common obesity variant near *MC4R* gene is associated with higher intakes of total energy and dietary fat, weight change and diabetes risk in women. *Human Molecular Genetics, 17*(22), 3502-3508. https://doi.org/10.1093/hmg/ddn242
35. Koochakpoor, G., Hosseini-Esfahani, F., Daneshpour, M. S., Sedaghati-Khayat, B., & Mirmiran, P. (2023). Investigation of the interaction between dietary fat quality indices and *MC4R* gene

in relation to metabolic syndrome. *Scientific Reports, 13,* 12345. https://doi.org/10.1038/s41598-023-38988-9

36. Corella, D., Ortega-Azorín, C., Sorlí, J. V., Covas, M. I., Buckland, G., González, J. I., ... Ordovás, J. M. (2012). Statistical and biological gene-lifestyle interactions of *MC4R* and *FTO* with diet and physical activity on obesity: New effects on alcohol consumption. *PLoS ONE, 7*(12), e52344. https://doi.org/10.1371/journal.pone.0052344
37. Farooqi, I. S., & O'Rahilly, S. (2006). *Leptin* and *Leptin* receptor mutations in rodents and humans: Insights into the pathophysiology of obesity. *Endocrine Reviews, 27*(3), 304-318. https://doi.org/10.1210/er.2005-0026
38. Considine, R. V., Sinha, M. K., Heiman, M. L., Kriauciunas, A., Stephens, T. W., Nyce, M. R., ... Caro, J. F. (1996). Serum immunoreactive-*Leptin* concentrations in normal-weight and obese humans. *New England Journal of Medicine, 334*(5), 292-295. https://doi.org/10.1056/NEJM199602013340503
39. Mammès, O., Betoulle, D., Aubert, R., Herbeth, B., Siest, G., & Fumeron, F. (1998). *Leptin* receptor gene variation and obesity in the French population. *Obesity Research, 6*(2), 122-126. https://doi.org/10.1002/j.1550-8528.1998.tb00321.x
40. Montague, C. T., Farooqi, I. S., Whitehead, J. P., Soos, M. A., Rau, H., Wareham, N. J., ... O'Rahilly, S. (1997). Congenital *Leptin* deficiency is associated with severe early-onset obesity in humans. *Nature, 387*(6636), 903-908. https://doi.org/10.1038/43185
41. Chagnon, Y. C., Rankinen, T., Snyder, E. E., Weisnagel, S. J., Perusse, L., & Bouchard, C. (2003). *LEPR* gene polymorphisms are associated with obesity-related phenotypes: The HERITAGE Family Study. *International Journal of Obesity, 27*(5), 593-600. https://doi.org/10.1038/sj.ijo.0802261
42. Quinton, N. D., Lee, A. J., Ross, R. J., Eastell, R., & Blakemore, A. I. (2001). A single nucleotide polymorphism (SNP) in the *Leptin* receptor gene is associated with obesity and the metabolic syndrome in a UK Caucasian population. *Diabetologia, 44*(3), 222-229. https://doi.org/10.1007/s001250051601
43. Heo, M., Leibel, R. L., Fontaine, K. R., Boyer, C., Chung, W. K., & Koulu, M. (2002). A meta-analysis of genome-wide association studies of obesity in different populations. *American Journal of Clinical Nutrition, 75*(6), 972-979. https://doi.org/10.
44. Link, A., Balaguer, F., & Goel, A. (2013). Cancer chemoprevention by dietary polyphenols: Promising role for epigenetics. *Biochemical Pharmacology, 85*(9), 1266–1276. https://doi.org/10.1016/j.bcp.2013.02.011.
45. Denver, R. J., Bonett, R. M., & Boorse, G. C. (2011). Evolution of *Leptin* structure and function. *Neuroendocrinology, 94*(1), 21–38. https://doi.org/10.1159/000328435.

FOOD INTOLERANCE, FOOD SENSITIVITY AND FOOD ALLERGY

Introduction

Individual responses to food vary widely due to a combination of environmental influences and genetic factors. Advances in nutrigenetics and nutrigenomics have highlighted the role of genetic polymorphisms in determining susceptibility to food intolerance, sensitivity, and allergy. These genetic variations can alter enzyme activity, immune function, and metabolic pathways, affecting food digestion, nutrient absorption, and immune responses.

Food-related reactions are broadly classified into food allergy, food intolerance, and food sensitivity — each characterized by distinct mechanisms, causes, and health implications. A clear understanding of these differences is essential for accurate diagnosis and effective dietary management.

Classification of Food-Related Reactions

Food Allergy

This is an **immune system reaction** triggered by a specific food protein. Even small amounts of the allergen can cause **severe or life-threatening reactions** (anaphylaxis). Food allergies typically involve **IgE-mediated immune responses** and require **strict avoidance of the allergen**.

Food Intolerance

Unlike allergies, **food intolerance does not involve the immune system**. Instead, it results from an **enzyme deficiency, chemical sensitivity, or gastrointestinal disorder**, leading to symptoms like bloating, diarrhea, or abdominal pain. Individuals with food intolerance may tolerate small amounts of the food without severe reactions.

Food Sensitivity

Food sensitivity, although sometimes used interchangeably with intolerance, generally refers to non-IgE immune-mediated responses, often involving delayed reactions. These responses may include IgG-mediated inflammation, leading to symptoms such as headaches, joint pain, fatigue, skin issues, or digestive disturbances.

Comparison Table of Food Allergy, Sensitivity, and Intolerance

Category	Definition	Immune System Involvement	Symptoms	Common Examples	Severity & Management
Food Allergy	An immune reaction to a specific food protein.	Yes (IgE-mediated)	Hives, swelling, difficulty breathing, anaphylaxis	Peanuts, shellfish, milk, eggs	Severe; requires strict avoidance & emergency treatment (e.g., epinephrine)
Food Sensitivity	A delayed immune response that causes inflammation and discomfort.	Yes (Non-IgE mediated, often IgG)	Headaches, joint pain, bloating, fatigue	Gluten, dairy, food additives (e.g., MSG)	Moderate; symptoms may appear hours to days later, and elimination diets are used for management.
Food Intolerance	A non-immune reaction due to enzyme deficiency or chemical intolerance	No	Bloating, diarrhea, gas, nausea	Lactose (dairy), histamine (aged foods), sulfites (wine, dried fruits)	Mild to moderate; small amounts may be tolerated depending on sensitivity

Common Types of Food Allergy, Sensitivity, and Intolerance

Category	Examples	Description
Food Allergies	**Peanut Allergy**	Severe immune response to peanut proteins, often leading to anaphylaxis.
	Shellfish Allergy	Common in adults, can trigger life-threatening reactions.
	Milk Allergy	Different from lactose intolerance; immune response to milk proteins (casein, whey).
Food Sensitivities	**Gluten Sensitivity**	Non-celiac reaction to gluten, causing gastrointestinal and inflammatory symptoms.
	Dairy Sensitivity	Reaction to milk proteins without IgE-mediated allergy may cause digestive discomfort.
	Histamine Sensitivity	Reaction to histamine-rich foods (e.g., fermented foods, aged cheese) causes varied symptoms.
Food Intolerances	**Lactose Intolerance**	Deficiency of the lactase enzyme leads to difficulty digesting lactose.
	Fructose Malabsorption	Inability to properly absorb fructose, causing bloating and digestive discomfort.
	Sulfite Sensitivity	Sensitivity to sulfite preservatives in wine, dried fruits, and processed foods.

Understanding Wheat: A Foundation for Gluten Intolerance

Introduction

Wheat has been a cornerstone of human civilization for over 10,000 years, serving as a staple food across cultures and continents. Its domestication in the Fertile Crescent marked the beginning of widespread cultivation, with early farmers adapting wheat to diverse environments worldwide. Today, wheat remains one of the most extensively grown cereal crops due to its high yield, storage stability, and adaptability to various climatic conditions.

Wheat's genetic diversity — encompassing over 25,000 varieties of *Triticum aestivum L.* — enables its cultivation across temperate, Mediterranean, and subtropical regions.

Wheat is classified based on its sowing time:

- **Winter wheat**: Sown in autumn and requiring a period of low temperatures (0–5°C) during the vegetative phase. This variety accounts for approximately 80% of global wheat production.
- **Spring wheat**: Planted in spring and harvested in late summer or fall, especially in South Asian and North African countries.

Progressive domestication led to significant morphological changes, such as the restructuring of the rachis and glumes, converting brittle wild wheat ears into non-brittle, bare-grained cultivated varieties. These changes facilitated large-scale cropping, greatly increasing wheat's economic significance.

Nutritionally, wheat is a primary source of carbohydrates (mainly starch) and contributes substantially to dietary protein intake. Of particular significance are the endosperm storage proteins — **prolamins** — which are categorized into **gliadins and glutenins.** These proteins form the gluten network when wheat flour is mixed with water, giving rise to the viscoelastic properties essential for dough formation. The balance between glutenins (providing strength and elasticity) and gliadins (contributing to dough extensibility) varies among wheat varieties and directly influences their suitability for different culinary applications such as bread, cakes, pasta, and biscuits.

Additionally, wheat quality for commercial use is determined by factors such as grain protein content and hardness, which influence processing characteristics and end-use performance. Global market demands have driven extensive breeding programs aimed at enhancing both yield and functional protein quality to meet industry needs.

This chapter provides an overview of the history and unique characteristics of wheat, laying the groundwork for a deeper understanding of gluten's role in food production. This knowledge is essential for exploring the pathophysiology and management of gluten intolerance in subsequent sections.

Origin and Evolution of Wheat

Wheat cultivation originated in the Fertile Crescent, a region encompassing modern-day Jordan, Palestine, Lebanon, Syria, Turkey, Iraq, and Iran. It was among the earliest crops domesticated by humans, laying the foundation for agricultural societies. The first cultivated wheat species included einkorn (*Triticum monococcum*), emmer (*Triticum dicoccum*), and spelt (*Triticum spelta*), which gradually evolved into the modern wheat varieties consumed today.

How Wheat Evolved

Wheat has gone through multiple evolutionary changes, mainly through a process called **polyploidization**—a natural genetic combination where different wheat species merged to form new varieties with better adaptability and higher yield.

- **First Evolutionary Event**: Two wild diploid wheat species combined their genomes to create tetraploid wheat, known as **wild emmer wheat (Triticum dicoccum)**. This new wheat was more resilient and had better yields than its ancestors.
- **Second Evolutionary Event**: Wild emmer wheat later combined with another wild grass, **Aegilops tauschii**, forming the modern **hexaploid wheat (Triticum aestivum)**—which is the most commonly cultivated wheat today.

Why These Changes Matter

Each stage of wheat's evolution improved its adaptability to diverse environmental conditions, increased grain yield, and facilitated more efficient harvesting techniques. However, domestication also reduced genetic diversity, rendering modern wheat more susceptible to pests, diseases, and environmental stressors.

Types of Wheat

Ancient Wheats

1. **Einkorn (Triticum monococcum)** - One of the oldest wheat varieties, known for its high protein and antioxidant content.
2. **Emmer (Triticum dicoccum)** - An early cultivated wheat that is rich in fiber and still used in some traditional foods.
3. **Spelt (Triticum spelta)** - Popular for its high mineral content and nutty flavor.

Modern Wheats

1. **Durum Wheat (Triticum durum)** - Used primarily for pasta, couscous, and semolina products.
2. **Bread Wheat (Triticum aestivum)** - The most commonly consumed wheat, used in bread, pastries, and processed foods.

Wheat Production and Consumption

Wheat is a staple food worldwide, with **China, India, Russia, the USA, and France** as the top producers. It is categorized as either **winter wheat** (planted in autumn) or **spring wheat** (planted in spring), based on climatic adaptation.

Green Revolution and High-Yield Varieties

The **Green Revolution** in the 1960s introduced high-yield wheat varieties, accompanied by increased use of chemical fertilizers and pesticides. The introduction of **dwarfing genes (Rht1 and Rht2)** from the Japanese variety 'Norin 10' improved yield potential but also increased reliance on agrochemicals.

Nutritional Composition of Wheat

Wheat is composed of carbohydrates, proteins, fats, vitamins, and minerals. The endosperm, germ, and bran contribute to its nutritional profile:

- **Carbohydrates:** Predominantly starch, serving as a major energy source.
- **Proteins:** Includes gluten-forming proteins — gliadins and glutenins — essential for dough elasticity and baking quality.
- **Lipids:** Present in small amounts, contributing to cellular structure and function.
- **Micronutrients:** Rich in iron, zinc, B-vitamins, and antioxidants, particularly in whole grain forms where the bran and germ are retained.

Gluten: The Key to Wheat's Versatility

Structure and Function

Gluten is a protein complex formed by the interaction of two main components—**gliadins and glutenins**—found in wheat endosperm. This network is essential for the unique viscoelastic properties of wheat-based dough. Gliadins are responsible for dough extensibility (stretchiness), while glutenins provide elasticity and structural strength. Together, they form the gluten matrix, which traps gas during fermentation and gives baked products their structure and chewiness.

Variability in Gluten Content

Gluten strength and quantity vary across wheat species, influencing their culinary applications:

- **Bread wheat (Triticum aestivum):** Contains high-gluten strength, ideal for leavened products such as bread and rolls.
- **Durum wheat (Triticum durum):** Has lower gluten elasticity, making it suitable for firm pasta and semolina-based dishes.

- **Ancient wheats (spelt, emmer):** Contain gluten but in lower concentrations and with different protein compositions. Despite lower gluten content, they remain unsuitable for individuals with gluten-related disorders.

Wheat in Human Health

Digestive Properties

Wheat digestion begins in the gastrointestinal tract, where enzymes break down proteins. However, gluten is particularly rich in proline and glutamine, making it resistant to complete enzymatic degradation. This incomplete digestion leads to the formation of gluten peptides, which may provoke immune or inflammatory responses in genetically predisposed individuals.

Gluten-Related Disorders

1. **Non-Celiac Gluten Sensitivity (NCGS)** - Characterized by gastrointestinal and extra-intestinal symptoms following gluten ingestion, without the autoimmune markers or intestinal damage seen in celiac disease.
2. **Celiac Disease** - A chronic autoimmune condition where ingestion of gluten leads to immune-mediated damage to the small intestinal lining, resulting in nutrient malabsorption and systemic effects.
3. **Wheat Allergy** - An IgE-mediated allergic reaction to wheat proteins, including but not limited to gluten, leading to symptoms such as hives, respiratory distress, or anaphylaxis in severe cases.

Understanding Non-Celiac Gluten Sensitivity

Imagine you eat a slice of pizza and, a few hours later, you feel bloated, tired, and have a headache. You might think it's the cheese or the grease, but for some people, the culprit is **gluten**—a protein found in wheat, barley, and rye. However, unlike **celiac disease**, which involves an autoimmune reaction, and **wheat allergy**, which is an allergic response, **NCGS** is a different condition with its own unique mechanisms.

NCGS is defined as *a condition where individuals experience gastrointestinal and extra-intestinal symptoms triggered by gluten intake, without having celiac disease or wheat allergy.* To be classified as NCGS, a patient **must not test positive for celiac disease (CD) or wheat allergy (WA)** but should still report **relief of symptoms** upon **eliminating gluten** from their diet.

Since **no specific biomarker exists**, diagnosing NCGS requires:

1. **Ruling out Celiac Disease**
    - Negative for **anti-tissue transglutaminase (tTG-IgA) and anti-endomysial (EMA) antibodies**.
    - No evidence of intestinal damage (**villous atrophy**) on biopsy

2. **Ruling out Wheat Allergy**
   - Negative for **IgE-mediated allergy tests**.
3. **Observing Symptoms**
   - Symptoms improve **after removing gluten** from the diet and reappear **when gluten is reintroduced**.

Due to the lack of standardized diagnostic criteria, many cases remain undiagnosed or are misclassified, often as irritable bowel syndrome (IBS).

Epidemiology: How Common is NCGS?

The prevalence of NCGS **varies widely** depending on how it is diagnosed:

- **Survey-based studies** (self-reported gluten sensitivity) estimate NCGS affects **0.49% to 14.9% of the population**.
- The **true prevalence** is **unknown** because there are **no standardized diagnostic criteria**.
- It **appears more common in women** than men, particularly in **young to middle-aged adults**.

While **celiac disease** occurs in about **1% of the population**, **NCGS may be much more common**, but **many cases are misdiagnosed as IBS**.

Pathogenesis of NCGS

Step 1: The Gut Reacts—But Differently Than in Celiac Disease

In celiac disease, gluten triggers the immune system to **attack the gut lining**, causing serious damage. In NCGS, the innate immune system—the body's first line of defense—is triggered instead, without causing permanent harm to the gut.

- Inflammatory molecules like interleukins and tumor necrosis factor alpha (TNF-α) are released, causing temporary irritation.

Mild intestinal inflammation may occur, but villous atrophy, as seen in celiac disease, is absent.

Example: Think of it like a mild food poisoning episode—you don't feel well after eating certain foods, but your gut isn't permanently harmed.

Step 2: The Gut Barrier Gets Weakened

Your intestines have a **protective barrier** that decides what enters your bloodstream. In NCGS, this barrier becomes "leaky," allowing particles that should stay out to slip through.

- This increased intestinal permeability (commonly called "leaky gut") allows partially digested food or microbes to cross into the bloodstream.

This breach triggers localized and systemic inflammation.

Example: Imagine your gut as a coffee filter. Normally, it only lets coffee through, keeping the grounds out. In NCGS, it's like the filter has holes, so bits of coffee grounds get into your cup, making the coffee taste strange and triggering a reaction.

Step 3: The Brain and Body React

Because of the **gut-brain connection**, when the gut is irritated:

- People experience **brain fog, headaches, fatigue, and even mood changes**.
- Some also get **joint pain, skin issues, and muscle aches**, making it seem like a **whole-body problem**.

Example: Think of it like an allergic reaction where, instead of just a rash, you also get headaches, stomach pain, and fatigue.

Other Suspects: It's Not Just Gluten!

Emerging research shows that gluten may not be the sole culprit in NCGS. Other components in wheat, like:

1. **FODMAPs** – Short-chain carbohydrates that can cause bloating and discomfort.
2. **Amylase-Trypsin Inhibitors (ATIs)** – Proteins in wheat that may **trigger inflammation**.
3. **Microbiome Changes** – Some people have gut bacteria that react badly to wheat, leading to digestive distress.

Example: Imagine you think you're allergic to a certain perfume, but in reality, it's the mix of chemicals inside it, not just one ingredient.

Symptoms of NCGS

People with Non-Celiac Gluten Sensitivity (NCGS) experience a range of **gastrointestinal** and **extra-intestinal** symptoms, often making diagnosis difficult.

Gastrointestinal Symptoms

These symptoms mimic **irritable bowel syndrome (IBS)** and include:

- **Bloating**
- **Abdominal pain**
- **Diarrhea or constipation**
- **Nausea and acid reflux**

B. Extra-Intestinal Symptoms

NCGS can also affect **the brain, immune system, and nervous system**, leading to:

- **Headaches and migraines**
- **Fatigue and brain fog**
- **Joint and muscle pain**
- **Depression or mood swings**
- **Eczema or rashes**

The symptoms **appear within hours or days** after gluten consumption and **disappear upon gluten elimination**.

Diagnosis: How is NCGS Identified?

Because there is **no specific test**, doctors diagnose NCGS by:

- **Excluding Celiac Disease and Wheat Allergy**
- **Observing Symptom Relief on a Gluten-Free Diet**
- **Performing a "Gluten Challenge"** (Reintroducing gluten to see if symptoms return)

Challenges in Diagnosis:

- Many NCGS patients self-diagnose and **do not undergo proper testing**.
- **Placebo effect** plays a role—some people **feel better just by avoiding gluten**, even if it's not the real cause.

Management of NCGS

The **primary treatment** for NCGS is **a gluten-free diet (GFD)**.

A. Gluten-Free Diet (GFD)

- **Avoid** wheat, barley, rye, and processed foods containing gluten.
- **Focus on** naturally gluten-free foods like **rice, quinoa, fruits, vegetables, and lean proteins**.
- **Monitor nutrient intake**, as GFD can lead to **deficiencies in fiber, iron, and B vitamins**.

B. Low-FODMAP Diet (For Some Patients)

- Some patients improve **more on a low-FODMAP diet** than a gluten-free diet.
- Low-FODMAP diets reduce **bloating and digestive issues** caused by wheat carbohydrates.

C. Reintroduction Phase

- **Unlike celiac disease, NCGS may not require a lifelong gluten-free diet**.
- **Some patients** can tolerate small amounts of gluten over time.

Future Research and Unanswered Questions

Researchers are still trying to understand:

- What are the **genetic factors** influencing NCGS?
- Are there **specific biomarkers** for diagnosis?
- Is NCGS **a separate disease** or a symptom of another condition?
- Can some NCGS patients safely **reintroduce gluten**?

As research progresses, better **diagnostic tests and treatment options** may emerge.

A Growing Concern for Nutritionists

NCGS is a **real but poorly understood condition** that affects **many people**. Since **no specific test** exists, diagnosis relies on **eliminating gluten and observing symptom relief**.

As awareness increases, nutritionists are key in helping individuals navigate NCGS:

- Understand the **difference between NCGS, celiac disease, and wheat allergy**.
- Follow a **proper elimination diet** to determine **true gluten sensitivity**.
- Ensure a **balanced diet** to prevent nutritional deficiencies.

With informed care and continued research, those affected by NCGS can achieve better health outcomes and improved quality of life.

Understanding Celiac Disease

Celiac disease is a chronic autoimmune disorder triggered by the ingestion of gluten. Unlike non-celiac gluten sensitivity (NCGS), celiac disease involves a specific immune-mediated attack on the small intestine, which, if unmanaged, can lead to serious long-term health complications.

Pathogenesis of Celiac Disease

The **development** of celiac disease is a complex process involving **genetic predisposition, immune activation, and environmental triggers**.

Step 1: Genetic Susceptibility

- Nearly all individuals with celiac disease have the **HLA-DQ2 or HLA-DQ8** genes, which help the immune system recognize gluten as an antigen.
- However, **not everyone with these genes develops celiac disease**, meaning environmental factors play a crucial role.

Example: The HLA-DQ2/DQ8 genes act like a lock. Gluten is the key that fits and opens the door to immune activation—but only in genetically predisposed individuals.

Step 2: Gluten Exposure and Immune Activation

- When **gluten enters the digestive system**, it is broken down into **gliadin** and **glutenin** peptides.
- In people with celiac disease, gliadin peptides are only partially digested, allowing them to cross the intestinal lining, triggering the immune system.
- An enzyme called **tissue transglutaminase (tTG)** modifies gliadin peptides, making them more visible to immune cells.
- This leads to **T-cell activation**, which releases **inflammatory cytokines** (IL-15, IFN-γ), leading to **intestinal damage**.

Example: Imagine the immune system as a fire alarm system. In celiac disease, the system **mistakenly detects gluten as fire**, setting off alarms and sending firefighters (immune cells) to attack the intestines.

Step 3: Villous Atrophy and Malabsorption

- The immune response leads to **chronic inflammation**, damaging the **villi**—tiny, finger-like projections responsible for absorbing nutrients in the small intestine.
- Over time, the **villi flatten** (villous atrophy), reducing the ability to absorb essential nutrients like **iron, calcium, and vitamins**.

Example: Think of the villi as a sponge that absorbs water. In celiac disease, the sponge is flattened, preventing proper absorption of nutrients.

Step 4: Systemic Effects

- As a result of **intestinal damage**, people with celiac disease may experience:
    - **Digestive symptoms**: Diarrhea, bloating, abdominal pain.
    - **Nutritional deficiencies**: Anemia (due to iron deficiency), osteoporosis (due to calcium and vitamin D malabsorption).
    - **Neurological symptoms**: Brain fog, depression, headaches.
    - **Skin manifestations**: **Dermatitis herpetiformis**—a chronic, itchy rash linked to celiac disease.

Example: Some individuals experience fatigue and headaches instead of digestive symptoms, making diagnosis difficult.

Epidemiology and Prevalence of Celiac Disease

Celiac disease is a **global health concern**, affecting millions of people. However, **prevalence varies by region, genetics, and environmental factors**.

Global Prevalence

- The prevalence of celiac disease is estimated to be **1% of the global population**.
- **Many cases remain undiagnosed**, as symptoms can be subtle or mistaken for other conditions like irritable bowel syndrome (IBS).

Prevalence by Region

- **Highest Prevalence**: Found in populations with **European ancestry**, especially in **North America, Europe, and Australia** (~1-2%).
- **Lower Prevalence**: Less common in **East Asia, sub-Saharan Africa, and Japan**, likely due to lower frequencies of HLA-DQ2/DQ8 genes.
- **Middle Eastern and South Asian Populations**: Show a **moderate prevalence** but often underdiagnosed due to low awareness.

Risk Factors Influencing Prevalence

1. **Genetics**: First-degree relatives of celiac patients have a **10-15% higher risk** of developing the disease.
2. **Gluten Consumption**: Early or excessive gluten introduction during infancy may increase the risk of triggering celiac disease in genetically susceptible children.
3. **Gut Microbiome**: Imbalances in gut bacteria may play a role in triggering celiac disease.
4. **Environmental Triggers**: Certain infections and stressors may **initiate immune dysregulation** in genetically predisposed individuals.

Example: In Scandinavian countries, studies have shown a higher incidence of celiac disease in children with early gluten exposure and higher dietary gluten intake.

Understanding Wheat Allergy

Wheat allergy is an adverse immune response to proteins found in wheat, leading to allergic reactions that can range from mild to severe. This condition is distinct from celiac disease and non-celiac gluten sensitivity, involving different immune mechanisms.

Pathogenesis

Wheat allergy arises when the immune system mistakenly identifies certain proteins in wheat as harmful, triggering an allergic reaction. This response can be mediated by immunoglobulin E (IgE) antibodies or involve non-IgE mechanisms:

- **IgE-Mediated Reactions**: Upon exposure to wheat proteins, the immune system produces IgE antibodies, leading to immediate allergic reactions. These can manifest as hives, swelling, respiratory issues, or even anaphylaxis—a severe, life-threatening reaction. For instance, a child consuming a wheat-containing cookie might develop hives and breathing difficulties within minutes.
- **Non-IgE-Mediated Reactions**: These involve chronic immune responses, such as eosinophilic esophagitis, characterized by inflammation of the esophagus, leading to difficulty swallowing and food impaction. Symptoms typically develop over hours to days, making diagnosis more challenging.

Epidemiology and Prevalence

Wheat allergy is relatively uncommon, with prevalence varying by age and region:

- **Children**: More commonly affected, with prevalence rates ranging from 0.4% to 1%. Many children outgrow the allergy by school age.
- **Adults**: Less commonly affected, with prevalence rates around 0.1% to 0.3%. In adults, wheat allergy can be associated with occupational exposure, such as in bakers, leading to respiratory symptoms known as baker's asthma.

Diagnosis

Accurate diagnosis involves a combination of clinical evaluation and testing:

1. **Medical History**: Documenting symptoms, their onset relative to wheat exposure, and any family history of allergies.
2. **Skin Prick Test**: Introducing small amounts of wheat protein into the skin to observe for allergic reactions.
3. **Specific IgE Testing**: Measuring IgE antibodies against wheat proteins in the blood.
4. **Oral Food Challenge**: Under medical supervision, the patient consumes increasing amounts of wheat to monitor for reactions.

For non-IgE-mediated allergies, endoscopic evaluation and biopsies may be necessary to assess inflammation in the gastrointestinal tract.

Treatment

Management focuses on avoidance and preparedness:

- **Wheat Avoidance**: Eliminating wheat-containing foods from the diet. This requires careful reading of food labels and awareness of potential cross-contamination. For example, individuals must avoid products like bread, pasta, and certain sauces that may contain wheat.
- **Emergency Preparedness**: Patients at risk for severe reactions should carry an epinephrine auto-injector (e.g., EpiPen) to treat anaphylaxis. Education on recognizing early symptoms and proper use of emergency medication is crucial.
- **Occupational Measures**: For those with occupational exposure, such as bakers, implementing workplace modifications like proper ventilation and personal protective equipment can reduce the risk of respiratory symptoms.

Single Nucleotide Polymorphisms (SNPs) Associated with Gluten-Related Disorders

Condition	SNP (rsID)	Gene	Risk Allele	Normal Allele
Celiac Disease	rs2187668	HLA-DQA1	T	C
Celiac Disease	rs7454108	HLA-DQB1	C	T
Celiac Disease	rs13119723	IL21	G	A
Celiac Disease	rs6822844	IL21	T	C
Gluten Sensitivity	rs2187668	HLA-DQA1	T	C
Gluten Sensitivity	rs7454108	HLA-DQB1	C	T
Wheat Allergy	rs9275596	HLA-DQA1	A	G
Wheat Allergy	rs2858331	HLA-DQB1	T	C

Non-HLA Genes Associated with Celiac Disease

Beyond the well-established HLA-DQ2/DQ8 associations, several non-HLA genes have been implicated in the pathogenesis of celiac disease. These genes influence immune signaling, cytokine response, and lymphocyte migration:

TAGAP (T-cell Activation RhoGTPase Activating Protein):

- **SNPs Identified:** Multiple single nucleotide polymorphisms (SNPs) within the TAGAP gene have been associated with CD.
- **Function:** TAGAP is involved in T-cell activation, a crucial process in the adaptive immune response.
- Association with CD: Variants in TAGAP may influence T-cell behavior, contributing to the inappropriate immune response to gluten observed in CD patients.

IL18R1 (Interleukin 18 Receptor 1):

- **SNPs Identified:** Specific SNPs within the IL18R1 gene have shown an association with CD.
- **Function:** IL18R1 encodes a receptor for interleukin 18, a cytokine involved in inflammatory responses.
- **Association with CD:** Genetic variations in IL18R1 may alter cytokine signaling pathways, leading to enhanced inflammatory responses in the intestinal mucosa of CD patients.

CCR9 (C-C Motif Chemokine Receptor 9):

- **SNPs Identified:** Several SNPs in the CCR9 gene have been linked to CD susceptibility.
- **Function:** CCR9 is a chemokine receptor that directs the migration of lymphocytes to the small intestine.

- **Association with CD:** Alterations in CCR9 may affect lymphocyte trafficking, contributing to the intestinal inflammation characteristic of CD.

IL2 and IL21 (Interleukin 2 and Interleukin 21):

- **SNP Identified:** rs13119723 has been associated with CD.
- **Function:** Both cytokines play roles in the regulation of immune responses.
- **Association with CD:** Variants near these genes may influence cytokine production, affecting the balance of immune regulation in the gut.

RGS21 (Regulator of G-protein Signaling 21):

- **SNPs Identified:** Specific SNPs within RGS21 have been associated with CD.
- **Function:** RGS21 modulates G-protein coupled receptor signaling, which is vital for various immune responses.
- **Association with CD:** Genetic variations in RGS21 may disrupt normal immune signaling pathways, contributing to CD pathogenesis.

PLEK (Pleckstrin):

- **SNPs Identified:** Certain SNPs in the PLEK gene have been linked to CD.
- **Function:** Pleckstrin is involved in actin cytoskeleton rearrangement during immune cell activation.
- **Association with CD:** Variants in PLEK may affect immune cell movement and function, playing a role in the development of CD.

Lactose Intolerance: A Genetic and Evolutionary Perspective

Lactose intolerance is a **condition where the body loses the ability to digest lactose**, the sugar found in milk and dairy products. It results from a **decline in the production of lactase**, the enzyme responsible for breaking down lactose into glucose and galactose for absorption. This leads to **digestive discomfort**, including bloating, diarrhea, and abdominal pain when consuming dairy.

The Role of Lactase and Genetic Evolution

Lactase persistence—the ability to digest milk beyond infancy—is a **recent evolutionary adaptation** in some human populations. The ability to digest lactose depends on the **LCT gene**, which encodes **lactase-phlorizin hydrolase**, the enzyme that breaks down lactose in the **small intestine**.

- In most mammals, **lactase production declines after weaning**, leading to lactose intolerance.
- However, some human populations have evolved **genetic mutations** that **keep lactase production active throughout life**, allowing them to consume dairy without issues.

How Does Lactose Intolerance Occur?

- In **lactose-intolerant individuals**, the undigested lactose **passes to the large intestine**, where gut bacteria ferment it.
- This fermentation process **produces gas and short-chain fatty acids**, leading to symptoms such as bloating, cramps, and diarrhea.

Real-Life Example:

Imagine drinking a glass of milk but experiencing severe stomach cramps and bloating soon after. This happens because your body **lacks lactase**, leaving lactose undigested in the gut, where bacteria break it down and release **gas and acids**, causing discomfort.

The Genetic Basis of Lactose Intolerance

Studies on **African populations, particularly pastoralist groups**, have revealed **multiple independent genetic mutations** associated with **lactase persistence**.

- In **Europe**, a **single mutation (C→T at rs4988235, located upstream of the LCT gene)** is responsible for lactase persistence.
- In **Africa**, multiple distinct **genetic mutations in non-coding regions** regulate lactase expression, allowing lactase persistence in **pastoralist communities** that rely on milk for nutrition.

These mutations are **an example of convergent evolution**—where different genetic changes lead to the same beneficial trait in different populations.

Real-Life Example:

A Maasai herder from East Africa drinks milk without discomfort due to inherited mutations that allow lifelong lactase production. In contrast, a person from West Africa may experience lactose intolerance due to the absence of these genetic variants.

Prevalence and Geographic Distribution

Lactose intolerance is **more common globally** than lactase persistence. The ability to digest milk as an adult **varies across populations** based on genetic and cultural factors.

Lactose Tolerance and Intolerance Across Global Populations

Region	Lactose Tolerance (%)	Lactose Intolerance (%)
Northern Europe	80-90%	10-20%
Southern Europe	50-70%	30-50%
West Africa	10-20%	80-90%
East Africa (Pastoralists)	50-80%	20-50%
East Asia	5-10%	90-95%
Native Americans	0-5%	95-100%

- **Europeans and East African pastoralists** have the highest prevalence of **lactase persistence** due to the historical dependence on dairy.
- **East Asians, Native Americans, and most West Africans** have **high rates of lactose intolerance**, as dairy was not a staple part of their ancestral diet.

Diagnosis of Lactose Intolerance

To determine if a person is lactose intolerant, doctors use **several diagnostic tests**:

Lactose Tolerance Test

- The patient drinks a lactose solution, and blood glucose levels are monitored.
- If glucose **does not rise**, it indicates that **lactose is not being broken down**.

Hydrogen Breath Test

- After lactose consumption, the patient breathes into a device that measures hydrogen levels.
- High hydrogen levels indicate fermentation of undigested lactose by gut bacteria—confirming lactose malabsorption.

Genetic Testing

- Identifies specific mutations associated with lactase persistence or non-persistence, particularly in the MCM6 regulatory region near the LCT gene.
- Useful in determining inherited lactose intolerance, especially in asymptomatic individuals or in populations with a known genetic predisposition.

Evolutionary and Cultural Significance

Lactase persistence is a striking example of gene-culture co-evolution, where human genetic adaptation aligns with long-term dietary practices. In populations that relied on dairy products for nutrition and hydration, especially in environments where other food sources were scarce or vitamin D synthesis was limited, natural selection favored individuals who could digest lactose into adulthood.

Key Evolutionary and Cultural Insights:

- Northern Europeans developed high levels of lactase persistence due to the need for dietary calcium and vitamin D in regions with limited sunlight.
- East African pastoralists consumed milk regularly as both a nutritional and hydration source, leading to genetic adaptations that promote lactase persistence.
- West African, East Asian, and Native American populations traditionally consumed little or no dairy. Consequently, lactase non-persistence remained the ancestral and prevalent trait in these regions.

This adaptation showcases **how human evolution is shaped by dietary practices and environmental conditions**.

Genetic Basis of Lactose Intolerance and Lactase Persistence

Lactose intolerance, also known as **lactase non-persistence (LNP)**, is a condition where individuals lose the ability to digest lactose—the sugar found in milk—due to a decline in lactase enzyme production after weaning. The ability to digest lactose in adulthood, known as **lactase persistence (LP)**, is determined by specific genetic variants upstream of the **LCT gene**, which encodes the lactase enzyme. These regulatory variants are located in the **MCM6 gene**, which modulates **LCT** expression. The two primary variants responsible for lactase persistence or non-persistence are **LCT -13910C>T (rs4988235)** and **LCT -22018G>A (rs182549)**.

Key Genetic Variants Associated with Lactase Persistence and Intolerance

Variant (rsID)	Genomic Location	Associated Trait	Alleles	Functional Effect	Common in Populations
rs4988235	-13,910 bp upstream of LCT (MCM6)	Lactase Persistence (European)	C (intolerance), T (persistence)	T allele allows continued lactase expression	High in Europeans
rs182549	-22,018 bp upstream of LCT (MCM6)	Lactase Persistence (African/Asian)	G (intolerance), A (persistence)	A allele supports extended lactase production	Moderate in East Africans and some Asians

Population Distribution and Evolutionary Adaptation

The **T allele of LCT -13910C>T** is most prevalent in **Northern and Central European populations**, where dairy farming has been a key part of human evolution. This allele frequency is highest in

Scandinavia (>90%), and it gradually declines in **Southern Europe, the Middle East, and Central Asia**. In contrast, the **C allele**, associated with lactase non-persistence, dominates in **East Asian, African, and Indigenous American populations**, where **historical reliance on dairy was minimal**, leading to higher rates of lactose intolerance.

Similarly, the **A allele of LCT -22018G>A** is found more frequently in **Middle Eastern, South Asian, and some East African populations**, suggesting **a separate evolutionary event that favored lactase persistence**. In **Sub-Saharan Africa**, different **SNPs (-13907C>G, -13915T>G, and -14010G>C)** have been linked to lactase persistence in **pastoralist communities**, emphasizing how genetic adaptation to dairy consumption evolved in multiple regions independently.

The persistence of lactase production into adulthood is considered **a classic example of gene-culture co-evolution**, where human dietary habits influenced **natural selection**. Societies that relied on dairy for nutrition retained genetic mutations that allowed **continued lactase expression**, while populations with limited dairy consumption did not experience **selection pressure** for lactase persistence.

Molecular Mechanism of Lactase Regulation

The LCT gene is not self-regulated but is controlled by enhancer elements located within the MCM6 gene, which lies upstream of LCT. These enhancer regions act as molecular switches:

- In individuals with the T allele (rs4988235) or A allele (rs182549), the enhancers remain active into adulthood, allowing continuous transcription of the LCT gene and persistent lactase production.
- In individuals with the C or G alleles, enhancer activity declines after weaning, leading to epigenetic silencing of the LCT gene and a natural drop in lactase levels, a trait typical of most mammals.

This "switch-off" mechanism represents the ancestral state. Mutations that maintain enhancer activity represent a genetic override, allowing lifelong digestion of lactose in populations where dairy was a key food source.

Clinical and Nutritional Implications

Genetic testing for **LCT -13910C>T and LCT -22018G>A** can provide **valuable insights** into an individual's ability to digest lactose. **Screening for these variants** can help:

1. **Identify individuals with lactose intolerance** and recommend appropriate dietary modifications.
2. **Guide precision nutrition strategies**, ensuring adequate calcium and vitamin D intake for those avoiding dairy.

3. **Assist in differential diagnosis** for gastrointestinal disorders, distinguishing lactose intolerance from conditions like **irritable bowel syndrome (IBS) or inflammatory bowel disease (IBD)**.

For **lactase non-persistent individuals**, dietary adjustments can help **mitigate symptoms** of lactose intolerance. Some effective strategies include:

- **Switching to lactose-free dairy products** like almond milk, soy milk, or lactose-free cow's milk.
- **Taking lactase enzyme supplements** before consuming dairy to aid digestion.
- **Consuming fermented dairy products** (e.g., **yogurt, kefir, aged cheese**) that naturally contain lower levels of lactose.
- **Ensuring adequate calcium and vitamin D intake** through non-dairy sources like leafy greens, nuts, seeds, and fortified foods to prevent deficiencies.

Conclusion

The **LCT -13910C>T (rs4988235) and LCT -22018G>A (rs182549)** variants are the primary **genetic determinants of lactase persistence and lactose intolerance**. These SNPs **regulate lactase expression**, influencing an individual's ability to digest lactose throughout adulthood.

Population differences in lactase persistence highlight the role of **evolutionary adaptation**, where **historical reliance on dairy shaped genetic selection**. **Understanding these genetic variants** enables **personalized dietary recommendations**, improving health outcomes for those with **lactose intolerance**. Genetic screening for **lactase persistence markers** helps in **precision nutrition planning**, optimizing diet choices based on individual genetic profiles.

Caffeine Sensitivity

Caffeine is one of the most widely consumed psychoactive substances in the world. Found in coffee, tea, chocolate, and energy drinks, caffeine is part of daily life for billions of people. Whether it's the smell of freshly brewed coffee in the morning or the ritual of sipping tea in the evening, caffeine plays a major role in our dietary and cultural habits.

However, individuals react to caffeine very differently. One person might enjoy a double espresso late at night and fall asleep with ease, while another may experience a racing heart and hours of restlessness after a single afternoon cup. Why such differences? The answer lies in our genes.

Caffeine sensitivity is the degree to which an individual responds to caffeine. It is influenced by several factors—most importantly, genetic variations in how our body processes caffeine. In this chapter, we will explore the history of caffeine, common dietary sources of caffeine, and how our genetic makeup determines our caffeine sensitivity.

History of Caffeine

Ancient Beginnings

The story of caffeine begins thousands of years ago. Some of the earliest records of caffeine consumption date back to ancient China and Ethiopia.

- **Tea in China (around 2737 BCE):** According to legend, Emperor Shen Nong discovered tea when leaves from a wild tree blew into his pot of boiling water. The infusion produced a pleasant aroma and a stimulating effect, leading to the early use of tea as a medicinal drink.
- **Coffee in Ethiopia (9th Century CE):** In another legend, a goat herder named Kaldi noticed that his goats became unusually energetic after eating berries from a certain tree. Curious, Kaldi tried the berries himself and experienced a similar boost. These berries were the seeds of the coffee plant.

Spreading Across the World

Caffeine-rich drinks like coffee and tea eventually made their way around the globe:

- **Middle East and Europe:** By the 15th century, coffee was being consumed in the Arab world, especially in Yemen, where Sufi monks drank it to stay awake during prayers. It reached Europe in the 17th century and quickly became popular in coffee houses, earning the nickname "penny universities" because of the intellectual discussions they hosted.
- **Asia and the Americas:** Tea traveled from China to Japan, then to Europe, and finally became an essential part of British culture. It was also introduced to India by the British East India Company. Meanwhile, in the Americas, cacao—another natural source of caffeine—was cultivated and consumed by the Mayans and Aztecs in ceremonial and daily life long before European colonization.

Modern Day

Today, caffeine is an integral part of everyday life. It is consumed through traditional sources like coffee, tea, and chocolate, as well as in soft drinks, energy drinks, and over-the-counter medications. The global coffee industry alone is valued at over $100 billion, and caffeine remains the most widely used psychoactive substance in the world.

Foods and Beverages Rich in Caffeine

Caffeine is naturally found in a variety of plants and is widely consumed through both food and beverages. Recognizing these sources is especially important for individuals with caffeine sensitivity, as intake can quickly accumulate throughout the day.

1. Coffee

Coffee is one of the most concentrated and commonly consumed sources of caffeine.

- **Caffeine content:** ~95 mg per 8 oz (240 ml) cup of brewed coffee.
- **Types of coffee:**
    - *Espresso* (one shot ~63 mg)
    - *Instant coffee* (~60 mg per cup)
    - *Decaf coffee* (not caffeine-free—still contains ~2-5 mg per cup)

Example: A 16 oz brewed coffee from a café chain may deliver over 180 mg of caffeine in a single serving.

2. Tea

Tea contains varying levels of caffeine depending on the type and preparation.

- **Black tea:** ~47 mg per cup
- **Green tea:** ~28 mg per cup
- **Oolong tea:** ~30–50 mg per cup
- **Matcha:** Higher caffeine content due to powdered whole leaf (~70 mg per serving)

Example: A cup of black tea in the morning may feel gentler compared to coffee, but drinking multiple cups can still lead to high caffeine intake.

3. Chocolate and Cocoa Products

Caffeine is naturally present in cocoa beans, with content varying by product.

- **Dark chocolate (70–85% cacao):** ~23 mg per 1 oz
- **Milk chocolate:** ~6 mg per 1 oz
- **Hot cocoa:** ~5 mg per 8 oz cup

Example: Enjoying a few squares of dark chocolate after dinner could disrupt sleep for caffeine-sensitive individuals.

4. Soft Drinks and Colas

These beverages often contain added caffeine, though less than coffee or energy drinks.

- **Coca-Cola (12 oz can):** ~34 mg
- **Pepsi (12 oz):** ~38 mg
- **Diet versions:** Slightly different but comparable levels

Example: Kids who drink cola with dinner may stay awake longer than usual due to the caffeine content.

5. Energy Drinks

Marketed for alertness and performance, energy drinks are among the most concentrated caffeine sources.

- **Red Bull (8.4 oz):** ~80 mg
- **Monster (16 oz):** ~160 mg
- **Bang Energy (16 oz):** ~300 mg

Example: A teenager drinking two cans of Monster may be consuming over 300 mg of caffeine—equivalent to three cups of coffee.

6. Medications and Supplements

Caffeine is commonly included in over-the-counter drugs and dietary aids.

- **Headache medications** (like Excedrin)
- **Weight loss supplements**
- **Alertness tablets** (e.g., NoDoz)

Example: Taking a caffeine-containing pain reliever along with coffee could unintentionally double caffeine intake.

7. Lesser-Known Sources

Some natural or supplemental products also contribute to caffeine intake.

- **Guarana:** A plant native to the Amazon with high caffeine content, often found in energy drinks.
- **Yerba mate:** A South American tea-like drink with ~85 mg of caffeine per cup.
- **Green coffee bean extract:** Used in weight loss supplements.

Caffeine Metabolism: How the Body Processes Caffeine

Caffeine metabolism refers to the way our body breaks down and eliminates caffeine from the bloodstream. Understanding this process is essential because it helps explain why people react differently to the same amount of caffeine. Some feel alert and focused, while others may get anxious, jittery, or struggle with sleep.

This variation largely depends on **how quickly or slowly our liver enzymes break down caffeine**—and that's where genetics comes in.

What Happens When You Drink Caffeine?

When you consume caffeine—whether it's through coffee, tea, chocolate, soda, or an energy drink—it is **rapidly absorbed** in the stomach and small intestine. Within **30 to 45 minutes**, caffeine reaches its peak levels in the blood.

From there, it **travels to the brain**, where it binds to specific receptors, temporarily blocking a chemical called **adenosine**, which normally promotes sleep and relaxation. This is why caffeine makes you feel more awake and alert.

However, the duration and intensity of these effects vary depending on how efficiently your body processes caffeine.

The Role of the Liver: *CYP1A2* Enzyme

The liver is the central processing unit for caffeine metabolism. The **main enzyme responsible** for this task is **Cytochrome P450 1A2**, commonly called ***CYP1A2***.

This enzyme breaks down caffeine into **three major metabolites**:

Metabolite	% of Total Metabolism	Effects
Paraxanthine	~84%	Increases lipolysis (the breakdown of fats), which elevates free fatty acid levels in the blood. It may also modestly raise blood pressure.
Theobromine	~12%	A mild vasodilator (widens blood vessels) and diuretic. It is naturally found in chocolate and contributes to its mild stimulant effect.
Theophylline	~4%	Relaxes smooth muscles in the airways and has been used in medications for asthma and other respiratory conditions.

The balance and clearance of these metabolites influence how caffeine affects the body overall.

Genetic Influences on Caffeine Sensitivity: An Integrated Review

While lifestyle factors—such as coffee consumption habits or smoking—do affect how the body processes caffeine, **genetic makeup has a powerful influence**. Some people are genetically "wired" to break down caffeine quickly and feel little effect, while others metabolize it slowly and may experience anxiety, palpitations, or insomnia even after a small cup.

Let's explore the key **genetic variants** identified in recent studies and what they mean for caffeine sensitivity.

Recent advances in nutrigenetics have revealed that individual responses to caffeine are governed by complex interactions between multiple genes, affecting both **metabolism** and **neurological sensitivity**. Genome-wide association studies (GWAS) and targeted genetic research have provided a clearer picture of the genetic variants that determine caffeine sensitivity, particularly those influencing how caffeine is metabolized and how it affects the brain and sleep.

1. Genetic Variation in Caffeine Metabolism

The ***CYP1A2*** gene is the most well-established genetic determinant of how quickly caffeine is broken down in the liver. This gene encodes the enzyme cytochrome P450 1A2, responsible for metabolizing nearly 95% of ingested caffeine. A well-studied single nucleotide polymorphism (SNP), **rs762551**, alters enzyme activity and divides individuals into **fast** or **slow metabolizers**:

- **AA genotype (fast metabolizers):** Individuals with this variant break down caffeine quickly, resulting in shorter exposure and fewer physiological effects. These individuals can often tolerate higher caffeine intake with minimal adverse reactions.
- **AC or CC genotypes (slow metabolizers):** These variants slow caffeine metabolism, prolonging its presence in the bloodstream and increasing the likelihood of side effects such as anxiety, insomnia, and elevated blood pressure.

This variation has clinical relevance. Slow metabolizers have been shown to be more susceptible to **caffeine-induced hypertension**, particularly with habitual high intake (>3 cups/day). This genotype–environment interaction highlights that caffeine is not universally harmful or safe; its effects depend on how your body handles it at the molecular level.

Further upstream, **AHR (Aryl Hydrocarbon Receptor)**—a gene that regulates the expression of *CYP1A2*—also influences caffeine metabolism indirectly. Variants in AHR may reduce enzyme expression, slowing caffeine breakdown even if the *CYP1A2* gene itself is unaffected.

2. Genetic Influence on Caffeine's Neurological Effects

Beyond metabolism, **how your brain responds to caffeine** is equally important in determining overall sensitivity. Caffeine works by **blocking adenosine receptors** in the brain, particularly those encoded by the **ADORA2A** gene. Adenosine is a neurotransmitter that promotes sleep and relaxation; caffeine inhibits it, promoting alertness.

A specific variant in ADORA2A, **rs5751876**, plays a critical role in how caffeine affects the central nervous system:

- Individuals with the **CC genotype** tend to be more sensitive to caffeine's neurostimulatory effects, often experiencing **increased anxiety**, nervousness, and **disrupted sleep** even at modest doses.
- The **TT genotype** is associated with a lower risk of these side effects, indicating reduced sensitivity to caffeine's effects on the brain.

Interestingly, these effects are **most pronounced in people who are not regular caffeine consumers**, suggesting that genetic sensitivity may be partially masked or altered by tolerance in habitual users.

Moreover, studies have shown that **caffeine can interfere with sleep architecture**, particularly in genetically sensitive individuals. This is because genetic variants in ADORA2A, and other sleep-related genes, influence how adenosine receptors regulate **slow-wave sleep** (deep, restorative sleep). People with caffeine-sensitive genotypes often report lighter sleep, more awakenings, and reduced sleep efficiency, even if caffeine is consumed in the early afternoon.

3. Genetic Factors Shaping Caffeine Consumption Behavior

Interestingly, the same genes that influence caffeine metabolism and response also affect **how much caffeine people naturally consume**. Fast metabolizers (with *CYP1A2* AA genotypes) tend to consume more caffeine, perhaps because they experience fewer side effects and require higher intake to feel alert.

Genome-wide association studies have also identified several other genes associated with habitual caffeine intake, including:

- **BDNF (Brain-Derived Neurotrophic Factor):** This gene plays a role in mood regulation and cognitive function. Variants may influence how positively individuals perceive caffeine's cognitive-enhancing effects, thus affecting consumption.
- **SLC6A4 (Serotonin Transporter Gene):** Involved in serotonin reuptake, this gene may influence caffeine-related mood effects—either enhancing mood or increasing anxiety—thereby affecting an individual's caffeine-seeking behavior.

These findings support the view that caffeine consumption is not solely a matter of personal preference or cultural exposure, but is also partially genetically driven, shaped by both metabolic and neurological factors.

4. Caffeine, Gene–Environment Interaction, and Personalized Nutrition

Together, these studies highlight the importance of **gene–environment interaction** in determining caffeine sensitivity. It's not just the presence of a specific genetic variant that determines sensitivity, but how that variant functions in combination with lifestyle habits, dietary choices, and caffeine exposure.

For instance:

- A **slow metabolizer (carrying the *CYP1A2* C allele)** who regularly consumes multiple cups of coffee may have an elevated risk of adverse cardiovascular outcomes, such as increased blood pressure or palpitations.
- An individual with a **sensitive ADORA2A genotype** may experience insomnia or anxiety even after a single afternoon coffee, reflecting heightened neurological sensitivity to caffeine.
- Meanwhile, a **fast metabolizer with low ADORA2A sensitivity** may tolerate and even benefit from higher caffeine consumption, experiencing increased alertness and mental clarity without adverse effects.

These insights form the basis of **nutrigenetics-based caffeine recommendations**, allowing individuals to tailor their caffeine intake to suit their unique genetic profile.

Conclusion

Caffeine sensitivity is a complex trait influenced by multiple genes that affect both its metabolism in the liver and its effects in the brain. Variants in ***CYP1A2***, **AHR**, **ADORA2A**, and other related genes shape not only how caffeine is processed but also how it makes us feel—calm and focused, or restless and wired.

Understanding these genetic influences empowers individuals to make more informed choices about caffeine consumption, optimizing its benefits while minimizing potential health risks. As part of personalized nutrition, **genetic testing for caffeine sensitivity** can help guide dietary advice in clinical settings and public health nutrition, especially in populations with diverse caffeine habits and genetic backgrounds.

Nutrigenetic Overview of Caffeine Sensitivity: Key SNPs and their Effects

Gene Name	SNP (rsID)	Risk Allele/ Normal Allele	Inference/Effect	Population Affected	Reference
CYP1A2	rs762551	A = Normal (Fast metabolizer) C = Risk (Slow metabolizer)	Influences rate of caffeine metabolism. C/C genotype = slow clearance, increased sensitivity to caffeine, higher risk of hypertension with high caffeine intake.	Common across populations. C allele frequency ~30–50% in Europeans, Asians.	Cornelis et al., 2006; Nehlig, 2016
AHR	rs4410790	T = Normal C = Risk	Regulates *CYP1A2* expression. The C allele is associated with lower *CYP1A2* activity, slower caffeine metabolism.	Variable across ethnic groups.	Cornelis et al., 2011
ADORA2A	rs5751876	T = Normal C = Risk	Affects caffeine-induced anxiety and sleep disturbance. C/C genotype associated with higher anxiety response to caffeine.	Higher C allele frequency in East Asians and Europeans.	Childs et al., 2008; Rogers et al., 2010
POR (Cytochrome P450 oxidoreductase)	*rs1057868*	T = Normal C = Risk	Affects electron transfer to *CYP1A2*, influencing caffeine metabolism indirectly.	Present across populations; less studied than *CYP1A2*.	Pandey & Flück, 2013
CYP2A6	*rs1801272*	T = Normal A = Reduced activity	Impacts nicotine and caffeine metabolism. Low activity can slow caffeine clearance.	More prevalent in Asians.	Fukami et al., 2005

BDNF	*rs6265* (Val66Met)	Val (G) = Normal Met (A) = Risk	May influence caffeine's effects on mood and cognition; interaction with ADORA2A.	Common in Asians (~20–50%)	Terracciano et al., 2017
PDSS2	*rs17070145*	T = Normal C = Risk	Associated with caffeine consumption behavior; C allele linked to reduced caffeine intake.	Observed in European populations.	Cornelis et al., 2016

Factors Beyond Genetics: Environmental and Physiological Influences on Caffeine Sensitivity

While genetics plays a central role in determining how the body processes caffeine, it is only part of the story. **Environmental, lifestyle, and physiological factors** can significantly modify how caffeine is metabolized and experienced—even in individuals with the same genetic background.

Think of your **genes as the blueprint**, but your **lifestyle and health status as the tools** you use to follow that blueprint. In this section, we'll explore how common factors such as smoking, age, hormonal changes, liver function, and diet interact with the body's caffeine metabolism.

1. Smoking

Effect: Speeds up caffeine metabolism.

Mechanism: Cigarette smoke contains compounds that induce the activity of the ***CYP1A2*** enzyme in the liver—the main enzyme responsible for caffeine breakdown. As a result, smokers tend to metabolize caffeine faster than non-smokers.

Real-life impact: A smoker may need to drink more coffee to feel the same stimulating effects, while a non-smoker might feel jittery with a smaller dose.

Note: This enzyme-inducing effect can mask genetic caffeine sensitivity in smokers who are otherwise slow metabolizers.

2. Oral Contraceptives

Effect: Slows down caffeine metabolism.

Mechanism: Estrogen-containing birth control pills **inhibit *CYP1A2* activity**, meaning caffeine stays in the bloodstream longer.

Real-life impact: A woman on oral contraceptives might experience **stronger or prolonged effects** from caffeine—such as increased alertness, anxiety, or insomnia—even with a standard dose.

Example: If both partners drink coffee after dinner, the woman on oral contraceptives might still feel wired at bedtime, while her partner falls asleep easily.

3. Pregnancy

Effect: Slows down metabolism significantly— especially in the third trimester.

Mechanism: During pregnancy, hormonal changes—particularly elevated estrogen and progesterone—**reduce liver enzyme activity**, including that of *CYP1A2*.

Real-life impact: Pregnant individuals are **more sensitive to caffeine** and may experience palpitations, nausea, or insomnia with doses they previously tolerated. Moreover, **caffeine crosses the placenta**, and the fetus cannot metabolize it efficiently, raising concerns about fetal health.

Clinical advice: Most guidelines recommend limiting caffeine intake to **<200 mg/day** during pregnancy (roughly one 12-oz cup of brewed coffee).

4. Liver Function and Liver Disease

Effect: Impaired caffeine clearance.

Mechanism: The liver is the main site for caffeine metabolism. In conditions such as **hepatitis, cirrhosis, or non-alcoholic fatty liver disease**, *CYP1A2* enzyme activity is often reduced.

Real-life impact: Individuals with liver dysfunction may experience **exaggerated effects** from even small amounts of caffeine—such as tremors, restlessness, or prolonged wakefulness.

Note: Caffeine is sometimes used clinically as a marker of liver function due to its reliance on hepatic clearance.

5. Age

Effect: Caffeine metabolism is slower in **infants** and may decline in **older adults**.

Mechanism:

- **In infants**, the *CYP1A2* enzyme system is underdeveloped. Caffeine clearance is very slow, and half-life can exceed 80 hours in newborns.
- **In older adults**, age-related changes in liver function, kidney function, and body composition may reduce caffeine clearance.

Real-life impact:

- Infants exposed to caffeine through breast milk may experience irritability or poor sleep.
- Older adults may find themselves more sensitive to caffeine over time, even if they were previously tolerant.

6. Diet and Nutrients

Certain foods and nutrients can influence caffeine metabolism by **modulating enzyme activity** or competing for metabolic pathways. These interactions are especially relevant for individuals who experience strong effects from caffeine or consume it regularly.

a. Cruciferous Vegetables (e.g., broccoli, Brussels sprouts, cabbage)

- **Effect:** Increase *CYP1A2* activity, **speeding up caffeine metabolism**.
- **Mechanism:** These vegetables contain compounds like **indole-3-carbinol** that induce phase I detoxification enzymes in the liver.

b. Char-grilled Meats

- **Effect**: May enhance caffeine metabolism.
- **Mechanism**: Cooking meats at high temperatures produces polycyclic aromatic hydrocarbons (PAHs), which can also induce *CYP1A2* activity.

c. Grapefruit Juice

- **Effect:** May slightly reduce caffeine metabolism.
- **Mechanism:** Grapefruit juice is known to inhibit liver enzymes, especially CYP3A4. Though CYP3A4 is not the main enzyme for caffeine, its inhibition can indirectly interfere with liver metabolism and reduce overall clearance efficiency.

d. Supplements and Herbs

- **St. John's Wort:** May induce liver enzymes, increasing caffeine clearance.
- **Echinacea:** May alter liver enzyme activity and affect caffeine metabolism.

7. Physical Activity and Sleep Deprivation

- **Sleep Deprivation:** Acute lack of sleep can heighten caffeine sensitivity, amplifying its stimulating effects. People who are sleep-deprived may feel jittery or anxious even at usual doses.
- **Physical Activity:** Regular exercise may improve caffeine tolerance over time. This could be due to enhanced liver metabolism, better energy utilization, or increased adenosine receptor plasticity in the brain.

Summary Table: Environmental and Physiological Factors that Influence Caffeine Metabolism

Factor	Effect on Caffeine Metabolism
Smoking	Speeds up metabolism (induces *CYP1A2* enzyme)
Oral contraceptives	Slows down metabolism (inhibits *CYP1A2*)
Pregnancy	Slows down metabolism significantly

Liver disease	Reduces caffeine clearance
Age (infants, elderly)	Slower metabolism; infants have very limited clearance
Cruciferous vegetables	May induce *CYP1A2* activity, increasing clearance
Char-grilled meats	Induces liver enzymes; speeds up metabolism
Grapefruit juice	May reduce metabolism by interfering with liver enzymes
St. John's Wort	May increase caffeine clearance

Real-Life Examples of Caffeine Sensitivity

Example 1: The Night Owl vs. The Early Bird

Priya and Rahul are siblings. Priya can drink a cup of coffee at 9 PM and still fall asleep by 10. Rahul, on the other hand, avoids coffee after 2 PM—otherwise, he tosses and turns all night.

Genetic testing later revealed the reason behind their contrast: Rahul has a slow-metabolizing variant of the ***CYP1A2*** gene, which means caffeine lingers in his system longer. Priya, on the other hand, carries the fast-metabolizing variant, allowing her body to break down caffeine quickly and avoid sleep disruption.

Example 2: The Anxiety Link

Maya, a college student, relies on caffeine to stay alert during exam week. After three cups of coffee in one day, she starts feeling jittery, her heart races, and she experiences a wave of anxiety. Her friend Ritu drinks the same amount and feels completely fine.

The difference might lie in their genes. Maya could have a specific variation in the ***ADORA2A*** gene, which makes her more neurologically sensitive to caffeine. This gene affects how caffeine interacts with adenosine receptors in the brain—people with this variant are more likely to feel anxious or overstimulated after caffeine intake.

Conclusion

Although genetics sets the foundation for how our body metabolizes and responds to caffeine, many **external and physiological factors** can alter this response significantly. From lifestyle habits like smoking to biological states like pregnancy or aging, these influences can **either amplify or dampen** caffeine's effects.

For truly personalized nutrition guidance, it's important to consider both **genetic predisposition** and **current lifestyle or health context**. This holistic approach ensures that caffeine intake recommendations are tailored, safe, and effective for each individual.

Questions

1. What is gluten?
2. Which condition is triggered by an autoimmune reaction to gluten?
3. What is non-celiac gluten sensitivity?
4. What test confirms celiac disease?
5. What is lactose intolerance?
6. Which sugar in milk causes lactose intolerance symptoms?
7. Name one common symptom of lactose intolerance.
8. Which enzyme is lacking in lactose intolerance?
9. What is caffeine sensitivity?
10. Which organ metabolizes caffeine?
11. Which gene is most studied in caffeine sensitivity?
12. What are typical effects of caffeine on the body?
13. What symptom can occur if a caffeine-sensitive person drinks coffee late in the evening?
14. What is the recommended treatment for lactose intolerance?
15. Which beverage contains caffeine naturally—milk, coffee, or orange juice?
16. How does gluten trigger an immune response in individuals with celiac disease?
17. What genetic markers are strongly associated with celiac disease?
18. How is non-celiac gluten sensitivity different from wheat allergy?
19. What role does the microbiome play in gluten sensitivity?
20. Explain the difference between primary and secondary lactose intolerance.
21. How do genetic variations in the LCT gene affect lactose tolerance?
22. What diagnostic test is used to confirm lactose intolerance?
23. Why do some lactose-intolerant individuals tolerate yogurt better than milk?
24. How does the *CYP1A2* gene affect caffeine metabolism?
25. What health risks are linked to slow caffeine metabolism?
26. How does caffeine affect adenosine receptors in the brain?
27. Why might caffeine sensitivity vary between individuals despite similar caffeine intake?
28. What is the relationship between caffeine, sleep, and anxiety disorders?
29. How does lactose intolerance prevalence vary across populations?
30. How can personalized nutrition address gluten, lactose, and caffeine sensitivity?

Answers

1. Gluten is a protein complex found in wheat, barley, and rye that gives dough elasticity.
2. Celiac disease.
3. A condition where people experience gluten-related symptoms without celiac disease or wheat allergy.
4. Serologic testing (anti-tTG antibodies) and small intestinal biopsy.
5. The inability to digest lactose due to reduced lactase enzyme activity.
6. Lactose.
7. Bloating, diarrhea, abdominal cramps, or gas.
8. Lactase.
9. A condition where individuals metabolize caffeine slowly, leading to stronger or prolonged effects.
10. The liver.
11. *CYP1A2*.
12. Increased alertness, stimulation of the central nervous system, elevated heart rate.
13. Insomnia or disturbed sleep.
14. Reducing lactose intake or using lactase enzyme supplements.
15. Coffee.
16. Gluten peptides are presented by HLA-DQ2/DQ8 molecules, activating T-cells and causing villous atrophy.
17. HLA-DQ2 and HLA-DQ8 haplotypes.
18. NCGS involves symptoms without immune markers or intestinal damage, while wheat allergy is IgE-mediated.
19. Gut bacteria influence gluten peptide breakdown and immune tolerance, potentially modulating sensitivity.
20. Primary: gradual lactase decline with age (genetic). Secondary: results from gut injury or disease.
21. Lactase persistence variants in the LCT gene allow continued lactase production into adulthood.
22. Hydrogen breath test or lactose tolerance blood test.
23. Fermented dairy like yogurt contains bacterial lactase and lower lactose content.
24. Variants determine whether someone is a "fast" or "slow" caffeine metabolizer.
25. Increased risk of hypertension, heart disease, and sleep disturbances.
26. It blocks adenosine receptors, preventing drowsiness and promoting alertness.
27. Due to differences in *CYP1A2* and ADORA2A genes, liver enzyme activity, age, sex, and hormones.
28. Caffeine can worsen insomnia and anxiety in sensitive individuals due to nervous system overstimulation.
29. Highest in East Asian and African populations, lowest in Northern Europeans.
30. Through genetic testing (HLA, LCT, *CYP1A2*), dietary adjustments (gluten-free, lactose-free, reduced caffeine), and microbiome-based interventions.

References

1. Monsuur, A. J., de Bakker, P. I. W., Zhernakova, A., et al. (2008). Effective detection of human leukocyte antigen risk alleles in celiac disease using tag single nucleotide polymorphisms. *PLoS ONE, 3*(5), e2270. https://doi.org/10.1371/journal.pone.0002270
2. Cárdenas-Torres, F. I., Cabrera-Chávez, F., Figueroa-Salcido, O. G., & Ontiveros, N. (2016). Non-celiac gluten sensitivity: An update. In Feighery, C., & Murray, J. A. (Eds.), *Celiac disease and non-celiac gluten sensitivity*. National Center for Biotechnology Information (NCBI). https://www.ncbi.nlm.nih.gov/books/NBK441900/
3. Cárdenas-Torres, F. I., Cabrera-Chávez, F., Figueroa-Salcido, O. G., & Ontiveros, N. (2016). Non-celiac gluten sensitivity: An update. *Gastroenterology Research and Practice, 2016,* 5760724. https://doi.org/10.1155/2016/5760724.
4. Sapone, A., Bai, J. C., Ciacci, C., et al. (2012). Spectrum of gluten-related disorders: consensus on new nomenclature and classification. *BMC Medicine, 10*, 13. https://doi.org/10.1186/1741-7015-10-13.
5. Laaksonen, M. M. L., Mikkilä, V., Räsänen, L., Rontu, R., Lehtimäki, T. J., Viikari, J. S. A., & Raitakari, O. T.; Cardiovascular Risk in Young Finns Study Group. (2009). Genetic lactase non-persistence, consumption of milk products and intakes of milk nutrients in Finns from childhood to young adulthood. *British Journal of Nutrition, 102*(1), 8–17. https://doi.org/10.1017/S0007114508184677 PubMed
6. Lamri, A., Poli, A., Emery, N., Bellili, N., Velho, G., Lantieri, O., Balkau, B., & Marre, M., & Fumeron, F. (2013). The lactase persistence genotype is associated with body mass index and dairy consumption in the D.E.S.I.R. study. *Metabolism, 62*(9), 1323-1329. https://doi.org/10.1016/j.metabol.2013.04.006 PubMed
7. Peng, M.-S., He, J.-D., Zhu, C.-L., Wu, S.-F., Jin, J.-Q., Zhang, Y. P., et al. (2012). Lactase persistence may have an independent origin in Tibetan populations from Tibet, China. *Journal of Human Genetics, 57*(6), 394-397. https://doi.org/10.1038/jhg.2012.41
8. Nehlig, A. (2016). Interindividual Differences in Caffeine Metabolism and Factors Driving Caffeine Consumption. *Pharmacological Reviews*, 68(3), 1043–1079. https://doi.org/10.1124/pr.115.011288
9. Cornelis, M.C., & El-Sohemy, A. (2007). Coffee, caffeine, and coronary heart disease. *Current Opinion in Lipidology*, 18(1), 13–19. https://doi.org/10.1097/MOL.0b013e328011c6e1
10. Grosso, G., et al. (2016). Coffee, Caffeine, and Health Outcomes: An Umbrella Review. *Annual Review of Nutrition*, 36, 123–152. https://doi.org/10.1146/annurev-nutr-071715-050859
11. World Health Organization. (2020). *Caffeine in Food and Dietary Supplements: Examining Safety*.
12. Institute of Medicine (US) Committee on Military Nutrition Research. (2001). *Caffeine for the Sustainment of Mental Task Performance: Formulations for Military Operations*.
13. Higdon, J.V., & Frei, B. (2006). Coffee and health: a review of recent human research. *Critical Reviews in Food Science and Nutrition*, 46(2), 101–123.

14. Mayo Clinic. (2023). Caffeine content for coffee, tea, soda, and more.
15. Cornelis, M.C., et al. (2006). Genetic Polymorphisms of *CYP1A2* and Response to Caffeine. *Journal of Clinical Pharmacology*, 46(2), 142–150.
16. Cornelis, M. C., et al. (2006). Genetic polymorphisms of *CYP1A2* and response to caffeine. *Journal of Clinical Pharmacology*, 46(2), 142–150.
17. Nehlig, A. (2016). Interindividual differences in caffeine metabolism and factors driving caffeine consumption. *Pharmacological Reviews*, 68(3), 1043–1079.
18. Cornelis, M. C., et al. (2011). Genome-wide meta-analysis identifies regions on 7p21 (AHR) and 15q24 (*CYP1A2*) as determinants of habitual caffeine consumption. *PLoS Genetics*, 7(4), e1002033.
19. Childs, E., et al. (2008). Genetic variation in adenosine A2A receptor predicts caffeine-induced anxiety. *Neuropsychopharmacology*, 33(2), 279–289.
20. Rogers, P. J., et al. (2010). Association of the anxiogenic and alerting effects of caffeine with adenosine A2A receptor genotype. *Neuropsychopharmacology*, 35(9), 1973–1983.
21. Pandey, A. V., & Flück, C. E. (2013). NADPH P450 oxidoreductase: structure, function, and pathology of diseases. *Pharmacology & Therapeutics*, 138(2), 229–254.
22. Fukami, T., et al. (2005). A novel polymorphic allele of the CYP2A6 gene, CYP2A6*14, found in a Japanese population. *Drug Metabolism and Disposition*, 33(1), 118–122.
23. Terracciano, A., et al. (2017). BDNF Val66Met is associated with response to caffeine, mood, and cognitive function. *Psychopharmacology*, 234(2), 323–331.
24. Cornelis, M. C., et al. (2016). Genome-wide association study of caffeine intake among UK Biobank participants. *Human Molecular Genetics*, 25(24), 5492–5502.
25. Palatini, P., et al. (2012). *CYP1A2* genotype modifies the association between coffee intake and the risk of hypertension. *Journal of Hypertension*, 30(7), 1342–1349. https://pubmed.ncbi.nlm.nih.gov/22336631/
26. Rogers, P. J., et al. (2010). Association of the anxiogenic and alerting effects of caffeine with adenosine A2A receptor genotype. *Neuropsychopharmacology*, 35(9), 1973–1983. https://pmc.ncbi.nlm.nih.gov/articles/PMC2745641/
27. Southward, K., et al. (2020). Genetics of habitual caffeine consumption and its association with performance in endurance athletes. *Nutrients*, 12(12), 3701. https://pubmed.ncbi.nlm.nih.gov/31817803/
28. Bjorness, T. E., et al. (2020). Caffeine and adenosine receptors: Genetic and molecular pathways of sleep disruption. *Sleep Advances*, 1(1), zpaa004. https://pubmed.ncbi.nlm.nih.gov/32615857/

CHAPTER 7

HOMOCYSTEINE METABOLISM

Methylation and Homocysteine Metabolism – The Cellular Switches Behind Your Health

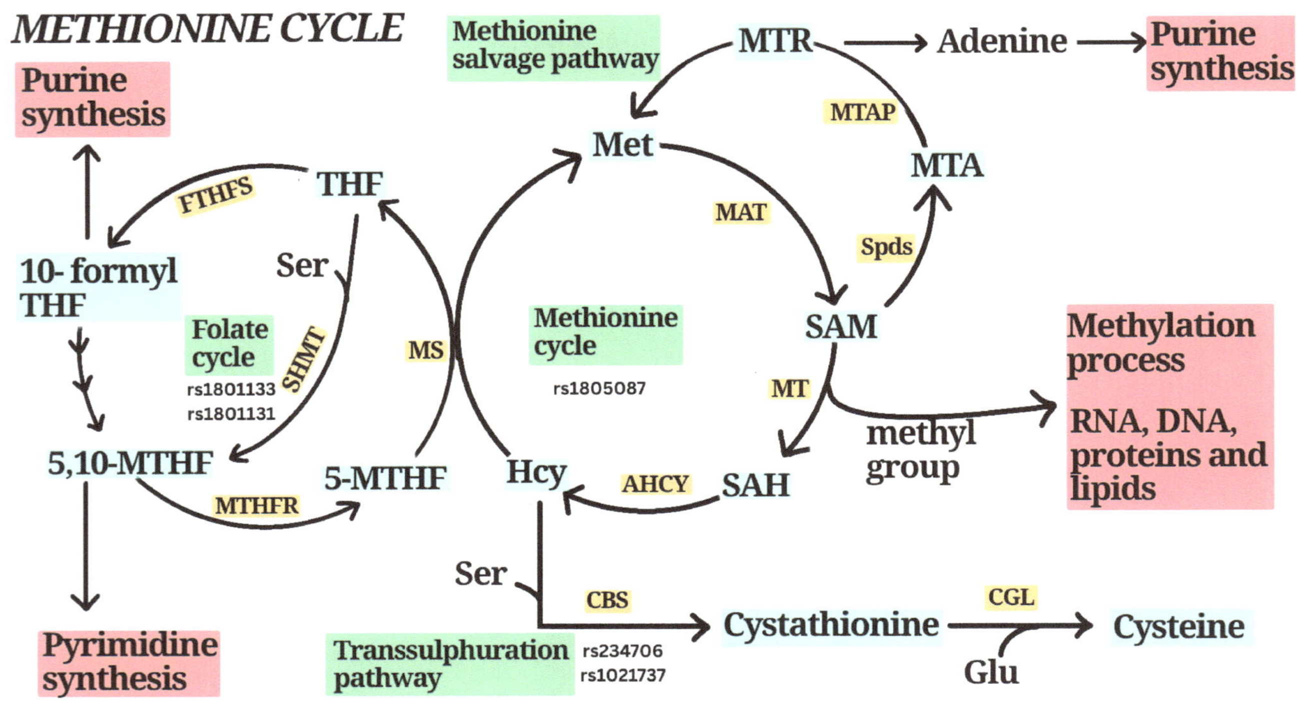

Imagine your body as a busy city, with countless workers keeping everything running smoothly—traffic lights guiding cars, signals telling machines when to start and stop, and workers following instructions to build and repair. One of the most important systems making sure all this works at a microscopic level is a process called **methylation**.

Methylation is like the body's master control switch. It involves attaching tiny chemical groups called **methyl groups** ($-CH_3$) to different molecules, including DNA, proteins, and neurotransmitters. These methyl groups act like traffic signals—telling your genes when to turn "on" or "off," guiding detoxification, supporting brain health, building neurotransmitters like serotonin and dopamine, and even helping you fight infections and maintain energy.

But for methylation to work properly, your body depends on a fine-tuned cycle of nutrients and enzymes—and one key player in this process is a compound called **homocysteine**.

What is Homocysteine?

Homocysteine is a natural byproduct that forms when our body breaks down an essential amino acid called **methionine**, which comes from protein-rich foods like meat, eggs, and fish. Under normal conditions, homocysteine is recycled into methionine or converted into another helpful compound called **cysteine**—but this only happens efficiently when your body has enough **vitamins B6, B12, folate (B9),** and certain enzymes that guide the process.

If this recycling doesn't happen well, homocysteine levels can rise in the blood, and this becomes a problem. **High levels of homocysteine are like factory waste that builds up when the machines are not working efficiently.** Over time, it can damage blood vessels, increase the risk of heart disease, stroke, dementia, pregnancy complications, and more.

The Two Main Pathways of Homocysteine Metabolism

Homocysteine doesn't just float around forever. Your body processes it using **two main pathways**:

1. Remethylation (Recycling Back to Methionine)

This is like the recycling plant of your cellular city.

- Homocysteine is converted back into methionine with the help of vitamin B12 (cobalamin) and folate (vitamin B9).
- The enzyme that facilitates this process is methionine synthase.
- 5-Methyltetrahydrofolate (5-MTHF), the active form of folate, donates the methyl group required for this conversion.
- A genetic variant in the MTHFR gene (commonly the C677T mutation, which reduces the enzyme's activity) can impair this process by limiting the availability of 5-MTHF.

Real-life example:

An IT professional, Arjun, started taking folic acid supplements after learning about high homocysteine levels in his blood. But his levels didn't improve. A genetic test revealed he had the MTHFR C677T mutation, making it hard for him to convert folic acid into active 5-MTHF. Once he switched to methylated folate, his homocysteine levels improved.

2. Transsulfuration (Conversion to Cysteine)

This is like sending homocysteine down the detoxification drain of your body.

- Homocysteine is first converted to cystathionine, then into cysteine, a building block for glutathione—a powerful antioxidant.
- This reaction relies on vitamin B6 and the enzyme cystathionine β-synthase (CBS).

Real-life example:

Radha, a woman with frequent fatigue and low immunity, was found to have low B6 levels and high homocysteine. Once she added **vitamin B6-rich foods** (like bananas, poultry, and chickpeas) and took a B-complex supplement, her energy and lab values improved.

Key Genetic Variants Influencing Homocysteine Metabolism and Methylation Efficiency

Gene	SNP (rsID)	Function	Normal/ Risk Allele	Inference	References
MTHFR	rs1801133 (C677T)	Converts 5,10-methylene-THF to 5-MTHF (active folate)	C = Normal, T = Risk	T allele reduces enzyme activity (up to 70% if homozygous TT); associated with elevated homocysteine, increased need for methylfolate	Frosst et al., 1995; Crider et al., 2012
MTHFR	rs1801131 (A1298C)	Modulates folate metabolism and methylation	A = Normal, C = Risk	C allele may reduce enzyme activity (less than C677T); combined effect with C677T may impair methylation	van der Put et al., 1998
MTR	rs1805087 (A2756G)	Encodes methionine synthase which remethylates homocysteine to methionine	A = Normal, G = Risk	G allele may reduce enzyme efficiency; increased need for B12	Harmon et al., 1999
MTRR	rs1801394 (A66G)	Regenerates methionine synthase; maintains B12-dependent remethylation	A = Normal, G = Risk	G allele linked to reduced MTRR activity; may raise homocysteine	Chen et al., 2001
CBS	rs234706 (844ins68)	Converts homocysteine to cystathionine (transsulfuration pathway)	Wild type = Normal, 68 bp insertion = Risk	Insertion variant may impair CBS activity; higher homocysteine, requires B6 support	Kraus et al., 1999
SHMT1	rs1979277	Affects interconversion of folate forms and supports methyl group availability	G = Normal, A = Risk	A allele may reduce folate cycle efficiency and impact homocysteine regulation	Skibola et al., 2002
BHMT	rs3733890	Involved in alternative remethylation pathway using betaine	G = Normal, A = Risk	A allele may reduce enzyme activity, higher homocysteine if folate/ B12 is low	Schwahn et al., 2003

Homocysteine and Heart Health: The Historical and Scientific Perspective

A Historical Breakthrough: Dr. Kilmer McCully's Discovery

In 1969, **Dr. Kilmer McCully**, a pathologist at Harvard Medical School, made a revolutionary connection that changed how we think about heart disease. He noticed that children with homocystinuria—a rare genetic disorder characterized by extremely high homocysteine levels—developed severe atherosclerosis and vascular disease at a young age.

McCully hypothesized that **even moderately elevated levels of homocysteine**—in individuals without this rare disorder—might contribute to **atherosclerosis and cardiovascular disease (CVD)** in the general population. At the time, his hypothesis was met with skepticism, and he faced significant academic backlash, including the loss of his position at Harvard. Despite these challenges, his persistence laid the foundation for what became known as the homocysteine hypothesis of cardiovascular disease, eventually earning him recognition and a nomination for the prestigious Lasker Award.

"In the long run, it is not the mainstream but the truth that matters." — Dr. Kilmer McCully

Observational Evidence: Epidemiological Support for the Hypothesis

Numerous observational and epidemiological studies later supported Dr. McCully's idea, consistently demonstrating that elevated plasma homocysteine levels are associated with increased risk for several cardiovascular conditions, including:

- Coronary artery disease (CAD)
- Ischemic stroke
- Peripheral arterial disease
- Aortic stiffness

Example: A 2002 meta-analysis by the Homocysteine Studies Collaboration showed that a **5 µmol/L increase in homocysteine** was associated with a **20% increased risk of ischemic heart disease** and a **32% increased risk of stroke**.

Randomized Controlled Trials (RCTs): Promising Biochemistry, Mixed Clinical Outcomes

Following promising epidemiological data, several RCTs explored whether lowering homocysteine through supplementation—primarily with folic acid, vitamin B6, and vitamin B12—could reduce the risk of cardiovascular events. While these trials consistently demonstrated reductions in homocysteine levels, the results for clinical outcomes were mixed.

Key Trials:

- **HOPE-2 (2006)**: Found a modest reduction in stroke incidence, but no significant impact on myocardial infarction or cardiovascular death.

- **NORVIT (2006)** and **VISP (2004)**: Despite lowering homocysteine levels, these trials did not show a significant reduction in recurrent cardiovascular events.

Inference: Although homocysteine-lowering therapy improves biochemical markers, it may not translate into immediate cardiovascular benefits—particularly in individuals with pre-existing vascular damage. These findings suggest that earlier intervention, longer follow-up periods, or additional therapeutic targets may be needed to see meaningful cardiovascular risk reduction.

Mendelian Randomization Studies

Mendelian randomization (MR) uses genetic variants as proxies to assess causality between homocysteine and CVD.

- Studies using **MTHFR C677T** variants showed that individuals with **TT genotypes** (associated with higher homocysteine levels) had an increased risk of stroke—but evidence for **coronary heart disease** remained inconsistent
- MR studies concluded that **homocysteine might be more causally associated with stroke than with heart disease**.

Genome-Wide Association Studies (GWAS)

GWAS identified several **SNPs affecting homocysteine metabolism**, including:

Gene	SNP	Effect
MTHFR	rs1801133 (C677T)	Reduced enzyme activity, increased homocysteine
CBS	rs234706	Affects transsulfuration
MTR, MTRR	Various	Affect remethylation via B12 pathway

Despite these associations with homocysteine levels, many of these SNPs have not shown consistent associations with coronary artery disease across diverse and large population cohorts.

Landmark Studies Linking Homocysteine to Cardiovascular Disease

Study Name/Year	Study Type	Primary Outcome	Secondary Outcome	Findings
McCully (1969)	Case study	Observation of vascular disease in homocystinuria	Hypothesis development	Homocysteine damages blood vessels
Homocysteine Studies Collaboration (2002)	Meta-analysis	Coronary artery disease	Stroke	Risk increases with homocysteine elevation
VISP (2004)	RCT	Stroke recurrence	Total mortality	No benefit from B-vitamin therapy

NORVIT (2006)	RCT	Recurrent MI	Stroke, death	No benefit, possible harm with high-dose vitamins
HOPE-2 (2006)	RCT	Major cardiovascular events	Stroke	Stroke risk reduced, no effect on MI or death
Meta-analysis by Clarke et al. (2012)	MR	Ischemic stroke	Coronary disease	MTHFR TT genotype linked to stroke, not CHD
van Meurs et al. (2013)	GWAS	Homocysteine levels	CAD	13 loci identified, no causal role in CAD

Homocysteine-Related SNPs and Cardiovascular Risk Across Populations

Gene	SNP (rsID)	Risk/Normal Allele	Populations Most Affected	Inferences	References
MTHFR	rs1801133 (C677T)	T = Risk, C = Normal	East Asians (~30–40% TT), South Asians (~10–20% TT), Hispanics (~20%)	T allele reduces enzyme activity → ↓ 5-MTHF → ↑ homocysteine → ↑ CVD, stroke risk	Frosst et al., 1995; Clarke et al., 2012
MTHFR	rs1801131 (A1298C)	C = Risk, A = Normal	Caucasians (~30–35% AC or CC), Middle Eastern populations	May lower MTHFR activity (less than 677T); additive risk with C677T	van der Put et al., 1998
MTR	rs1805087 (A2756G)	G = Risk, A = Normal	European populations (~20% G carriers)	Reduces methionine synthase efficiency → impaired remethylation → ↑ homocysteine	Harmon et al., 1999
MTRR	rs1801394 (A66G)	G = Risk, A = Normal	Globally distributed; higher in Europeans and Asians	Impairs regeneration of B12-dependent enzymes → ↑ homocysteine	Chen et al., 2001
CBS	rs234706 (844ins68)	Insertion = Risk, Wild type = Normal	Rare in general population; more frequent in some homocystinuria families	Reduces CBS enzyme activity → impaired transsulfuration pathway → ↑ homocysteine	Kraus et al., 1999
SHMT1	rs1979277	A = Risk, G = Normal	European and American populations (~20% AA)	Alters folate cycle flow → ↑ homocysteine; interacts with MTHFR SNPs	Skibola et al., 2002
BHMT	rs3733890	A = Risk, G = Normal	African Americans and Caucasians (~10–15%)	Affects alternative remethylation (via betaine) → ↑ homocysteine when folate is low	Schwahn et al., 2003

References

1. McCully, K.S. (1969). *Vascular pathology of homocystinuria: implications for the pathogenesis of arteriosclerosis*. Am J Pathol.
2. Homocysteine Studies Collaboration. (2002). *Homocysteine and risk of ischemic heart disease and stroke: a meta-analysis.* JAMA.
3. Lonn, E., et al. (2006). *HOPE-2 trial.* N Engl J Med.
4. Bonaa KH, et al. (2006). *NORVIT trial.* N Engl J Med.
5. Toole JF, et al. (2004). *VISP trial.* JAMA.
6. Clarke R, et al. (2012). *MTHFR and CHD: a meta-analysis of genetic studies.* BMJ.
7. van Meurs JBJ, et al. (2013). *GWAS of plasma homocysteine.* Hum Mol Genet.
8. Wald DS, et al. (2002). *Homocysteine and cardiovascular disease: evidence on causality.* BMJ.
9. Frosst P, et al. (1995). *A candidate genetic risk factor for vascular disease: a common mutation in methylenetetrahydrofolate reductase.* Nat Genet.
10. Crider KS, et al. (2012). *Folate and DNA methylation: a review of molecular mechanisms and the evidence for folate's role.* Adv Nutr.
11. van der Put NM, et al. (1998). *A second common mutation in the methylenetetrahydrofolate reductase gene.* Am J Hum Genet.
12. Harmon DL, et al. (1999). *Methionine synthase polymorphisms and homocysteine.* Clin Chem Lab Med.
13. Chen J, et al. (2001). *Methionine synthase reductase A66G polymorphism and risk of cardiovascular disease.* Circulation.
14. Kraus JP, et al. (1999). *Mutations in the CBS gene and homocystinuria.* Hum Mutat.
15. Skibola CF, et al. (2002). *Polymorphisms in SHMT1 and risk of adult acute leukemia.* Cancer Epidemiol Biomarkers Prev.
16. Schwahn B, et al. (2003). *Betaine-homocysteine methyltransferase (BHMT) polymorphisms: determinants of homocysteine levels.* Clin Chem.

Homocysteine Metabolism and Infertility

Fertility is not only influenced by hormones and reproductive organs—it also depends on the **fine-tuned biochemistry inside our cells**. One such biochemical player is **homocysteine**, a sulfur-containing amino acid produced during methionine metabolism.

Although homocysteine is a normal intermediate in metabolism, when it **accumulates in excess**—a condition called **hyperhomocysteinemia**—it can cause **oxidative stress, inflammation, impaired blood flow, and DNA damage**, all of which can negatively impact reproductive health in both men and women.

Understanding the Connection: Homocysteine and Reproductive Health

In Women

1. **Egg Quality & Follicular Environment**

   Elevated homocysteine in **follicular fluid** can impair **oocyte maturation**, leading to poor egg quality and reduced fertilization rates.

2. **Implantation Failure**

   High homocysteine levels can impair **endometrial receptivity** by causing **vascular dysfunction** and **microthrombi formation**, leading to **implantation failure** and **early miscarriage**.

3. **Polycystic Ovary Syndrome (PCOS)**

   Women with PCOS often have **elevated homocysteine**, which worsens **insulin resistance** and **inflammation**, contributing to subfertility.

4. **Recurrent Pregnancy Loss (RPL)**

   Hyperhomocysteinemia is strongly linked with **recurrent miscarriages**, especially when combined with **MTHFR gene variants** and low folate/B12 levels.

In Men

1. **Sperm DNA Integrity**

   Homocysteine-induced **oxidative stress** can damage **sperm DNA**, leading to reduced sperm motility and increased fragmentation.

2. **Hormonal Imbalance**

   Elevated homocysteine can affect the **hypothalamic–pituitary–gonadal (HPG) axis**, disturbing testosterone production and spermatogenesis.

3. **Poor Semen Parameters**

   Studies have shown that men with high homocysteine levels often have **low sperm count**, **poor morphology**, and **reduced motility**.

Genetic Factors: MTHFR and Fertility

The **MTHFR (methylenetetrahydrofolate reductase) gene** is critical in converting folate into its active form (5-MTHF), which donates methyl groups for the remethylation of homocysteine to methionine.

Mutations like **C677T** and **A1298C** reduce enzyme activity and lead to **elevated homocysteine** and **methylation defects**, which can impair fertility by:

- Disrupting DNA methylation during gamete formation (spermatogenesis and oogenesis)
- Compromising embryo development and implantation success
- Increasing the risk of neural tube defects (NTDs) in developing fetuses when maternal folate metabolism is impaired.

Nutritional and Clinical Management

Addressing elevated homocysteine and supporting methylation pathways can improve fertility outcomes, especially in individuals with MTHFR variants. A targeted nutritional approach involves increasing intake of key cofactors and methyl donors through diet and supplementation.

Nutritional Strategies to Lower Homocysteine

Nutrient	Role	Sources
Folate (B9)	Required for methylation of homocysteine	Leafy greens, legumes, methylfolate supplements
Vitamin B12	Works with folate in remethylation	Animal products, dairy, fortified cereals
Vitamin B6	Converts homocysteine to cysteine	Bananas, poultry, chickpeas
Betaine (TMG)	Alternative methyl donor	Beets, spinach, whole grains
Zinc & Magnesium	Cofactors in enzymes	Nuts, seeds, seafood

Key Research Studies Linking Homocysteine to Fertility Outcomes

A growing body of clinical research highlights the association between elevated homocysteine levels and impaired reproductive outcomes. The following studies demonstrate how homocysteine impacts fertility across various populations and conditions.

Study/Year	Population	Findings	Outcome
Berker et al., 2009	Women undergoing IVF	Higher follicular homocysteine = poor embryo quality	↓ Fertility success
Murto et al., 2013	Women with PCOS	Elevated homocysteine levels in PCOS	Associated with ovulatory dysfunction
Li et al., 2019	Men with infertility	Higher homocysteine = lower sperm motility and DNA damage	↓ Male fertility
Nelen et al., 2000	Women with RPL	High homocysteine linked to pregnancy loss	↑ Miscarriage risk
Ebisch et al., 2006	Couples with subfertility	MTHFR 677TT associated with higher homocysteine and poor fertility outcomes	↓ Reproductive success

Homocysteine-Related SNPs and Infertility Across Populations

Several single nucleotide polymorphisms (SNPs) in genes regulating homocysteine metabolism have been linked to infertility through impaired methylation, oxidative stress, and altered gamete quality. The table below summarizes key SNPs, their population prevalence, and reproductive health implications.

Gene	**SNP (rsID)**	**Risk/Normal Allele**	**Populations Most Affected**	**Inferences in Infertility**	**References**
MTHFR	rs1801133 (C677T)	T = Risk, C = Normal	High in East Asians (30–40% TT), South Asians (10–20% TT), Hispanics (~20%)	T allele → ↓ MTHFR activity → ↑ homocysteine → poor egg quality, RPL, implantation failure, sperm DNA damage	Forges et al., 2007; Nelen et al., 2000; Li et al., 2019
MTHFR	rs1801131 (A1298C)	C = Risk, A = Normal	Common in Caucasians (~30–35% AC/CC)	Reduces methylation efficiency; with 677T compound heterozygosity increases infertility risk	Ebisch et al., 2006
MTR	rs1805087 (A2756G)	G = Risk, A = Normal	More prevalent in European populations (~20%)	Affects remethylation of homocysteine; linked to poor methylation → miscarriage, male subfertility	Murphy et al., 2007
MTRR	rs1801394 (A66G)	G = Risk, A = Normal	Found globally; common in Asians & Europeans	Impaired regeneration of methionine synthase → ↑ homocysteine → implantation failure	Forges et al., 2007

CBS	rs234706 (844ins68)	Insertion = Risk	Rare; higher in families with homocystinuria	Impaired transsulfuration → toxic homocysteine levels; linked with early miscarriage, male infertility	Kraus et al., 1999
BHMT	rs3733890	A = Risk, G = Normal	Caucasians and African Americans (~10–15%)	Affects alternative methylation via betaine; associated with methylation errors → infertility, low embryo viability	Schwahn et al., 2003

Nutritional Interventions and the MTHFR C677T Polymorphism: Insights from Meta-Analyses and Studies

Numerous studies have explored the association between the MTHFR C677T polymorphism and metabolic health, particularly its effects on metabolic syndrome (MS), obesity, and sarcopenia. The MTHFR C677T polymorphism, which impairs folate metabolism, has been linked to elevated homocysteine levels, a known risk factor for cardiovascular disease, and other health issues. However, the relationship between this genetic variant and nutritional interventions has been highlighted more comprehensively through meta-analysis studies, which synthesize the findings of multiple studies to provide robust conclusions.

Meta-Analysis on MTHFR C677T and Folate Metabolism

A meta-analysis study focusing on the MTHFR C677T polymorphism and its impact on blood folate concentrations revealed a clear pattern of reduced folate levels in individuals with the TT genotype compared to those with the CC genotype. This study demonstrated that individuals with the T allele of the MTHFR polymorphism have significantly lower blood folate levels, which can lead to increased homocysteine concentrations, contributing to cardiovascular and other metabolic disorders. The analysis emphasized the additive effect of the MTHFR variant, suggesting that blood folate concentrations follow a pattern where CC > CT > TT, with TT carriers having the lowest levels of folate.

The findings from this meta-analysis support the need for targeted dietary interventions, particularly for individuals with the TT genotype, who are at higher risk for complications due to inadequate folate metabolism. These results underscore the importance of adequate folate intake, either through diet or supplementation, to mitigate the risk of elevated homocysteine and related health issues.

Another study explored the relationship between the MTHFR C677T polymorphism and blood folate concentrations, focusing particularly on how this genetic variation impacts folate metabolism and, by extension, health outcomes like cardiovascular disease and neural tube defects. The primary objective of the study was to evaluate whether the MTHFR C677T polymorphism affects the concentration of folate in the blood, as well as its implications for neural tube defect (NTD) prevention, which is highly dependent on folate status during pregnancy.

Key Findings

1. **Lower Folate Concentrations in TT Genotype Carriers:**
    - The study found that individuals with the **TT genotype** (homozygous for the T allele) had **significantly lower folate concentrations** in their blood compared to individuals with the **CC genotype** (homozygous for the C allele). This result is consistent with the known effect of the MTHFR 677C>T polymorphism on the **MTHFR enzyme activity**. The TT genotype leads to reduced MTHFR enzyme activity, which in turn impairs the conversion of homocysteine to methionine. This biochemical dysfunction leads to lower overall folate levels, as MTHFR plays a crucial role in folate metabolism.
2. **Elevated Homocysteine Levels:**
    - As a consequence of lower folate levels in TT carriers, the study indicated that **homocysteine levels** tend to be higher in individuals with the TT genotype. Elevated homocysteine is a known risk factor for cardiovascular diseases, including **stroke, heart disease, and peripheral vascular disease**. Homocysteine is also associated with other health issues such as osteoporosis, cognitive decline, and even certain cancers.
3. **Impact on Neural Tube Defect (NTD) Prevention:**
    - One of the major implications of this study is its focus on **neural tube defects** (NTDs), which are congenital abnormalities of the brain and spinal cord that occur in early pregnancy. Folate is essential for proper neural tube closure during pregnancy, and low levels of folate are a significant risk factor for NTDs.
    - The study underscored that **women with the TT genotype** are particularly at risk for low folate levels, which could increase the likelihood of having children with NTDs, as the body may not be able to maintain sufficient folate concentrations to meet the demands of pregnancy.
    - Folate supplementation, particularly **L-methylfolate** (the active form of folate), is highlighted as **crucial** for women with the TT genotype. This form of folate bypasses the defective MTHFR enzyme, providing the necessary folate to prevent NTDs.
4. **Importance of Adequate Folate Intake:**
    - The study strongly emphasized that individuals with the TT genotype **require higher folate intake**, either through **dietary sources or supplements**. Adequate folate intake is essential not only for preventing neural tube defects in pregnant women but also for reducing the elevated homocysteine levels associated with cardiovascular risks.
    - It is particularly important for **women of reproductive age** to be aware of their folate status and the potential need for **folic acid supplementation**. The study suggested that standard folic acid supplementation (400 µg/day) may be insufficient for individuals with

the TT genotype, and higher doses or the active form of folate (L-methylfolate) might be more beneficial.

5. **Implications for Public Health and Personalized Nutrition:**
    - Based on the study's findings, **public health guidelines** for folic acid supplementation may need to take genetic factors like the MTHFR C677T polymorphism into account. This is particularly relevant for women in countries with **folic acid fortification programs**, where the impact of genetic variations on folate status is not always considered in population-wide recommendations.
    - This study supports the idea of **personalized nutrition**, where genetic testing could guide more tailored dietary recommendations for individuals, particularly those with known MTHFR polymorphisms.

Nutritional Interventions for MTHFR C677T Carriers

Given the findings of the meta-analysis and various studies, nutritional interventions have been proposed to manage the effects of the MTHFR C677T polymorphism. These interventions focus primarily on addressing folate deficiency, reducing homocysteine levels, and improving overall metabolic health:

1. **Folate Supplementation and Diet:**
    - Individuals with the TT genotype are advised to increase their folate intake through both dietary sources and supplementation. Folate-rich foods, such as leafy greens, legumes, and fortified cereals, can help reduce the risk of elevated homocysteine levels.
    - **Supplementation**: L-methylfolate, the biologically active form, is particularly beneficial for TT carriers as it bypasses the compromised MTHFR enzyme. A dosage of 800–1000 µg/day is often recommended, especially for women of reproductive age, to prevent complications such as neural tube defects.
2. **Omega-3 Fatty Acids:**
    - Omega-3 fatty acids, found in fish and plant-based sources such as flaxseeds and walnuts, have been shown to reduce inflammation and lower triglyceride levels, which are critical in managing metabolic syndrome.
    - Increased omega-3 intake (2–4 grams per day) is especially beneficial for T(+) carriers, who may be at higher risk for cardiovascular diseases.

3. **Protein Intake:**
    - Adequate protein consumption is essential to preserve lean body mass and prevent sarcopenia, especially in individuals with the MTHFR C677T polymorphism.
    - Protein intake should be tailored to individual needs, with recommendations around 1.2–1.5 grams of protein per kilogram of body weight per day. This is particularly important for individuals undergoing weight loss interventions, as maintaining muscle mass is key to overall health.
4. **Mediterranean Diet:**
    - The Mediterranean diet, rich in monounsaturated fats, omega-3 fatty acids, and fiber, has been shown to benefit individuals with metabolic syndrome and obesity.
    - For individuals with the MTHFR C677T polymorphism, this diet can help manage inflammation, improve body composition, and support cardiovascular health.
5. **B-Vitamins and Magnesium:**
    - B-vitamins—especially B6 and B12—play essential roles in homocysteine metabolism. Alongside folate, these vitamins help convert homocysteine to methionine or cysteine, thus lowering its concentration in the body.
    - Magnesium, a cofactor in many enzymatic reactions, also contributes to homocysteine regulation and supports energy metabolism. Ensuring sufficient intake of these micronutrients—either through diet or supplements—can enhance the efficacy of folate interventions.

Summary of MTHFR C677T Polymorphism, Enzyme Activity, and Folate-Related Considerations (India and Global)

Genotype (MTHFR C677T)	Approx. enzyme activity vs wild type	Folate RDA anchors (India/ global)*	Typical folate/folic-acid practice (India & global)	Potential role of 5-MTHF (active folate)**	Key clinical/ population notes	Key references
CC (wild type)	~100% activity; normal conversion of folic acid → 5-MTHF	India: Men 300, women 220, pregnancy 570, lactation 330 µg/ day. Global: Adults 400, pregnancy 600, lactation 500 µg DFE/day	Standard practice: ≥400 µg/day folic acid for women planning pregnancy; IFA tablets during pregnancy; many countries fortify cereals/flour	Standard folic acid is generally adequate; 5-MTHF ~400 µg/ day can substitute when desired	CC is baseline genotype. In India, folate/ B12 insufficiency can still elevate homocysteine even without SNP variation	ICMR–NIN 2020; NIH/ODS folate sheet; Indian periconceptional folate guidelines; global NTD-prevention literature
CT (heterozygous)	~60–70% activity; mild reduction in 5-MTHF production; homocysteine can rise when folate/B12 are low	Same formal RDAs as above (no genotype-based adjustments)	Managed like general population: ~400 µg/day folic acid periconceptionally; similar preventive doses worldwide	5-MTHF 400–800 µg/day may be helpful if homocysteine remains high despite folic acid or when other one-carbon SNPs (MTR/ MTRR) co-occur	CT increases vulnerability under low folate/ B12 conditions. Common in India and globally; strongest functional impact seen when B12 is also low	PNAS/NEJM homocysteine–folate research; Indian CAD/RPL studies on C677T; Li et al., 2015 (Nutrients)
TT (homozygous variant)	~20–30% activity; markedly reduced ability to convert folic acid to 5-MTHF; highest tendency to hyper homocyste in aemia	Same RDAs on paper; in practice TT carriers benefit from consistently achieving RDA-level intake and avoiding marginal folate/B12	India: routine 400–500 µg/day folic acid in pregnancy; 4 mg/day only for very high-risk NTD history (not genotype-specific). Globally: 400 µg/ day preconception; higher doses in specific clinical indications	TT is the clearest case where 5-MTHF 400–800 µg/day is mechanistically preferred, as it bypasses the impaired MTHFR step and can normalise methylation more efficiently than folic acid	TT is associated with higher NTD risk when folate/B12 are low; combined deficiency (folate + B12) is common in India, increasing functional impact; global effect varies by population	Meta-analyses of MTHFR C677T and NTDs; global CAD/ homocysteine papers; Indian pregnancy-loss and vascular-risk studies; Qin et al., 2012; Zhang et al., 2013

Summary of MTR (A2756G) and MTRR (A66G) Polymorphisms, Enzyme Activity, and Folate-Related Considerations (India and Global)

Gene/SNP & Genotype	Approx. enzyme activity vs wild type	Folate RDA anchors (India/global)*	Typical folate/folic-acid practice (India & global)	Potential role of 5-MTHF (active folate)**	Key clinical/population notes	Key references
MTR A2756G – AA (wild type)	~100% activity; normal methionine synthase function	**India**: Men 300, women 220, pregnancy 570, lactation 330 µg/day. **Global:** Adults 400, pregnancy 600, lactation 500 µg DFE/day	India and globally: standard preconception/antenatal folic acid ≈400 µg/day; many countries fortify flour/cereals	Folic acid usually adequate; 5-MTHF ~400 µg/day can substitute in settings concerned about unmetabolised folic acid or multiple one-carbon variants	Acts as baseline genotype; homocysteine risk mainly driven by low folate/B12, not by the SNP itself	ICMR–NIN 2020; NIH ODS folate sheet; Klerk et al., 2003; Li et al., 2015 (Nutrients)
MTR A2756G – AG (heterozygous)	~80–90% activity; mild tendency to higher homocysteine if folate/B12 marginal	Same numeric RDAs as above (no genotype-specific values)	Managed like general population: IFA or folic acid 400 µg/day in India; similar preventive doses and fortification globally	5-MTHF 400–800 µg/day may be considered if homocysteine remains elevated despite folic acid and adequate B12 or if other risk SNPs (MTHFR/MTRR) are present	Contributes modestly to hyperhomocysteinaemia, CAD/NTD risk when combined with low folate/B12; emphasis is on status correction, not higher RDA	PLOS One meta-analyses on MTR A2756G; Zhang et al., 2013; Li et al., 2015
MTR A2756G – GG (homozygous variant)	~60–70% functional activity; more sensitive to low folate/B12	RDAs unchanged on paper; in practice, better to keep intake at or above RDA, especially in vegetarians/low-B12 settings	Folic-acid dosing is risk- and indication-based (e.g., NTD prevention, homocysteine lowering), not genotype-based; typical ranges 0.4–1 mg/day (higher in some therapeutic uses)	5-MTHF 400–800 µg/day is mechanistically attractive for high homocysteine, vascular or pregnancy risk, especially with combined MTHFR/MTRR variants	Part of a polygenic homocysteine-risk profile; effect becomes clinically relevant with low folate/B12 and other one-carbon variants	Qin et al., 2012; Klerk et al., 2003; Li et al., 2015; Indian CAD/RPL homocysteine studies

Gene/SNP & Genotype	Approx. enzyme activity vs wild type	Folate RDA anchors (India/ global)*	Typical folate/folic-acid practice (India & global)	Potential role of 5-MTHF (active folate)**	Key clinical/population notes	Key references
MTRR A66G – AA (wild type)	~100% activity; normal regeneration of methionine synthase	Same RDAs as above (India and global)	Standard folic-acid protocols: 400 µg/day periconceptionally; IFA in India; fortification plus 400 µg/day supplements in many countries	Folic acid or 5-MTHF can be used; genotype does not drive choice	Reference group; risk determined more by folate/B12 status, other SNPs and clinical context than by A66G alone	ICMR–NIN 2020; NIH/ EFSA folate guidance; Zhang et al., 2013; Li et al., 2015
MTRR A66G – AG (heterozygous)	~70–80% activity; modest homocysteine elevation when folate/ B12 are marginal	RDAs unchanged; functionally, AG may benefit from reliably meeting or slightly exceeding RDA, especially where B12 intake is low	No genotype-specific change to folic-acid dose; same antenatal and vascular-risk regimens as general population	5-MTHF 400–800 µg/ day is an option if homocysteine remains high despite standard folic acid and B12, particularly in carriers of multiple one-carbon variants	Common globally and in India; associated with higher homocysteine, NTD or cleft-risk in some studies when maternal folate/B12 are low	Murthy et al. (Indian cleft-lip studies); Ouyang et al., 2013; Wang et al., 2015; Li et al., 2015
MTRR A66G – GG (homozygous variant)	Often <60–70% of wild-type activity; consistently associated with higher homocysteine and greater methylation demand	Same formal RDAs; practically, GG carriers should avoid low folate/B12 and maintain at least RDA-level intakes	Folic-acid dosing guided by clinical indications (NTD history, vascular disease, hyperhomocysteinaemia). Doses ~0.4–1 mg/day common; higher in some therapeutic contexts	Strong candidate for preferential use of 5-MTHF 400–800 µg/day (often with B12/B6) when homocysteine is elevated despite folic acid, or in highly fortified settings where unmetabolised folic acid is a concern	Recognised as part of a higher-risk one-carbon profile for folate deficiency, NTDs and vascular events, particularly when combined with low folate/B12 or other pathway SNPs; no agency has yet adopted genotype-specific RDAs	Li et al., 2015 (folate-deficiency risk); Li et al., 2020 (stroke); Zhang et al., 2013; global reviews on one-carbon polymorphisms and 5-MTHF vs folic acid

Conclusion

Evidence from numerous studies, including large-scale meta-analyses, underscores the significant role of the MTHFR C677T polymorphism in shaping metabolic health and influencing individual responses to dietary interventions. Carriers of the TT genotype are particularly vulnerable to folate deficiency and elevated homocysteine levels—both of which are associated with increased risks for cardiovascular disease, metabolic syndrome, and other chronic conditions.

Personalized nutritional strategies, such as L-methylfolate supplementation, increased intake of omega-3 fatty acids, and adequate protein consumption, offer effective tools for mitigating these risks. These targeted interventions not only support better metabolic outcomes and improved body composition but also reflect a broader move toward precision nutrition—an approach that integrates genetic insights into dietary planning.

Incorporating genotype-specific recommendations into public health and clinical nutrition practices represents a promising step forward in optimizing long-term health and preventing disease.

Questions

1. What is homocysteine?
2. Which amino acid is homocysteine derived from?
3. Name the two major metabolic pathways of homocysteine.
4. Which vitamin is required for remethylation of homocysteine to methionine?
5. Which enzyme converts homocysteine to cystathionine?
6. Which cofactor is needed by cystathionine β-synthase (CBS)?
7. High levels of homocysteine in blood are termed what condition?
8. Name one genetic mutation commonly associated with elevated homocysteine levels.
9. Which B-vitamin deficiency can impair methionine synthase activity?
10. What is the normal plasma concentration range of homocysteine in adults?
11. Elevated homocysteine is associated with which cardiovascular condition?
12. Which nutrient directly lowers homocysteine by promoting methylation—folate, iron, or vitamin C?
13. Homocysteine can be measured in which biological sample: blood, urine, or saliva?
14. What is the effect of vitamin B6 deficiency on homocysteine levels?
15. Name one lifestyle factor that can increase homocysteine levels.
16. Explain the role of folate and vitamin B12 in the remethylation cycle of homocysteine.
17. How does the MTHFR C677T polymorphism contribute to hyperhomocysteinemia?
18. Describe the mechanism by which homocysteine induces vascular endothelial damage.
19. Why is homocysteine considered a risk factor for neural tube defects in pregnancy?
20. Compare the effects of folate deficiency versus vitamin B6 deficiency on homocysteine metabolism.
21. Discuss how homocysteine levels influence DNA methylation and epigenetic regulation.
22. Explain the connection between homocysteine and Alzheimer's disease risk.
23. How does homocysteine accumulation affect oxidative stress in cells?
24. What is the difference between homocystinuria and hyperhomocysteinemia?
25. How can elevated homocysteine impair fertility in both men and women?
26. Discuss the role of homocysteine in thrombosis and stroke development.
27. Why might supplementation with folate alone sometimes fail to lower homocysteine effectively?
28. Explain the biochemical link between homocysteine, S-adenosylmethionine (SAM), and methylation reactions.
29. Describe the role of renal function in regulating plasma homocysteine levels.
30. How does the balance between remethylation and transsulfuration determine homocysteine homeostasis?

Answers

1. Homocysteine is a sulfur-containing non-protein amino acid.
2. Derived from methionine.
3. Remethylation and transsulfuration.
4. Folate (via 5-methyl-THF) and vitamin B12.
5. Cystathionine β-synthase (CBS).
6. Vitamin B6 (pyridoxal phosphate).
7. Hyperhomocysteinemia.
8. MTHFR C677T.
9. Vitamin B12.
10. 5–15 μmol/L.
11. Atherosclerosis and cardiovascular disease.
12. Folate.
13. Blood (plasma or serum).
14. It increases homocysteine due to impaired transsulfuration.
15. Smoking, coffee intake, alcohol, sedentary lifestyle.
16. Folate donates a methyl group (via 5-methyl-THF) and vitamin B12 acts as a cofactor for methionine synthase.
17. The mutation reduces enzyme activity, impairing 5-methyl-THF formation, leading to poor remethylation of homocysteine.
18. Homocysteine generates reactive oxygen species, promotes endothelial dysfunction, and reduces nitric oxide availability.
19. High homocysteine interferes with folate metabolism and DNA methylation, affecting neural tube closure.
20. Folate deficiency impairs remethylation (methionine synthase), while B6 deficiency impairs transsulfuration (CBS).
21. Homocysteine levels regulate SAM and SAH ratios, influencing global DNA methylation.
22. Elevated homocysteine contributes to neurotoxicity, oxidative stress, and vascular impairment in the brain.
23. It auto-oxidizes to form reactive oxygen species, increasing oxidative stress.
24. Homocystinuria is a rare inborn error with very high levels, while hyperhomocysteinemia is a milder, acquired or genetic elevation.
25. In women, it increases miscarriage risk; in men, it reduces sperm motility and DNA integrity.
26. Elevated homocysteine promotes platelet activation, clot formation, and vascular damage.
27. Because vitamin B12 and B6 deficiencies can also impair metabolism, folate alone may not correct levels.
28. Homocysteine is a precursor to SAM, the universal methyl donor; imbalances affect methylation capacity.
29. Kidneys help clear homocysteine; renal insufficiency leads to accumulation.
30. Remethylation reduces homocysteine by recycling it, while transsulfuration eliminates it into cysteine; balance maintains normal levels.

References

1. Berker, B., Kaya, C., Aytac, R., Satiroglu, H., & Atabekoglu, C. S. (2009). Homocysteine concentrations in follicular fluid are associated with poor oocyte and embryo quality in IVF patients. *Human Reproduction, 24*(5), 1024–1028. https://doi.org/10.1093/humrep/dep011
2. Crider, K. S., Yang, T. P., Berry, R. J., & Bailey, L. B. (2012). Folate and DNA methylation: A review of molecular mechanisms and the evidence for folate's role. *Advances in Nutrition, 3*(1), 21–38. https://doi.org/10.3945/an.111.000992
3. Ebisch, I. M. W., Thomas, C. M. G., Peters, W. H. M., Braat, D. D. M., & Steegers-Theunissen, R. P. M. (2006). Homocysteine, folate, and sperm quality. *Fertility and Sterility, 86*(3), 718–722. https://doi.org/10.1016/j.fertnstert.2006.01.034
4. Forges, T., Monnier-Barbarino, P., Alberto, J.-M., Guéant-Rodriguez, R.-M., Daval, J.-L., & Guéant, J.-L. (2007). Impact of folate and homocysteine metabolism on human reproductive health. *Human Reproduction Update, 13*(3), 225–238. https://doi.org/10.1093/humupd/dml063
5. Frosst, P., Blom, H. J., Milos, R., Goyette, P., Sheppard, C. A., Matthews, R. G., ... Rozen, R. (1995). A candidate genetic risk factor for vascular disease: A common mutation in methylenetetrahydrofolate reductase. *Nature Genetics, 10*(1), 111–113. https://doi.org/10.1038/ng0595-111
6. Friso, S., & Choi, S. W. (2002). Gene–nutrient interactions and DNA methylation. *The Journal of Nutrition, 132*(8 Suppl), 2382S–2387S. https://doi.org/10.1093/jn/132.8.2382S
7. Goyette, P., Frosst, P., Rosenblatt, D. S., & Rozen, R. (1998). Gene structure of human methylenetetrahydrofolate reductase (MTHFR) and identification of two missense polymorphisms. *American Journal of Human Genetics, 62*(5), 1258–1265. https://doi.org/10.1086/301860
8. Goyette, P., Sumner, J. S., Milos, R., Duncan, A. M., Rosenblatt, D. S., Matthews, R. G., & Rozen, R. (2001). Genetic determinants of elevated homocysteine levels and risk of cardiovascular disease. *Clinical Chemistry and Laboratory Medicine, 39*(8), 725–733. https://doi.org/10.1515/CCLM.2001.118
9. Homocysteine Studies Collaboration. (2002). Homocysteine and risk of ischemic heart disease and stroke: A meta-analysis. *JAMA, 288*(16), 2015–2022. https://doi.org/10.1001/jama.288.16.2015
10. Li, Z., Gu, L., Yang, L., Yin, Y., & Guo, R. (2019). Association between serum homocysteine and semen parameters and sperm DNA damage in infertile men. *Andrologia, 51*(7), e13291. https://doi.org/10.1111/and.13291
11. McCully, K. S. (1996). Homocysteine and vascular disease. *Nature Medicine, 2*(4), 386–389. https://doi.org/10.1038/nm0496-386
12. Mudd, S. H., Levy, H. L., & Kraus, J. P. (2001). Disorders of transsulfuration. In C. R. Scriver, A. L. Beaudet, W. S. Sly, & D. Valle (Eds.), *The metabolic and molecular bases of inherited disease* (8th ed., pp. 2007–2056). McGraw-Hill.

13. Murphy, M. M., Scott, J. M., Arija, V., Molloy, A. M., & Fernandez-Ballart, J. D. (2007). Effect of folate and vitamin B12 on reproduction: A review. *Food & Nutrition Research, 51*(4), 1806. https://doi.org/10.3402/fnr.v51i4.1806
14. Murto, T., Bjuresten, K., Landgren, B.-M., & Stavreus-Evers, A. (2013). Elevated serum homocysteine in women with polycystic ovary syndrome: A prospective study and meta-analysis. *Fertility and Sterility, 100*(6), 1795–1801. https://doi.org/10.1016/j.fertnstert.2013.07.201
15. Nelen, W. L. D. M., Blom, H. J., Steegers, E. A. P., den Heijer, M., & Eskes, T. K. A. B. (2000). Hyperhomocysteinemia and recurrent early pregnancy loss: A meta-analysis. *Fertility and Sterility, 74*(6), 1196–1199. https://doi.org/10.1016/S0015-0282(00)01595-5
16. Obeid, R., & Herrmann, W. (2006). Mechanisms of homocysteine neurotoxicity in neurodegenerative diseases with special reference to dementia. *FEBS Letters, 580*(13), 2994–3005. https://doi.org/10.1016/j.febslet.2006.04.088
17. Refsum, H., Smith, A. D., Ueland, P. M., Nexo, E., Clarke, R., McPartlin, J., ... Scott, J. M. (2004). Facts and recommendations about total homocysteine determinations: An expert opinion. *Clinical Chemistry, 50*(1), 3–32. https://doi.org/10.1373/clinchem.2003.021634
18. Selhub, J. (1999). Homocysteine metabolism. *Annual Review of Nutrition, 19,* 217–246. https://doi.org/10.1146/annurev.nutr.19.1.217
19. Wan, L., Li, Y., Zhang, Z., Sun, Z., He, Y., & Li, R. (2018). Methylenetetrahydrofolate reductase and psychiatric diseases. *Translational Psychiatry, 8*, 242. https://doi.org/10.1038/s41398-018-0281-0
20. National Institutes of Health, Office of Dietary Supplements. (2023). *Folate: Fact sheet for health professionals.* https://ods.od.nih.gov/factsheets/Folate-HealthProfessional/
21. Centers for Disease Control and Prevention. (2023). *MTHFR gene variant and folic acid.* https://www.cdc.gov/folic-acid/data-research/mthfr/index.html
22. National Center for Biotechnology Information. (2023). *Dietary reference intakes: Appendix A – Folate intake table.* https://www.ncbi.nlm.nih.gov/books/NBK593620/table/appa.tab2/
23. Royal Australian College of General Practitioners. (2016). MTHFR genetic testing: Controversy and clinical implications. *Australian Family Physician, 45*(4), 237–240. https://www.racgp.org.au/afp/2016/april/mthfr-genetic-testing-controversy-and-clinical-imp
24. Carboni, L. (2022). Active folate versus folic acid: The role of 5-MTHF (methylfolate) in human health. *Integrative Medicine (Encinitas), 21*(3), 36–41. PMID: 35999905
25. Ledowsky, C. J., Schloss, J., & Steel, A. (2023). Variations in folate prescriptions for patients with the MTHFR genetic polymorphisms: A case series study. *Exploratory Research in Clinical and Social Pharmacy, 10*, 100277. https://doi.org/10.1016/j.rcsop.2023.100277
26. Prinz-Langenohl, R., Brämswig, S., Tobolski, O., Smulders, Y. M., Smith, D. E. C., Finglas, P. M., & Pietrzik, K. (2009). [6S]-5-methyltetrahydrofolate increases plasma folate more effectively than folic acid in women with the homozygous or wild-type 677C→T MTHFR polymorphism. *British Journal of Pharmacology, 158*(8), 2014–2021. https://doi.org/10.1111/j.1476-5381.2009.00492.x

27. U.S. Preventive Services Task Force. (2023). Folic acid supplementation to prevent neural tube defects: US Preventive Services Task Force reaffirmation recommendation statement. *JAMA, 330*(5), e231543. https://doi.org/10.1001/jama.2023.1543
28. Samaniego-Vaesken, M. L., Morais-Moreno, C., Carretero-Krug, A., Puga, A. M., Montero-Bravo, A. M., Partearroyo, T., & Varela-Moreiras, G. (2024). Supplementation with folic acid or 5-methyltetrahydrofolate and prevention of neural tube defects: An evidence-based narrative review. *Nutrients, 16*(18), 3154. https://doi.org/10.3390/nu16183154
29. Nair, R. R., Khanna, A., & Singh, K. (2012). MTHFR C677T polymorphism and recurrent early pregnancy loss risk in North Indian population. *Reproductive Sciences, 19*(2), 210–215. https://doi.org/10.1177/1933719111417888
30. Gupta, S. K., Kotwal, J., Kotwal, A., Dhall, A., & Garg, S. (2012). Role of homocysteine and MTHFR C677T gene polymorphism as risk factors for coronary artery disease in young Indians. *Indian Journal of Medical Research, 136*(4), 506–512.
31. Yadav, U., Kumar, P., & Rai, V. (2017). Methylenetetrahydrofolate reductase C677T polymorphism in Indian population: A revisit. *Indian Journal of Human Genetics, 23*(1), 1–10. https://doi.org/10.4103/ijhg.IJHG_32_16
32. EudraCT. (2006). *Clinical trial 2006-003242-42: [6S]-5-methyltetrahydrofolate vs folic acid in MTHFR genotypes.* https://www.clinicaltrialsregister.eu/ctr-search/trial/2006-003242-42

"The greatest medicine of all is teaching people how not to need it."

— Hippocrates

As we bring this textbook to a close, it is clear that **nutrigenetics** and **nutrigenomics** are no longer emerging sciences—they are foundational disciplines shaping the future of personalized healthcare. These fields offer a scientific framework to understand how individual genetic variations influence responses to nutrients, dietary patterns, and lifestyle factors. By integrating this knowledge into clinical and public health practice, we can move beyond the limitations of a one-size-fits-all model and embrace a truly personalized approach to nutrition—empowering individuals to prevent disease, enhance physical and cognitive performance, and promote long-term well-being.

Yet, our exploration of the interplay between genes, nutrition, and health is only at its beginning. The science is advancing rapidly, and its most meaningful applications are now unfolding across multiple clinical and performance domains. The next volume will take you there—translating mechanistic insight into practical, evidence-informed strategies.

Sports Genomics: Optimizing Performance and Recovery

In my next book, we will expand our focus to include several key domains where genomics is proving to be both clinically actionable and transformative. One of the most dynamic frontiers in this regard is **sports genomics**—a field dedicated to understanding how genetic differences influence athletic performance, physical potential, injury susceptibility, and recovery capacity.

Recent clinical trials and large-scale genome-wide association studies (GWAS) have uncovered genetic variants—such as *ACTN3*, *ACE*, and *PPARGC1A*—that influence traits like muscle fiber composition, power output, endurance, oxygen utilization, and metabolic flexibility. For example, the *ACTN3 R577X* polymorphism is associated with sprint and power-based performance due to its role in fast-twitch muscle function. In contrast, the *ACE I/I* genotype has been linked to improved endurance capacity through more efficient cardiovascular and pulmonary adaptations.

Beyond performance optimization, sports genomics is increasingly being used to **prevent injuries and enhance recovery**. Genetic variants in collagen-encoding genes such as *COL1A1* and *COL5A1* are associated with increased risk of tendon and ligament injuries. Awareness of these risk alleles allows trainers, coaches, and clinicians to develop more personalized training regimens and recovery protocols—maximizing results while minimizing harm.

For students of nutrigenetics and health sciences, the study of sports genomics is an exciting opportunity to see how theory meets practice. Whether you're supporting elite athletes or helping individuals achieve personal fitness goals, understanding the genetic factors behind physical performance provides a powerful tool to guide nutrition, supplementation, and training plans with precision.

Metabolic Health and Genomic Risk Stratification

In addition to sports genomics, the next volume will explore the **genetic foundations of metabolic health**, covering impactful and highly prevalent conditions such as cardiovascular disease, type 2 diabetes, hypertension, and osteoporosis. These are among the most widespread yet preventable chronic conditions globally. Understanding the **genetic architecture** of these diseases enables the development of personalized strategies for prevention, early detection, and targeted intervention.

- **Cardiovascular Disease (CVD):** Genes such as *APOE*, *LDLR*, and *PCSK9* play key roles in lipid metabolism, cholesterol transport, and inflammation. Genomic analysis can help identify individuals at higher risk for elevated LDL cholesterol or triglycerides, supporting early lifestyle interventions or nutraceutical strategies like omega-3 fatty acids or plant sterols.
- **Type 2 Diabetes (T2D):** Variants in genes like *TCF7L2*, *SLC30A8*, and *FTO* influence insulin secretion, pancreatic beta-cell function, and obesity risk. Nutrigenetic insights can be used to guide personalized carbohydrate intake and glycemic control strategies.
- **Hypertension:** Genes regulating sodium sensitivity (e.g., *ADD1*, *AGT*) and vascular tone (*NOS3*, *ACE*) impact how individuals respond to salt and potassium intake. These variations inform precision-based approaches for blood pressure management.
- **Bone Health:** Variants in genes such as *VDR*, *COL1A1*, and *LRP5* affect calcium absorption, bone mineral density, and fracture risk. With this knowledge, personalized recommendations for vitamin D, K2, calcium intake, and weight-bearing exercises can be developed.

By understanding these underlying genetic predispositions, students and clinicians can begin to think more precisely about long-term **metabolic health optimization** and preventive care.

Genomics of Mental Health and Nutrient-Mood Interactions

Mental health is increasingly recognized as a domain profoundly influenced by both genetics and nutrition. The next book will delve into how genetic variation affects brain chemistry, emotional resilience, and response to dietary interventions:

- **Neurotransmitter Function:** Genes like *COMT*, *MAOA*, *SLC6A4*, and *BDNF* influence the function of dopamine, serotonin, and norepinephrine—key neurotransmitters involved in mood, motivation, and stress response. Variations in these genes can predispose individuals to anxiety, depression, or altered emotional regulation.
- **Stress Resilience and Sleep:** Genetic polymorphisms in *FKBP5* and *CRHR1* impact the regulation of cortisol and the hypothalamic-pituitary-adrenal (HPA) axis. These pathways are central to stress response and circadian rhythm stability, offering potential targets for adaptogens and lifestyle-based stress interventions.
- **Nutrient-Mood Interactions:** Nutrients such as folate, B12, omega-3 fatty acids, magnesium, and zinc play critical roles in neurotransmitter synthesis and neuroplasticity. Genes like *MTHFR*, *FOLR1*, and *SLC19A1* affect folate metabolism and methylation pathways, which in turn influence mental well-being and cognitive health.

By connecting mental health to genomics and nutrition, students will develop a deeper and more **integrated understanding of psychonutrition**—a field that is rapidly evolving and becoming increasingly relevant in modern health practice.

Macro- and Micronutrient Metabolism: Designing Truly Individualized Nutrition

Another core component of the upcoming volume is **nutrient metabolism**, where we will explore how individual genetic profiles influence the way the body handles macro- and micronutrients:

- **Carbohydrate Metabolism:** Genes such as *TCF7L2*, *AMY1*, and *SLC2A2* affect insulin sensitivity, starch digestion efficiency, and glucose transport. Personalized carbohydrate recommendations can help mitigate postprandial glucose spikes and reduce diabetes risk.
- **Fat Metabolism:** Variants in *APOA2*, *FADS1/2*, and *PPARG* influence lipid synthesis, fatty acid metabolism, and body fat distribution. These can help guide dietary fat intake and choices of omega-3 vs. omega-6 supplementation.
- **Protein Utilization:** Genes such as *PEMT* and *MTHFR* affect amino acid metabolism and choline synthesis, both of which are vital for liver function, brain health, and detoxification pathways.
- **Micronutrient Requirements:** Individual SNPs in genes like *GC* (vitamin D binding), *SLC23A1* (vitamin C transport), *SLC52A1* (riboflavin transport), and *FUT2* (vitamin B12 absorption) impact the bioavailability and cellular utilization of essential vitamins and minerals. Personalized supplementation strategies become far more effective with this genomic knowledge.

This is precision nutrition elevated—not simply "more or less," but "right form, right dose, right person, right time."

This section will empower students to design **precision-based nutrition plans**—not just for disease treatment, but also for performance, energy optimization, and long-term health maintenance.

Epigenetics: The Future of Gene Expression Modulation

Finally, the book will explore one of the most promising areas of modern health science: **epigenetics**. Here, we will investigate how external factors—such as diet, physical activity, sleep, stress, and environmental exposures—can modify gene expression without changing the DNA sequence itself.

Through mechanisms such as DNA methylation, histone modification, and microRNA regulation, epigenetic changes can either enhance or suppress gene activity. These changes are reversible and offer enormous potential for intervention. Students will learn how to harness epigenetic science to delay aging, reduce chronic disease risk, and improve overall vitality—marking a paradigm shift from reactive care to proactive, precision health.

Together, these chapters in the next volume will move students beyond theory into the world of **practical, clinical, and performance-based genomics**. Whether your goal is to become a practitioner, researcher, health coach, or educator, understanding how genes influence metabolic pathways, nutrient interactions, mental health, and physical performance will be vital for the next generation of healthcare.

The future of precision health is being shaped right now—and your journey as a genomic health professional is only just beginning.

The Journey Continues: Where Science Meets Application

As you move forward—as a clinician, researcher, educator, coach, or innovator—remember that your capacity to integrate molecular insight with human context is what will define the future of practice. Precision health is no longer a distant vision; it is unfolding now, and you are part of the generation that will embed it into everyday care.

The future of precision health is being shaped right now—and your journey as a genomic health professional is only just beginning.

1000 Genomes Project

A large global research initiative that mapped human genetic variation to understand population-specific allele frequencies and rare variants.

Adipocytokines

Hormone-like signaling proteins released by adipose (fat) tissue that regulate appetite, inflammation, and metabolic processes.

Allele

Alternative forms of a gene found at the same locus on homologous chromosomes that produce variations in a trait.

Allele Frequency

The proportion of each genetic variant (allele) in a population, used to understand how common a SNP is across different ethnic groups.

Anaphase

A stage of mitosis where sister chromatids separate at the centromere and are pulled toward opposite poles of the cell by spindle fibers.

Anaphase I

A phase in meiosis I where homologous chromosomes are pulled to opposite poles, while sister chromatids remain together.

Anaphase II

A stage in meiosis II where sister chromatids separate and move toward opposite poles, becoming individual chromosomes.

Anticodon

A sequence of three nucleotides in tRNA that is complementary to an mRNA codon and ensures that the correct amino acid is added to the growing polypeptide chain.

Antiparallel Orientation

A structural feature of DNA in which the two strands run in opposite directions: one from 5′→3′ and the other from 3′→5′.

Appetite Regulation

The biological system that controls hunger and satiety through gut hormones, brain pathways, and energy needs.

Autosomal Dominant Inheritance

A pattern of inheritance in which only one copy of a mutant allele is needed for the trait or disorder to be expressed.

Autosomal Recessive Inheritance

An inheritance pattern where two copies of a mutant allele are required for a trait or disorder to appear.

Base Pairing

The specific hydrogen bonding between nitrogenous bases in nucleic acids: A pairs with T (or U in RNA) and G pairs with C.

BHMT (Betaine-homocysteine methyltransferase)

An enzyme that converts homocysteine into methionine using betaine as a methyl donor in the remethylation pathway.

BMI (Body Mass Index)

A numerical value calculated from height and weight used to classify underweight, normal weight, overweight, and obesity.

Cancer

A group of diseases characterized by uncontrolled cell division, invasion of surrounding tissues, and sometimes metastasis to distant sites.

Carrier

An individual who possesses one recessive allele for a trait but does not express it phenotypically.

CBS (Cystathionine beta-synthase)

An enzyme in the transsulfuration pathway that converts homocysteine into cystathionine, requiring vitamin B6.

Cell Cycle

A series of ordered stages that a cell passes through to grow, replicate its DNA, and divide into two daughter cells; essential for growth, development, and tissue repair.

Cell Cycle Checkpoints

Control points in the cell cycle (such as G_1, G_2, and M checkpoints) where the cell assesses DNA integrity, replication status, and spindle attachment before proceeding.

Celiac Disease

An autoimmune condition where consumption of gluten triggers immune-mediated damage to the small intestine in genetically susceptible individuals.

Chargaff's Rule

A principle stating that in DNA, the amount of adenine equals thymine and the amount of guanine equals cytosine.

Chiasma (plural: Chiasmata)

The visible site of crossing over where non-sister chromatids of homologous chromosomes have exchanged segments.

Chromatin

The complex of DNA and associated proteins (mainly histones) that packages genetic material in eukaryotic cells and condenses into chromosomes during division.

Chromosome

A highly condensed structure of DNA and associated proteins that carries genetic information; visible under a microscope during cell division.

Chromosome Location

The position of a SNP in the human genome, often expressed as chromosome number and nucleotide position.

ClinVar

A public database that reports clinically significant genetic variants and their associations with diseases and medical conditions.

Codominance

A type of inheritance where both alleles are fully and equally expressed in a heterozygous individual.

Codon

A sequence of three nucleotides in mRNA that specifies a particular amino acid or a stop signal during translation.

Complementary Strand

A nucleic acid strand formed based on base pairing rules, where each base matches its specific partner.

Consanguinity

A relationship between individuals who share a common biological ancestor.

Crossing Over

The exchange of genetic material between non-sister chromatids of homologous chromosomes during prophase I of meiosis, generating new allele combinations.

Cyclin-Dependent Kinases (CDKs)

Enzymes that, when bound to cyclins, phosphorylate target proteins to regulate progression through the cell cycle.

Cyclins

Regulatory proteins whose levels fluctuate during the cell cycle and which activate cyclin-dependent kinases (CDKs) to drive progression through different phases.

dbSNP (Database of Single Nucleotide Polymorphisms)

A central NCBI repository that stores SNPs and other small genetic variations such as indels, along with allele frequencies and genomic context.

Deoxyribonucleic Acid (DNA)

The molecule that stores genetic information in living organisms, composed of nucleotides arranged in a double helix.

Digenic/Polygenic Trait

A trait influenced by two or multiple genes rather than a single gene, important for understanding complex traits like obesity or vitamin metabolism.

Dihybrid Cross

A genetic cross examining the inheritance of two traits simultaneously, often demonstrating independent assortment.

Diploid (2n)

A cell or organism with two sets of chromosomes, one inherited from each parent.

DNA Ligase

The "molecular glue" enzyme that joins DNA fragments together by sealing breaks in the sugar–phosphate backbone.

DNA Polymerase

The enzyme that adds new nucleotides to a growing DNA strand using the original strand as a template, always synthesizing in the 5′ to 3′ direction.

DNA Replication

The process by which a cell makes an exact copy of its DNA before cell division, ensuring that each daughter cell receives the same genetic information.

Dopamine Reward System

A neural pathway in the brain that associates eating with pleasure, cravings, and motivation, influencing hedonic eating behavior.

Double Helix

The twisted ladder-like structure of DNA, consisting of two antiparallel strands wound around each other.

eQTL (Expression Quantitative Trait Loci)

Genetic variants that affect gene expression levels, used to identify whether a SNP influences how much of a gene product is produced.

Energy Balance

The relationship between calories consumed through food and calories expended through metabolism and physical activity.

Ensembl Genome Browser

An online genome visualization tool that provides detailed annotations of genes, SNPs, regulatory elements, and comparative genomics data.

Epigenetic Silencing

Suppression of gene expression due to changes such as DNA methylation or chromatin modification without altering the DNA sequence itself.

Epistasis

A form of gene interaction where one gene masks or modifies the expression of another gene.

Exon

A coding or functional sequence in eukaryotic pre-mRNA that is retained and joined together during splicing to form mature mRNA.

Expressivity

The degree to which a genotype is phenotypically expressed in an individual.

F_1 Generation

The first generation of offspring resulting from a genetic cross between parental organisms.

F_2 Generation

The second generation produced by selfing or crossing individuals from the F_1 generation.

Food Allergy

An immune-mediated adverse reaction to certain foods that may cause hives, swelling, gastrointestinal symptoms, breathing difficulty, or anaphylaxis.

Food Intolerance

A non-immune adverse reaction to food caused by difficulty digesting a component (e.g., lactose) due to enzyme deficiency.

Food Sensitivity

A delayed, non-allergic response to certain foods that may cause symptoms such as bloating, headaches, skin issues, or fatigue.

***FTO* Gene**

A gene strongly associated with appetite regulation, satiety, and obesity risk; certain SNPs (e.g., *rs9939609*) predispose individuals to increased food intake and weight gain.

Functional Variant

A genetic variant that directly influences biological outcomes (e.g., nutrient metabolism, disease risk, enzyme function).

G_1 Phase (First Gap Phase)

The phase of the cell cycle where the cell grows, synthesizes proteins, and produces organelles while checking whether conditions are suitable for DNA replication and division.

G_2 Phase (Second Gap Phase)

The phase following DNA replication where the cell continues to grow, synthesizes proteins needed for mitosis, and checks for DNA damage or replication errors.

Gametes

Reproductive cells (sperm and egg in humans) that contain one allele from each gene pair; they are haploid.

Gene

A segment of DNA that contains instructions for producing a specific protein or functional molecule.

Gene Expression

The process by which information encoded in DNA is used to produce RNA and proteins.

Gene Interaction

A situation in which multiple genes influence a single phenotype.

Genetic Diversity

Variation in the genetic makeup of individuals in a population, enhanced by meiosis and essential for evolution and adaptation.

Genetic Recombination

The production of new combinations of alleles through crossing over and independent assortment during meiosis.

Genotype

The genetic makeup of an organism, represented by alleles inherited from the parents.

Ghrelin

A hunger-stimulating hormone released mainly by the stomach that increases appetite and food intake.

***GHRL* Gene**

The gene that encodes the ghrelin protein and plays a role in regulating hunger, cravings, and reward-based eating.

GWAS (Genome-Wide Association Study)

A research method used to identify SNPs statistically associated with traits and diseases across large populations.

GWAS Catalog

A curated database containing results from published genome-wide association studies, linking SNPs with specific diseases and biological traits.

Haploid (n)

A cell with a single set of chromosomes, such as a gamete produced by meiosis.

Haplotye

A group of inherited genetic variants that tend to be passed together and are often studied when a trait cannot be explained by a single SNP.

HDAC (Histone Deacetylase)

A group of enzymes that remove acetyl groups from histones, tightening chromatin structure and generally reducing gene expression.

Helicase

An enzyme that unwinds and separates the two DNA strands by breaking hydrogen bonds between the bases.

Heterozygous

Having two different alleles for a particular gene.

Homocysteine

A sulfur-containing intermediate amino acid that must be recycled or converted; high levels are linked to cardiovascular, neurological, and reproductive risks.

Homologous Chromosomes

A pair of chromosomes (one from each parent) that are similar in size, shape, and gene content but may carry different alleles.

Homozygous

Having two identical alleles for a specific gene.

Hydrogen Bonds

Weak bonds that form between complementary nitrogenous bases in DNA and RNA, stabilizing their structure.

Independent Assortment

Mendel's principle stating that alleles for separate traits segregate independently during gamete formation; in meiosis, it refers to the random orientation of homologous chromosome pairs along the metaphase plate.

Indel (Insertion-Deletion Variant)

A small genetic alteration where nucleotides are inserted or deleted; stored alongside SNPs in many databases.

Inheritance Pattern

The manner in which genetic traits or disorders are passed from one generation to the next.

Initiation Factors

Proteins that help assemble the ribosome, mRNA, and initiator tRNA at the start codon to begin translation.

Intron

A non-coding sequence in eukaryotic pre-mRNA that is removed during RNA processing.

Lactase

An intestinal enzyme that breaks down the milk sugar lactose into glucose and galactose for digestion.

Lactose Intolerance

A condition caused by low lactase enzyme activity, leading to difficulty digesting lactose and symptoms like bloating, diarrhea, and gas.

Lagging Strand

The new DNA strand that is synthesized discontinuously in short segments (Okazaki fragments) opposite to the direction of fork movement.

Law of Segregation (Segregation)

Mendel's principle stating that allele pairs separate during gamete formation and reunite at fertilization.

Leading Strand

The new DNA strand that is synthesized continuously in the same direction as the replication fork movement.

***LEP* Gene (*Leptin* Gene)**

The gene that produces *Leptin*, a hormone that signals satiety to the brain and helps regulate energy balance.

***LEPR* Gene (*Leptin* Receptor Gene)**

The gene that encodes the *Leptin* receptor; variations may cause *Leptin* resistance and difficulty achieving satiety.

Leptin

A hormone produced by fat cells that decreases hunger and promotes fullness by acting on the hypothalamus.

Lethal Allele

An allele that causes death when present in a particular genotype, often in the homozygous state.

Licensing of Origins

The process of preparing replication origins in eukaryotic cells so that each is used only once per cell cycle, preventing re-replication.

LD (Linkage Disequilibrium)

A measure of how closely two SNPs are inherited together, helping identify tagging SNPs and haplotype blocks.

LDlink

A suite of online tools used to study linkage disequilibrium patterns and haplotype structures across populations.

M Phase (Mitotic Phase)

The phase of the cell cycle where the nucleus divides (mitosis) and the cytoplasm splits (cytokinesis), resulting in two genetically identical daughter cells.

***MC4R* Gene**

A gene central to appetite and energy regulation through the melanocortin pathway; certain variants are strongly linked to obesity risk.

Meiosis

A specialized type of cell division that reduces the chromosome number by half, producing four genetically unique haploid gametes from a diploid cell.

Meiosis I

The first division of meiosis in which homologous chromosomes pair, undergo crossing over, and are separated into two haploid cells.

Meiosis II

The second division of meiosis, similar to mitosis, in which sister chromatids are separated, producing four haploid gametes.

Messenger RNA (mRNA)

A type of RNA that carries the genetic code from DNA to ribosomes for protein synthesis.

Metaphase

A stage of mitosis where chromosomes align at the cell's equatorial plane (metaphase plate), attached to spindle fibers from opposite poles.

Metaphase I

A stage in meiosis I where paired homologous chromosomes align along the cell's equatorial plane.

Metaphase II

A stage in meiosis II where chromosomes align individually along the equatorial plane of each haploid cell.

Methionine

An essential amino acid that donates methyl groups needed for DNA methylation, detoxification, and cellular function.

Methionine Cycle

A biochemical process that converts methionine into homocysteine and back again, driven by methylation reactions.

Methylation

A biochemical process where methyl groups are added to DNA or proteins to regulate gene activity, detoxification, and cellular function.

Mismatch Repair

A post-replication repair system that detects and corrects base-pairing errors that escaped DNA polymerase proofreading.

Mitochondrial Inheritance

A pattern of inheritance where genes from mitochondrial DNA are passed exclusively from the mother to all offspring.

miRNA (MicroRNA)

Small regulatory RNA molecules that bind to mRNA and reduce gene expression by blocking translation or promoting mRNA degradation.

Mitosis

A type of cell division in which a diploid cell produces two genetically identical diploid daughter cells, used for growth, repair, and asexual reproduction.

MCM Helicase

The main helicase complex in eukaryotes that is loaded onto DNA at origins and unwinds the double helix during replication.

Monocistronic mRNA

An mRNA molecule (typical in eukaryotes) that encodes only a single protein product.

MTHFR Gene

A key gene in folate metabolism; variants can impair methylation efficiency and elevate homocysteine levels.

MTR/MTRR Genes

Genes that produce enzymes involved in remethylating homocysteine back into methionine, requiring vitamin B_{12} and folate.

Nitrogenous Bases

The components of nucleotides that form the rungs of DNA and RNA: adenine, thymine, guanine, cytosine, and uracil (in RNA).

Non-Celiac Gluten Sensitivity (NCGS)

A gluten-related condition where individuals develop symptoms similar to celiac disease but without autoimmune intestinal damage.

Nucleosome

The basic unit of chromatin, consisting of DNA wrapped around a core of histone proteins.

Nucleotide

The basic building block of DNA and RNA, consisting of a sugar, phosphate group, and nitrogenous base.

Okazaki Fragments

Short segments of DNA are synthesized on the lagging strand that are later joined together to form a continuous strand.

Origin of Replication

Specific site(s) on the DNA where replication begins and the double helix first unwinds.

Origin Recognition Complex (ORC)

A multi-protein complex in eukaryotic cells that binds to replication origins and marks them as starting points for DNA replication.

Pedigree Analysis

The study of inherited traits in families through diagrammatic family trees to predict inheritance patterns.

Peptide YY (PYY)

A satiety hormone released by the gut after meals that reduces appetite and slows gastric emptying.

Penetrance

The proportion of individuals with a specific genotype who actually express the associated phenotype.

Phenotype

The observable physical or biochemical traits of an organism resulting from its genotype and environment.

PhenoScanner

A database that integrates genotype–phenotype associations (SNPs, diseases, biomarkers, gene expression, methylation) from large studies.

Phosphodiester Bond

A strong covalent bond linking nucleotides together in DNA and RNA.

PKU (Phenylketonuria)

A rare inherited disorder in which the body cannot break down phenylalanine; requires lifelong dietary protein control.

Polycistronic mRNA

An mRNA molecule (common in prokaryotes) that carries coding information for more than one protein.

Precision Nutrition

Personalized nutrition strategies tailored to an individual's genetic makeup, lifestyle, and metabolic responses.

Primase

An enzyme that synthesizes short RNA primers to provide a starting point for DNA polymerase.

Prophase

The first stage of mitosis where chromatin condenses into visible chromosomes, the nuclear envelope breaks down, and the mitotic spindle begins to form.

Prophase I

The first stage of meiosis I where homologous chromosomes pair (synapsis), form tetrads, and crossing over occurs.

Prophase II

The first stage of meiosis II in which chromosomes re-condense and spindle fibers form in each haploid cell.

Proofreading

The ability of DNA polymerase to check and correct errors in newly synthesized DNA by removing and replacing incorrect nucleotides.

Promoter

A specific DNA sequence where RNA polymerase and associated factors bind to start transcription.

Punnett Square

A tool used to predict the possible genotypes and phenotypes resulting from a genetic cross.

Punnett Square Tools/SNP Query Tools

Software platforms embedded in some databases to explore SNP–trait associations, allele combinations, and statistical risk scores.

Purines

Double-ring nitrogenous bases (adenine and guanine).

Pyrimidines

Single-ring nitrogenous bases (cytosine, thymine, and uracil).

rRNA (Ribosomal RNA)

RNA that forms the core structural and catalytic components of ribosomes, the sites of protein synthesis.

Recessive Allele

An allele expressed only when two copies are present (homozygous state).

Regulatory Variant

A SNP that does not change protein structure but alters gene expression by affecting promoters, enhancers, or transcription factor binding.

RegulomeDB

A database that predicts whether a SNP lies in regulatory elements of the genome and whether it may influence gene expression.

Release Factors

Proteins that recognize stop codons during translation and promote release of the completed polypeptide from the ribosome.

Replication Fork

The Y-shaped region formed when the DNA double helix is unwound and the two strands are separated for replication.

Ribonucleic Acid (RNA)

A single-stranded nucleic acid involved in gene expression, protein synthesis, and regulation.

Ribosome

A large RNA–protein complex that reads mRNA and assembles amino acids into a polypeptide chain during translation.

RNA Folding

The ability of RNA to form secondary and tertiary structures, enabling diverse functional roles.

RNA Interference (RNAi)

A biological process where small RNAs (miRNA and siRNA) regulate gene expression by degrading mRNA or blocking translation.

RNA Polymerase

An enzyme that synthesizes RNA by using one strand of DNA as a template.

RNA Primer

A short stretch of RNA that serves as a starting point for DNA synthesis by DNA polymerase.

S Phase (Synthesis Phase)

The phase in which the cell replicates its DNA, producing identical copies of each chromosome so that each daughter cell can receive a complete genome.

Satiety

The feeling of fullness after eating that suppresses hunger and reduces further food intake.

Segregation (Law of Segregation)

(See **Law of Segregation**) Mendel's principle stating that allele pairs separate during gamete formation and reunite at fertilization.

Sex-Linked Inheritance (X-linked)

A pattern of trait inheritance involving genes located on the sex chromosomes, commonly the X chromosome.

Shine–Dalgarno Sequence

A ribosome-binding site in prokaryotic mRNA that helps align the ribosome with the start codon for translation.

Sigma Factor

A protein in prokaryotes that helps RNA polymerase recognize and bind to the correct promoter sequence.

Single-Strand Binding Proteins (SSBs)

Proteins that bind to separated DNA strands during replication to keep them apart and prevent them from re-annealing.

Single-Stranded Structure

A characteristic of RNA in which the molecule consists of only one nucleotide chain, unlike the double-stranded DNA.

siRNA (Small Interfering RNA)

Small RNA molecules that guide the degradation of specific mRNAs, often used in gene-silencing pathways.

snRNA (Small Nuclear RNA)

RNA molecules involved in splicing and processing of pre-mRNA within the nucleus.

SNP (Single Nucleotide Polymorphism)

A variation at a single DNA base that may influence traits, disease risk, and nutrient metabolism.

SNPedia

A wiki-style database summarizing known health, nutrition, and ancestry associations for specific SNPs.

Spindle Fibers (Mitotic Spindle)

Microtubule structures that extend from centrosomes and attach to chromosomes, helping to align and separate them during cell division.

Splicing

The process of removing introns and joining exons to produce a mature, functional mRNA.

Start Codon

The first codon recognized during translation (usually AUG), which codes for methionine and signals where protein synthesis begins.

Stop Codon

A codon (UAA, UAG, or UGA) that signals the end of translation and causes the release of the newly synthesized polypeptide.

Sugar-Phosphate Backbone

The alternating sugar and phosphate chain that forms the structural framework of DNA and RNA.

Synapsis

The close pairing of homologous chromosomes during prophase I of meiosis, allowing crossing over to occur.

TAGAP/IL18R1/CCR9/IL2/IL21

Non-HLA immune-related genes linked to increased susceptibility to celiac disease.

Telomere

A repetitive DNA sequence at the ends of linear chromosomes that protects them from degradation and loss of genetic information.

Telomerase

An enzyme that extends telomeres at chromosome ends, helping to solve the end-replication problem, especially in germ cells, stem cells, and many cancer cells.

Telophase

The final stage of mitosis where chromosomes decondense back into chromatin and new nuclear envelopes form around each set of chromosomes.

Telophase I and Cytokinesis

The completion of meiosis I where the cell divides into two haploid cells, each with a unique combination of chromosomes.

Telophase II and Cytokinesis

The final stages of meiosis where each of the two haploid cells divides again, producing four genetically distinct haploid gametes.

Trait

A characteristic or feature of an organism influenced by genetics, environment, or both.

tRNA (Transfer RNA)

An RNA molecule that delivers specific amino acids to the ribosome during translation and contains an anticodon that pairs with an mRNA codon.

Transcription

The process of copying a DNA sequence into RNA (usually mRNA) by RNA polymerase.

Transcription Factor

A protein in eukaryotes that binds DNA and helps RNA polymerase initiate transcription at the correct promoter.

Transsulfuration Pathway

A metabolic route that converts homocysteine into cysteine using CBS enzyme and vitamin B_6.

Translation

The process of decoding the information in mRNA to build a specific protein at the ribosome.

***UCP2* Gene**

A gene that influences appetite, metabolism, and fat oxidation through regulation of mitochondrial energy output.

Uncontrolled Cell Division

Cell proliferation that escapes normal cell cycle regulation, often leading to tumor formation and cancer.

Uracil (U)

A nitrogenous base found only in RNA, pairing with adenine.

Watson–Crick Model

The proposed structure of DNA as a right-handed double helix with complementary base pairing and antiparallel strands.

Wheat Allergy

An immune-mediated allergic reaction to wheat proteins that causes immediate hypersensitivity symptoms.

X-Ray Diffraction

A technique used to determine molecular structure by analyzing the pattern formed when X-rays interact with crystalline material.

www.ingramcontent.com/pod-product-compliance
Ingram Content Group UK Ltd.
Pitfield, Milton Keynes, MK11 3LW, UK
UKHW060019051026
15591UKWH00003B/283
* 9 7 9 8 9 0 1 7 6 7 3 8 2 *